Principles and Practice of Orthodontics

Churchill Livingstone Dental Series

Principles and Practice of Orthodontics

J. R. E. Mills

DDS, MSc, FDS, DOrth, RCS (Eng)
Professor of Orthodontics of London University at the Institute
of Dental Surgery; Honorary Consultant Orthodontist,
Eastman Dental Hospital, London and Queen
Elizabeth's Hospital for Children

SECOND EDITION

CHURCHILL LIVINGSTONE
EDINBURGH LONDON MELBOURNE AND NEW YORK 1987

CHURCHILL LIVINGSTONE
Medical Division of Longman Group UK Limited

Distributed in the United States of America by
Churchill Livingstone Inc., 1560 Broadway, New York,
N.Y. 10036, and by associated companies, branches
and representatives throughout the world.

First edition 1982
Second edition 1987

ISBN 0-443-03608-X

British Library Cataloguing in Publication Data
Mills, J.R.E.
    Principles and practice of orthodontics,
    — 2nd ed. — (Churchill Livingstone dental
    series).
    1. Orthodontics
    I. Title
    617.6'43   RK521

Library of Congress Cataloging in Publication Data
Mills, James Richard Ewart.
    Principles and practice of orthodontics.
    (Churchill Livingstone dental series)
    Includes bibliographies and index.
    1. Orthodontics.   I. Title.   II. Series.
[DNLM: 1. Orthodontics.   WU 400 M657p]
RK521.M55 1987   617.6'43   87-10291

Produced by Longman Singapore Publishers (Pte) Ltd.
Printed in Singapore

Preface

This book was primarily written for graduate students preparing for a higher degree or diploma in orthodontics, but in the preface to the first edition it was hoped that it would be of value to others with an interest in the subject, including undergraduate students, and this would seem to have been the case. For those proposing to specialise in orthodontics this can only be a supplement to the need for practical experience. For those aspiring to success in examinations each chapter concludes with a list of 'suggested reading'. This is not a conventional list of references, and articles mentioned in the text do not necessarily appear in the list or vice-versa. This is deliberate. If a published article makes a statement or illustrates a point and nothing else, this is repeated in the text, and there is little point in the student wasting his time in reading the original. Candidates for examinations are strongly advised to avoid the temptation to concentrate unduly on the 'small print', but rather to be selective and critical in their reading.

Some changes have been made in this second edition in order to keep abreast with recent advances in a rapidly developing specialty. In addition there is one new chapter covering the basic principles of appliance therapy, with a section on the properties or orthodontic alloys which has been included in response to requests. Otherwise I have attempted to avoid any great increase in size of the book, in the hope of keeping the price within the reach of students. This despite the criticism of an American reviewer that the book was unduly short; a sin seldom committed in North America.

Many of the photographs were taken and processed by the Photographic Department, the Eastman Dental Hospital; others by myself. In acknowledging the excellence of the former, I would not wish to transfer the blame for the latter.

Miss Janet Painter successfully interpreted my ravings into a tape-recorder and later interpreted my illegible writing. Without these efforts the first edition of the book would not have been produced.

My family have once again tolerated me, and once again I thank them for their forbearance.

London, 1986   J. R. E. Mills.

To
Margaret
Andrew
and
Jane

Acknowledgements

My thanks are acknowledged to many of my colleagues at the Eastman Dental Hospital, London, and elsewhere, who allowed me to use records of patients treated under their care, and have in some cases provided me with photographs, especially Professor C. F. Ballard, the late Dr W. R. Burston, Mr H. F. Fleming, Professor Malcolm Harris, Mrs E. N. Horrocks, Mr P. H. Morse, Mr R. T. Reed and Mrs K. W. L. Vig.

The cleft palate patients illustrated in Chapter 15 received surgical treatment by Mr R. P. G. Sandon, and the surgical cases in Chapter 16 by Mr Norman Rowe, with both of whom I have enjoyed many years of fruitful cooperation.

My thanks also to the publishers and where possible the authors of Figures 1.1, 1.2, 1.4, 1.5, 1.6, 1.8, and 2.2, the origins of which are indicated in the appropriate captions.

Several of the illustrations have previously been published in my own papers, and I am grateful to the publishers for allowing me to reproduce them here, as listed below:

Figures 3.2 and 3.11B are reproduced from Chapter 5 of "The Scientific Foundation of Dentistry", ed. B. Cohen and I. R. H. Kramer, London: William Heinemann Medical Books.

Figures 3.3, 3.7, 3.9A and B, and Fig. 3.10 from the Fortschritte der Kieferorthopaedie Band 30 (1969) Heft 1, pp. 72–81, Figures 1 to 7, by kind permission of Johann Ambrosius Barth, Leipzig, D.D.R.

Figures 3.14, 12.1, 12.6, 12.7 and 12.8 are reproduced from "An assessment of Class III malocclusion", Transactions of the British Society for the Study of Orthodontics.

Drs B. Holly Broadbent and W. H. Golden allowed me to use templates from their book 'Bolton Standards of Dentofacial Developmental Growth', St. Louis: C. V. Mosby, to prepare illustrations in Chapter 16.

To Professor A. Bjork for permission to use his template of average facial pattern in Figures 3.1 and 3.2, in addition to his illustrations elsewhere as indicated in their captions.

Finally, I would thank the numerous senior registrars, registrars and postgraduate students of the Eastman Dental Hospital, London, who carried out the day-to-day treatment of many of the cases illustrated, and apologise to anyone whose contribution I have overlooked.

Contents

1

Growth and development of the face and jaws

Orthodontic textbooks invariably commence with a chapter describing the normal development of the face, jaws and dentition. This book is no exception to the general rule, since it is important, before understanding the abnormal, to have a clear idea of the way in which the face and its component parts develop. It is proposed therefore to deal especially with those aspects of normal growth which are of particular interest to our specialty. Those interested in the subject as a whole are referred to the suggested reading at the end of the chapter.

PRENATAL DEVELOPMENT OF THE FACE

The development of the face commences at about the twenty-third day (or 10 somite stage) of intra-uterine life from the neural crest. This is, as its name suggests, a crest of ectoderm which develops to enclose the neural tube and from it processes of mesenchyme grow down to form the face. Certain facial syndromes, including Treacher-Collins syndrome and possibly some cases of facial clefts, are believed to arise at this early stage and are therefore termed neurocristopathies.

The embryo itself, at this stage, consists of a tube with the foregut separated from a depression in the surface ectoderm by the bucco-pharyngeal membrane. The breakdown of this membrane will form the future mouth. The mesenchymal processes from the neural crest form the branchial arches. The first arch numerically is also the first to form, and becomes the mandibular arch although the maxillary processes develop at an early stage from its upper surface. The two

mandibular arches grow forward and fuse with each other to separate the pericardium from the forebrain.

The frontal process grows down in mesenchyme over the forebrain. It is divided by the olfactory pit into the medial and lateral nasal processes. The maxillary process comes into contact with the lateral nasal process along the line of the future naso-lacrimal duct. It then goes on to join the median nasal process, and according to some authorities, continues to growth in front of the latter to join its fellow on the opposite side of the face at the end of the second month (Fig. 1.1A). A failure of fusion between the maxillary process and the lateral nasal process, gives rise to a lateral facial cleft, while failure of fusion between maxillary and mandibular processes, to a greater or lesser extent, causes macrostomia.

The fusion between maxillary and medial and lateral nasal processes forms the primary palate, that is, that part of the hard palate as far back as the future anterior palatine foramen (Fig. 1.1B). This part of the hard palate forms considerably earlier than the posterior or secondary palate and is also phylogenetically older, since fish and most reptiles do not possess a secondary palate. Fusion between the maxillary and median nasal process usually occurs about $4\frac{1}{2}$–6 weeks and a failure of this fusion (or of the mesenchyme to penetrate the ectoderm) will give rise to a cleft of the lip and primary palate.

Further posteriorly in the mouth, the posterior palate develops as a shelf arising from the medial side of each maxillary process (Fig. 1.1B) and lying vertically on each side of the tongue, which at this stage occupies most of the stomodaeum or primitive mouth cavity. During the third month

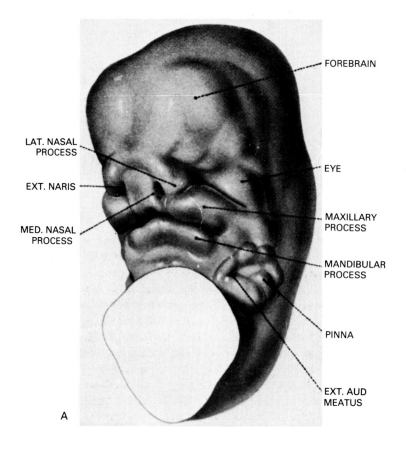

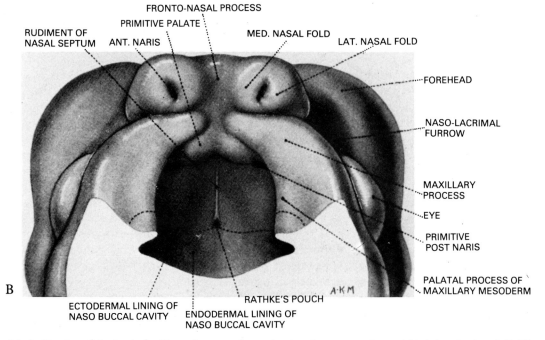

Fig. 1.1 A, Drawing of the head of a 14 mm human embryo, showing the processes from which it has developed. B, View of the roof of the stomodaeum at a slightly earlier stage. Note the primary palate and the beginning of the shelves which will later form the secondary palate. (From Hamilton W J, Boyd J D, Mossman H W 1944 Human embryology. Heffer, Cambridge.)

of intra-uterine life the face grows rapidly in the vertical dimension, and when this growth has been sufficient for the tongue to be accommodated in the lower part of the stomodaeum — the future mouth — the palatal shelves swing quite rapidly into the horizontal position and fuse with each other, with the nasal septum, and with the primary palate from before backwards. This change in position of the secondary palate apparently occurs very rapidly, certainly within 24 hours and probably less. Anything which prevents or delays this movement or prevents the fusion in the centre line will cause a cleft of the secondary or posterior palate.

DEVELOPMENT OF THE CRANIAL SKELETON

The skull may be divided both functionally and descriptively into two parts. The neuro-cranium is a box which protects the brain while the viscero-cranium supports the nose and mouth and in particular provides strength and rigidity for the jaws. The base of skull forms the junction between the two parts and has some characteristics of both of them. The calvaria develops in the membrane of the ectomeninx from one or more centres for each of the cranial bones. Ossification takes place from these centres and continues until the various bones meet each other in lines which form the sutures. These sutures are quite wide at birth so that the bones at this stage may slide over each other allowing the moulding of the cranium to make the actual process of birth easier. As the brain expands in size it would force the bones apart, and an actual separation of the sutures is prevented by deposition of further bone along the lines of the sutures, thus allowing for an increase in size of the calvaria. If the brain fails to develop then this part of the skull remains of its infantile size. This is a clear example of growth in sutures being secondary to an underlying growth process which would otherwise tend to separate the bones. The neurocranium, like the brain, develops early and growth is largely completed by the age of puberty. Growth of the visceral part of the skull, the face, is later and is fastest just before and during puberty.

The base of skull develops from areas of cartilage which form in front of and alongside the notochord, and around the developing organs of hearing and smell, in addition to the cartilaginous branchial arches. The whole of the base of skull is formed first in cartilage and this cartilage is later replaced by bone. Several small but important areas of cartilage remain. A synchondrosis exists between the two parts of the sphenoid bone until the first year of life. A similar synchondrosis between the sphenoid and occipital bones controls the growth of the posterior skull and growth here continues until adolescence. The mechanism in both these centres is for the cartilage to proliferate, thus tending to force apart the sutures which lie lateral to the synchondrosis, and bone is secondarily laid down in these sutures to prevent them springing apart.

In our primitive ancestors both upper and lower jaws were formed in cartilage. This can still be seen in a cartilaginous fish such as the shark or ray. It is represented in the developing fetus by the nasal capsule in the upper jaw and by Meckel's cartilage in the lower. The definitive human jaws do not develop in this cartilage but from membrane bones which develop on the lateral side of the nasal capsule and of Meckel's cartilage respectively. At most, these cartilaginous precursors may act as a template for the later bones. Ossification of the mandible commences in the angle between the incisal and mental branches of the inferior dental nerve at about the 18 mm stage. Bone grows upwards, backwards and inwards to enclose the nerve and then similarly grows around and encloses Meckel's cartilage (Fig. 1.2A). The latter is eventually resorbed and replaced by bone. The internal and external alveolar plates develop to enclose and support the tooth germs, so that at birth each of these tooth germs is lying in an open-topped box of bone. It is not at this stage attached to the alveolus, and if the mucous membrane is stripped from the bone in an infant cadaver the tooth germs will came away with mucous membrane. Posteriorly the deposition of bone grows up towards the base of skull and the traditional 'carrot-shaped mass' develops with its upper end in the position of the future condyle (Fig. 1.2B). This piece of cartilage is in no way related to Meckel's or other primitive

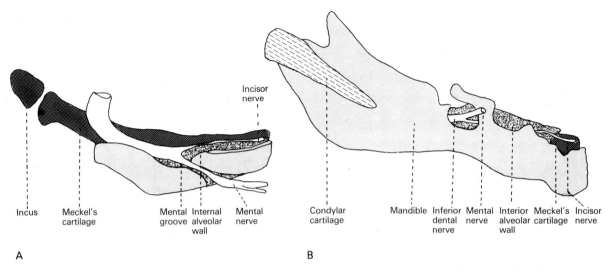

A

B

Fig. 1.2 A, View of the bony mandible developing alongside the inferior dental nerve and Meckel's cartilage. Seen from lateral side. B, The same at a somewhat later stage; note the 'carrot-shaped mass'. (Redrawn from Fawcett E 1924 in The growth of the jaws, normal and abnormal, in health and disease. Dental Board of the U.K., London.)

cartilages. It is a secondary structure to enable the laying down of a fairly bulky part of the mandible reasonably quickly. Before its formation is completed at the upper end, the pointed lower end is becoming calcified, resorbed and replaced by bone. A cap of this cartilage remains over the condyle and, as we shall see later, plays an important part in the overall growth of the mandible. Other secondary cartilages develop along the anterior margin of the coronoid process and in the chin region, although their presence is transitory.

The maxilla similarly ossifies laterally to the cartilaginous nasal capsule, again in the angle between two nerves. These are the infra-orbital and anterior-superior dental branches of the second division of the trigeminal nerve. Bony processes grow out to form the palate, and the frontal and zygomatic processes. Small islands of secondary cartilage may be found in the region of the zygmatic process. Alveolar processes again form on the buccal and lingual side of the developing tooth germs and a bridge forms between the germs so that each of these lies in its own bony box, as in the lower jaw. A depression, lined initially with cartilge of the nasal capsule, develops on the medial side of the maxilla and this is still present at birth, although no larger than half a pea. As the maxilla increases in size and particu-

larly in height, this depression develops into the maxillary antrum.

The premaxilla and palatine bones similarly develop in membrane on the lateral side of the cartilaginous nasal capsule. They are related to the anterior dental and spheno-palatine nerves respectively. These membrane bones, which now form our jaws, have developed phylogentically from the bony armour which covered the heads of primitive fishes. It is interesting that ontogenetically (and perhaps phylogenetically) both these and membrane bones of the calvaria develop initially to protect nervous tissues.

DEVELOPMENT OF MUSCLES OF THE FACE

There are three groups of muscles which are of importance in the areas surrounding the face: the muscles of mastication, the muscles of facial expression and the tongue. These all develop from the musculature of the branchial arches.

The muscles of mastication develop from a single mass which is the musculature of the first branchial arch. It is originally attached to Meckel's cartilage but the dividing muscles migrate for the most part to the bony mandible.

The exception is the tensor tympani which remains attached to the malleus — the original Meckelian condyle. The first muscle to split off is the internal pterygoid while the temporalis and masseter divide at a comparatively late stage. The lateral pterygoid muscle develops originally through the petro-tympanic fissure and is integral to the intra-articular disc, which develops when mesoderm is 'trapped' between the condyle and the glenoid fossa.

The muscles of facial expression are essentially second arch muscles which migrate up over the face. This is indicated by their nerve supply, which comes from the seventh (facial) nerve which is the nerve of the second arch. The tongue has a much more complicated origin. Sensation is provided by contributions from all the first four arches (the lingual branch of the fifth, chorda tympani branch of the seventh, together with branches from the glossopharyngeal and superior laryngeal nerves — the nerves of the third and fourth arches respectively). The muscles of the tongue however migrate down from the occipital myotomes and their nerve supply is therefore from the hypoglossal nerve.

In the fetus of any species the rates of development of different parts are not equal. Preference is given to those structures which need to function adequately immediately after birth. The newly born human baby has only two functions, it requires an ability to cry to attract attention to its hunger and an ability to suckle to satisfy it. The parts around the mouth therefore develop early, as we have already seen with the jaws. The same is true of the musculature. Already by 10 weeks musculature can be seen in the region of the obicularis oris and mentalis muscles, together with the tongue which is a very early structure to develop. It has been shown from work on aborted fetuses that stimulation of the perioral region will cause some response as early as $7\frac{1}{2}$ weeks, while by the end of 12 weeks, in a fetus only 5 cm long, stimulation around the mouth may cause deglutition. By 22 weeks a suctorial reflex is well developed. It should be borne in mind therefore, in considering the development of the face and jaws, that the bones grow within a 'field' of musculature which can, and probably does, function from a very early stage.

POSTNATAL GROWTH OF THE SKULL

Bone does not grow interstitially. There are therefore two mechanisms whereby bone generally may grow. Firstly, it may grow as a result of surface deposition by osteoblasts in the cellular layer of a periosteum. This can occur at a bony surface, in a suture or in a periodontal membrane. Secondly, it may grow through the intermediary of cartilage. In this case the cartilage proliferates — and cartilage, unlike bone, can grow interstitially — and the proliferating cartilage becomes calcified, is resorbed away, and is replaced by bone, which is again laid down by osteoblasts. Both mechanisms are found in the skull and face.

Base of skull

The cranial base may be divided into three areas:

1. The posterior part of the base of skull from the occiput to the sella turcica grows throughout the period of childhood and adolescence and as we have already seen, this occurs primarily at the spheno-occipital synchondrosis. This important growth centre has the effect of forcing apart the sutures which lie on its lateral sides, and an actual opening of the suture is prevented by deposition of bone within the sutures thus contributing to the overall growth in length of the skull.

2. The middle section from the sella turcica to the foramen caecum grows from a similar synchondrosis between the sphenoid and ethmoid bones. This growth of the anterior base of skull is more rapid than the posterior section in the fetus and early infancy, but this synchondrosis closes about the age of 7, after which the distance between the sella and foramen caecum does not increase. A cartilaginous growth area between the pre- and post-sphenoid closes before birth. There is also one between the body and greater wing of sphenoid which closes in the first year of life, and may have some effect in lateral growth.

3. The part anterior to the foramen caecum grows by deposition on the anterior surface of the frontal and nasal bones. An undue increase in bulk of this area is prevented to some extent by resorption on the inner surface and also by development of the frontal sinus, especially in the male. As we shall see later, this surface deposition in the

region of the fronto-nasal suture reduces the usefulness of the cephalometric point nasion in the analysis of lateral skull radiographs.

Bones of the upper jaw

These comprise the maxilla, premaxilla and palatine bones. The two former fuse at an early stage, with elimination of the suture on the facial surface of the bone, although remnants of it frequently remain in the palate. This suture therefore plays no part in the growth of the upper jaw during childhood in man, but it is of some interest that growth does occur here in the monkeys and apes, a point which may be borne in mind in interpreting the results of some animal experiments. Two obvious mechanisms are involved in the growth of this upper jaw. Surface deposition plays a part in the overall increase in size and this is especially true in the vertical dimension as a result, in the first place, of downward growth of the alveolus, which carries the teeth with it. This surface deposition is brought about not only by the alveolar periosteum, but also by that modified periosteum which we call the periodontal membrane. Surface deposition is not merely a mechanism to increase the bulk of the maxilla. It is co-ordinated with surface resorption of bone and is the principal mechanism whereby the shape of the bone is controlled. In this way as vertical growth of the maxilla proceeds, remodelling takes place so that the maxilla develops from its infantile to its adult shape. Indeed, some areas of both jaws may undergo an alternation of deposition and resorption by both periosteum and endosteum several times during their growth and it would seem that this remodelling process is the willing slave of whatever organising factor controls the final shape of the jaws.

As can be seen in Figure 1.3, the maxillae are surrounded by a complex system of sutures which may be divided into a horizontal group above the maxilla and a vertical group behind it. Growth at these two systems of sutures is associated with the propulsion of the maxilla downwards and forwards respectively. A mid-line suture contributes to lateral growth, and Sicher and Weinmann originally suggested that this element of growth was caused by an intrinsic forcing apart of the sutures

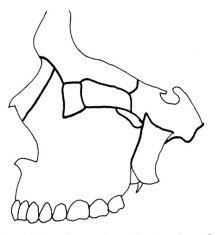

Fig 1.3 Lateral view of upper jaw and anteror base of skull. The heavy lines represent the principal sutures.

by the action of the osteoblasts in producing new bone. We have already seen, in the growth of the calvaria and base of skull, that the sutural system is essentially an in-filling process, the bones being forced apart in the one case by growth of the brain and in the other by growth at the synchondrosis. It therefore seems reasonable to believe that growth in the facial sutures is also in the nature of an in-filling mechanism. This would require some other force to carry the bones of the skull. While most authorities agree with this basic premise, there is controversy over the nature of the displacing force.

Cartilage is an obvious candidate for the honour. In embryonic development, the forming maxilla is carried downwards and forwards by the cartilaginous nasal capsule, of which the nasal septum forms a part which remains present after birth. Scott has suggested that this septum is responsible for the downwards and forwards displacement of the maxilla, at least in infancy, although the duration of such a mechanism is doubtful, Latham confining it to the first 18 months of life. Doubt has been cast on this theory by the fact that the maxilla will grow fairly normally in the absence of a cartilaginous septum. Vertical growth of the upper jaw includes a large element of surface deposition on its lower surface, and there is a strong tendency in the face for compensation by one form of growth when another fails.

Moss has put forward a theory, suggesting originally that facial growth was guided by the functional matrix, later divided into periosteal and capsular matrices. The shape of the bones was produced by the periosteal matrix and their translation, as they grow downwards and forwards by the capsular matrix. The former is to some extent well established. The coronoid process does not develop appreciably in the absence of the temporal muscle, the alveoli depend on teeth for their presence, while the muscles of the lips and cheeks, opposed by the tongue, probably guide their shape.

Moss draws attention to the calvaria, whose shape and size is largely determined by the matrix of the brain, while the orbit similarly has the eye for its matrix. He claims that the matrix for the rest of the face is the spaces within it — the nose, mouth and presumably, the antra. Growth is brought about by the expansion of these spaces. The causative agent is somewhat obscure but Moss speaks of growth of the spaces being controlled by that of the lining epithelium, the latter in turn stimulated by trophic mechanisms passing down the appropriate nerves. He is the author of numerous papers on the subject and the reader is directed to those in the suggested reading at the end of this chapter, together with the review article by Johnston in 'Factors affecting growth of the midface'.

A number of other mechanisms have been suggested for growth of the upper jaw, of which the most interesting is probably that of Azuma and co-workers from Enlow's laboratory. They identify a form of fibroblast, which they call myofibroblasts, in the periodontal membrane and also in certain sutures of the face. These have some of the characteristics of smooth muscle cells and it is claimed that, by attaching themselves to the collagen fibres of the periodontal membrane, they pull the root of the tooth upwards and thus cause its eruption. The same mechanism, they claim, is responsible for causing one bone to slide against its neighbour in the suture, so that growth is brought about, not by sutures forcing bones apart but by those at right angles to these, causing a lateral sliding of the one bone against its neighbour. These various theories are discussed in detail in the monograph 'Factors affecting the

growth of the midface', listed at the end of this chapter.

There is no doubt that the bony structures of the face have a considerable ability for compensatory growth to overcome, at least partly, the effects of genetic or environmental shortcomings. The jaws will do their best to work. However small may be one's mandible, it is never too narrow for the condyles to fit into the glenoid fossae. Nevertheless, it is difficult to believe that the resemblance between close relatives is entirely due to the similarity of their facial function. It is also difficult to believe that function is responsible for the production of some of the gross skeletal abnormalities which are seen by orthodontists.

Growth of the mandible

The mandible consists of a single bone after the fusion of the two halves during the first year of life. It can therefore grow only by surface deposition of bone, with its shape maintained and modified to adult form by deposition where required. As with the maxilla, some areas may undergo an alteration of deposition and resorption during its development.

The classical picture of growth is illustrated in Figure 1.4, and has been described by Enlow from histological studies and also by Björk. The latter has studied the growth of children by means of

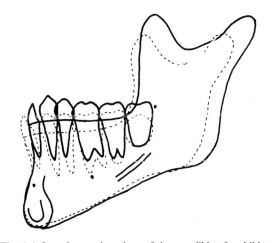

Fig. 1.4 Superimposed tracings of the mandible of a child at different ages superimposed on metal implants, to show areas of deposition and resorption of bone (From Björk A 1963 Journal of Dental Research 42: 400–11.)

small metal implants inserted into the growing child. Where three or four of these are inserted it is possible to superimpose lateral radiographs and to identify areas of superimposition and resorption. It will be seen later that the classical picture requires some modifications but the basic principle remains. There is deposition of bone on the upper surface of the body, as the teeth develop and erupt upwards, and also on the posterior border of the vertical ramus and lateral border of both rami. There is some resorption on the anterior border of the vertical ramus and inner side of the whole mandible, although in both cases less than one might think. This is, however, an over-simplification since, because of its slightly oblique position, the vertical ramus may at times show resorption on its lateral side and deposition on the medial, as it 'migrates' posteriorly. A somewhat surprising finding is that there is only very slight bony deposition on the bony chin, while the area labial to the roots of the incisors is usually resorptive.

The bony deposition in the mandible is produced by the osteoblasts of the periosteum with a notable exception. The condyle is covered by a layer of cartilage, the remnant of the 'carrot-shaped mass' of the fetal state. As already indicated, this is not homologous with the primary cartilage of an epiphysis of a long bone or of the base of the skull, and its properties are in some way intermediate between those of true cartilage and periosteum. Its importance lies in the fact that it is the part of the mandible which comes into close contact with the base of the skull. Since there is little growth at the chin, growth at the condyle is responsible for overall growth in length of the mandible, even though its actual contribution in volume is less than that of the periosteum.

The obvious belief is that the mandible is propelled downwards and forwards from the base of the skull by this cartilage, in a manner analogous to the epiphysis of a long bone, under genetic influences. This is not universally accepted and another school, essentially following Moss's hypothesis, consider that the growth at the condyle is an 'in-filling' process, analogous to that in a suture, with the mandible carried downwards and forwards by the mystical forces of the functional, or capsular, matrix.

GROWTH AS AN INTEGRAL PROCESS

So far in this chapter we have attempted to describe the processes whereby the tissues of the face grow. To describe, that is, *how* the face grows. In this section we shall consider the pattern of facial growth, *where* the face grows. Much work has been carried out on the growth of the human face, mostly by orthodontists. Earlier investigators, broadly before the Second World War, did this by making measurements on dried skulls or on the heads of living children. The former have the disadvantage that only cross-sectional studies were possible, comparing the skulls of young children with those of another group of older children. While longitudinal investigations could be carried out by direct measurements of live children, few if any such studies were made and here again they were usually of a cross-sectional nature. Generally, these early investigators found that the head and face grew in a regular fashion maintaining its infantile shape apart from certain changes which could be predicted. It was particularly noticeable that the face grew in height at a more rapid rate than in width or depth. Faces get longer as we pass from infancy into adulthood. They apparently grow in depth, antero-posteriorly, to a greater extent than in width, but the difference between these two dimensions is not great. Secondly, it was found that the angles between the various facial planes tend to decrease with age. The lower border of the mandible tends to become more horizontal and its angle more prominent. The changes which take place are different between the two sexes after puberty, with the male having a more angular face and noticeable development of the chin, nose and supra-orbital ridge. It was also noted that growth does not continue at the same pace throughout life, but there is a marked spurt around the age of puberty, with a smaller spurt at the time of first molar eruption. Brash, in an extensive review of the available facts, pointed out that in the newborn baby the face forms only $\frac{1}{8}$ of the total volume of the skull, whereas in the adult it forms approximately $\frac{1}{2}$ (Fig. 1.5). In other words the face grows considerably more than the brain case and in many ways the story of facial growth is the story of the migration of the face forwards and down-

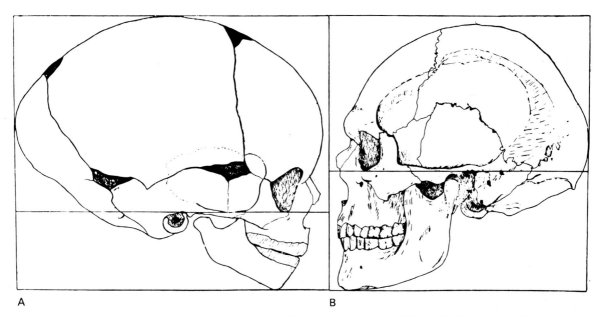

Fig. 1.5 Skulls of a child and of an adult. The child's skull is magnified twice that of the adult. Note that the face in the adult forms a much larger part of the whole than in the child. (From Brash, J C 1924 in The growth of the jaws, normal and abnormal, in health and disease. Dental Board of the U.K., London.)

wards from under the brain case as it becomes more prominent.

The development of the cephalostat by Broadbent in about 1930 gave a great impetus to growth studies although it has always had a tendency to make us believe that the human face has only two dimensions. Broadbent himself used this piece of apparatus to collect serial radiographs of a considerable number of children living in an institution, so that, by the time of his principal publications, he had these radiographs extending over a period of about 8 years. From his investigations he made a number of subjective statements suggesting that the face grew in a remarkably regular and unaltering fashion, with the shape hardly changing as the size increased. Brodie, in 1941, used Broadbent's radiographs to study the growth of children in more detail between 3 months and 8 years of life. His principal findings were of average changes although he made some reference to individual cases. He found once again, that there was remarkably little change in facial pattern during growth apart from the obvious one of increase in size. This study, of course, ended well before puberty, and a later

investigation, carrying on up to the age of 15 years, showed greater change occurring during the pubertal period together with considerable increase in variation between individuals when compared with mean. Nevertheless, the early findings by Broadbent and Brodie died hard, and for many years it was believed that the facial pattern did not change during growth. Björk and other investigators showed that there was a marked tendency for the face to swing forward during growth, as Brash had implied, and for both jaws to become more prognathous. The bases of the jaws, as represented by anterior nasal spine and chin point, come forward more than the alveolar portion and teeth. Moreover, the chin comes forward more than the anterior nasal spine, that is most people tend to become more Class III and less Class II. The average picture as indicated by Björk is shown in Figure 1.6 which is taken from one of his papers.

This author also showed that in addition to average changes there were individual variations. These were usually slight so that the facial appearance of children did not change very much apart from those changes resulting from growing up.

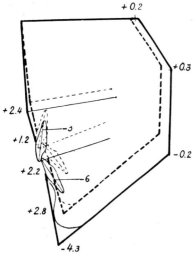

Fig. 1.6 Diagram to show the difference in facial pattern of 12-year old Swedish boys and 20–21-year-old Swedish adults. (From Björk A 1951 Dental Record 71: 197–208.)

Occasionally however an individual was seen in whom the facial pattern changed very much more than the average (Fig. 1.7).

We have already mentioned more recent work carried out by Björk using small metal implants

in the mandible (and, indeed, elsewhere in the skull). The situation shown in Figure 1.4, while clarifying the classical picture of growth of the mandible, is in fact an over-simplification. A more typical picture of mandibular growth, as shown by this method, is seen in Figure 1.8A, while an extreme example is seen in Figure 1.8B. These diagrams would seem to show that, while the pattern of bone deposition posteriorly, and at the alveolar margin is true as a generalisation, details

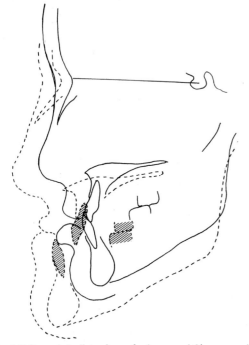

Fig. 1.7 Lateral skull tracings of a boy, aged 9½ years and 16 years, superimposed to show abnormal growth pattern.

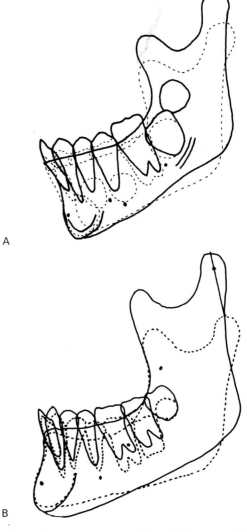

A

B

Fig. 1.8 Two tracings of mandible of children at different ages, superimposed to show areas of bone deposition and resorption. A, A typical case. B, An extreme case. (From Björk A 1963 Journal of Dental Research 42: 400–11.)

differ between individuals. The pattern shown in Figure 1.8B is clearly not what we expect to see in real life. Björk has also drawn attention to certain structures within the mandible which do not appreciably change their position during growth, and which may therefore serve as points of superimposition, in the same way as his metal implants. These are shown in Figure 1.9A by heavy lines and comprise the inner outline of the compact bone at the lower border of the symphysis menti, the labial outline above the most anterior point of the chin and the inferior dental canal below the molar teeth.

Figure 1.9A shows the superimposed lateral skull tracings of a boy with a very deep overbite and small lower facial height. The tracings have been superimposed conventionally on the anterior base of skull, and the two radiographs are separated by a period of about 10 years. Growth is apparently regular, with the shape remaining reasonably constant, although with some increase in overbite and with the lower border of the mandible becoming rather more horizontal. In Figure 1.9B we see the same radiographs superimposed on Björk's structures, as described above, in the mandible. The picture is very different. The whole face appears to rotate forward to an extreme extent. This rotation of the upper face is, of course, relative to the mandible and does not indicate that the individual now spends his life looking downwards. It is equally true, and more logical, to look upon this as rotation of the mandible forwards and upwards relative to the rest of the skull, rather than vice versa. The mandible appears to maintain its original shape in

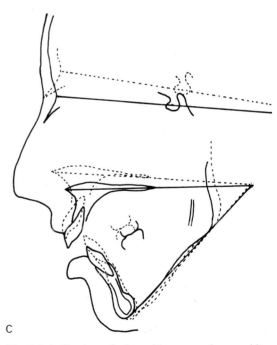

Fig. 1.9 A, Tracings of a boy with a severe deep overbite, at age of 9 and 16 years, superimposed on the anterior base of skull. B, Tracings of the same boy superimposed on structures in mandible, as suggested by Björk. C, Tracings of a girl with a reduced overbite, similarly superimposed on mandibular structures.

Figure 1.9A because of compensatory deposition and resorption, with massive resorption below the angle and deposition behind it. This masks the rotation to a large extent, although not completely. It can still be recognised by the reduction in the mandibular angle and, as we shall see later, by the apparent lingual movement of the lower incisors.

The body of the bone thus rotates forwards in this type of case. In a more recent paper. Björk and Skieller (1983) describe this as corpus rotation. The lower border of the mandible also rotates but a substantial proportion of this is disguised by appropriate deposition and resorption of bone. The rotation of the external surface of the bone is referred to as matrix rotation and is probably due to migration of muscle insertions. It should be noted that the idea of a matrix used here is not that employed by Moss.

Figure 1.9C shows a rather different picture in a patient with an abnormally long face. Here again the superimposed tracings cover a period of several years and it will be seen that in this case, when superimposed on the mandible, the face appears to rotate upwards and backwards. Again this is a relative movement, and if we were able to superimpose on the upper face, we could see that it is in fact the mandible which rotates downwards and backwards, producing a reduced overbite or even an anterior open bite. In this case the change in mandibular position is more apparent, since surface remodelling is less successful in masking it, so that the lower border of the mandible becomes much steeper. This downward and backward rotation is much less frequently seen than the forward and upward rotation, a mild form of which is in fact seen in ideal growth, producing the picture seen in Figure 1.8A. Backwards rotation is not usually masked, to any great extent, by surface remodelling.

The reason for this rotation is not fully understood. It is obviously associated with an imbalance in vertical growth of the vertical ramus of the mandible on one hand and molar region of the maxilla on the other but association does not necessarily imply cause and effect. It has been suggested by Møller that forward rotation is associated with a more powerful contraction of the mandibular elevator muscles than is backward rotation. Proffit, using strain gauges attached to the teeth, while confirming this difference in muscular force in adults, was unable to find any difference between the two facial patterns in children.

In further work, Björk has shown that similar rotation takes place in the maxilla relative to the base of skull during growth and that this again is variable. It is however usually much less marked in degree.

We have therefore a fairly clear idea of the pattern of facial growth. Most children remain recognisably unchanged apart from those changes which are a feature of development from the childish to the adult face. These involve an increase in the proportion of the skull which is occupied by the face, an increasing prominence of the chin, especially in the male, and an increased prominence of the jaws with a more horizontal lower border to the mandible. The nose also develops its adult form. Most individuals will depart to some extent from the average growth pattern and a small proportion of children will do so to a fairly extreme extent, but there is no evidence that the skeletal pattern can be changed substantially by conventional orthodontic treatment to any clinically useful extent.

WHY DOES THE FACE GROW?

Although we appear to have a fairly clear idea of how the face grows, and of where it grows, we have little idea of why it grows. We do not fully understand the factors which control the amount and direction of growth. Moss has sought to explain it by his concept of the 'functional matrix'. His hypotheses are not easy to understand but his theories would seem to represent something of an over-simplification. The giving of a long and erudite name to a process does not necessarily explain it.

There is no doubt that the face has a powerful tendency to grow to a predetermined size and shape. We tend to resemble our close relatives and to a decreasing extent, members of our own family, race and species. A Chinese baby brought up in the environment of an English family and functioning as an English child nevertheless develops into a Chinese adult. He would still bear a fairly close resemblance to his original Chinese parents and not to his English foster parents. Facial shape must be under basic genetic control. If however something occurs to interfere with the natural growth pattern, then nature has a considerable ability to compensate. If one epiphyseal cartilage in a long bone is destroyed the cartilage at the other end of the bone will overproduce in an effort, not completely successful, to maintain the full growth of the bone. Similarly if the condylar growth cartilage is destroyed, surface apposition will attempt to make up for the deficiency, albeit inadequately. Mandibular width is always the first priority and the intercondylar width always increases sufficiently to maintain the condyles in the glenoid fossae. The lower incisors will procline as will the anterior alveolus in an effort to bring the incisors into functional contact, probably under the influence of the soft tissues. Similarly, in a gross Class III skeletal pattern the lower incisors and associated alveolus lean lingually to bring the incisal edges of the lower incisors as close as possible to those of the upper teeth. This may well be the result of the pressure exerted from the soft tissues and in this sense the function is indeed the matrix.

Quite clearly there is a genetic influence which produces the right bone in the right place: a mandible in the lower part of the face and not a femur. It is well known that simpler bones can develop from limb buds *in vitro*. The genes having produced an assortment of bones (and also of other structures including muscles and other soft tissues) nature has then to put them together in a manner which will produce a functional individual. It would seem that perhaps the amount of bone is inherited but this may be adapted where necessary to make the best of the inheritance, for example, a large maxilla and a small mandible. There is a factor which brings this about but the nature of this factor is not at present understood and it is idle to pretend otherwise.

THE PREDICTION OF GROWTH

In recent years a considerable interest has been aroused by the possibility of predicting facial growth, since this might well, if successful, help in the planning of orthodontic treatment. The human face has already achieved about 75 per cent of its adult size by the age of 2 years and approximately 85 per cent by the age of 9. A fairly substantial error in predicting the final 15 per cent will not be too noticeable since the original 85 per cent will still be there. A number of individuals have put forward methods of prediction and these all involve the addition of average increments in growth to a limited number of points on the original lateral tracing, the intermediate regions being interpolated. One of the better known techniques is that of Lysle Johnston which is based on predicting six points, using a grid. The increments vary for each point both in amount and direction, and allowance is made for the pubertal growth spurt by the addition of extra increments. Figure 1.10A shows a prediction carried out by this technique. On the left is the tracing of the child at the age of 9 and on the right, 5 years later. The dotted outline shows the predicted growth using Johnston's method and it will be seen that a reasonably close approximation to the final shape has been achieved although it is by no means exact. It is generally found that this technique is more accurate for the maxilla than for the mandible. Figure 1.10B shows an attempt at prediction in the case of abnormal growth previously shown in Figure 1.7. Here, where prediction would be most valuable it does nothing to help.

Ricketts has evolved the technique further and has taken into account the forward rotation of the mandible which is seen in many individuals. He therefore adds his increments for the lower jaw not along a straight line but along a curved arc and he calls the method an arcial technique. He has inspired the use of a computer as a commercial service for forecasting growth, and this computer makes some allowance for a limited number of racial differences and for variations in the initial type of face. It may be that in the long term modifications to the computer program, resulting from experience, will enable this to become acceptably accurate, but at present the computer technique would seem to be no more accurate over a short period of 2 years than Johnston's manual method (and of course much more expensive), and only marginally more accurate in the long term. The technique produced by Popovich at the

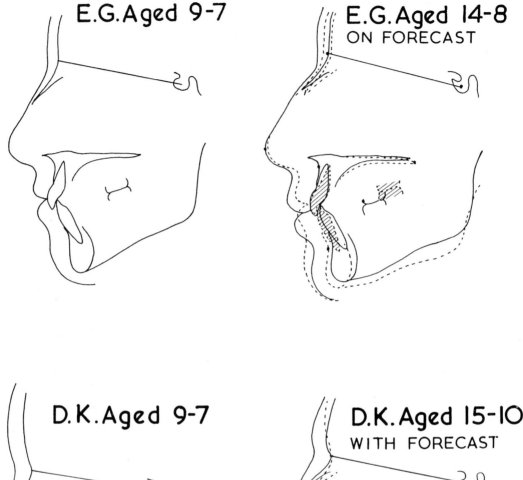

A

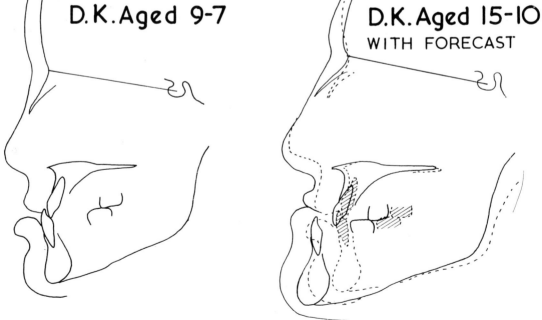

B

Fig. 1.10 A, Tracing of E.G. at the age of 9 years (*left*) with a tracing of the same boy at age 14 (*right*). The broken outline shows the situation as predicted according to the methods of Lysle Johnston. B, Similar tracings, at the ages of 9 and 15 years, of the boy shown previously in Fig. 1.7.

Burlington Growth Centre in Toronto would seem to be essentially similar except that some allowance is made both in amount and direction of predicted growth according to the age of the patient and the basic type of growth seen in the past.

It is not very difficult to visualise what a child of 10 will look like in 4 years time. In general he will be a little bigger. His chin is likely to be somewhat more prominent, especially if he is a boy. Occasionally, his growth pattern will depart considerably from the average and if it were possible to predict this it might tell us that orthodontic treatment would be particularly successful or alternatively, particularly unsuccessful. Unfortunately, at present prediction falls down just in those cases where this is needed most.

SUGGESTED READING

Björk A 1947 The face in profile. Svensk Tandlakare Tidskrift 40, Suppl. 5B

Björk A, Skieller V 1972 Facial development and tooth eruption. American Journal of Orthodontics 62: 339–83

Björk A, Skieller V 1976 Growth of the maxilla in three dimensions as revealed radiographically by the implant method. British Journal of Orthodontics 4: 53–64

Brodie A G 1941 On the growth pattern of the human head from the third month to the eighth year of life. American Journal of Anatomy 68: 209–62

Brodie A G 1953 Late growth changes in the human face. Angle Orthodontist 23: 146–57

Enlow D H 1966 A morphogenetic analysis of facial growth. American Journal of Orthodontics 52: 283–99

Greenberg L Z, Johnston L E 1975 Computerized prediction: the accuracy of long-range forecasts. American Journal of Orthodontics 67: 243–52

Johnston L E 1975 A simplified approach to prediction. American Journal of Orthodontics 67: 253–7

Lande M J 1952 Growth behaviour of the human bony facial profile as revealed by serial cephalometric roentgenograms. Angle Orthodontist 22: 78–90

McNamara J A (ed.) 1975 Determinants of mandibular form and growth. Monograph No. 4, Center for Human Growth and Development. Michigan, Ann Arbor

McNamara J A (ed.) 1976 Factors affecting growth of the midface. Monograph No. 6, Center for Human Growth and Development. Michigan, Ann Arbor

Mills J R E 1983 A clinician looks at facial growth. British Journal of Orthodontics 10: 58–72

Moss M L 1968 The primacy of the functional matrices in oro-facial growth. Transactions of the British Society for the Study of Orthodontics 54: 107–15

Moss M L 1975 Neurotrophic regulation of craniofacial growth. In: McNamara J A (ed.) Control mechanisms of craniofacial growth. Center for Human Growth and Development. Michigan, Ann Arbor

Moss M L 1981 Genetics, epigenetics and causation. American Journal of Orthodontics 80: 366–75

Schulhof E J, Bagha L 1975 A statistical evaluation of the Ricketts and Johnston growth-forecasting methods. American Journal of Orthodontics 67: 258–76

Scott J H 1966 The embryology of cleft palate and hare lip. British Dental Journal 120: 17–20

Sperber G H 1973 Craniofacial embryology. Wright, Bristol

2

Development of the dentition

It is obviously important for an orthodontist to recognise a malocclusion, and he can only do this by comparison with the ideal dentition for a child of the appropriate age. In this chapter it is not proposed to give a detailed account of the development and eruption of the two dentitions. This can be acquired from an undergraduate textbook. It is the intention rather, to draw attention to those aspects of the ideal occlusion which might be of particular interest to the orthodontist.

The first sign of the future deciduous teeth comprises a thickening of the oral ectoderm at about the thirty-fourth day of intra-uterine life. This is about the stage at which the mandibular arches fuse and before Meckel's cartilage is laid down. By the time that the embryo is 25 mm (1 inch) in length the 'bell' stage of the enamel organs is present and the inner and outer alveolar plates are growing up from their bony bases to support them. At birth all the deciduous teeth are calcified to some extent, the entire crown of the incisors but only the tips of the cusps of the deciduous and often first permanent molars. These tooth germs lie within the developing alveolar bone but are not attached to it.

The germs of all the successional teeth have formed on the lingual side of their deciduous predecessors. Thus the upper permanent canine germ begins to calcify, lingually to the deciduous canine, in the first year of life. At this stage the maxilla is very shallow with little or no antrum. The canine is immediately below the floor of the orbit. At 3–4 years it passes over the line of the deciduous anterior teeth and comes to lie on the labial side above the root of the lateral incisor. From here it moves downwards and distally to erupt in the line of the arch at 12 years (Fig. 2.1)

Since it erupts after its immediate neighbours, it is particularly liable to be the victim of crowding. It may indeed fail to cross the line of the deciduous roots and its displacement may therefore be either palatal or labial.

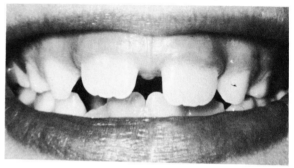

A

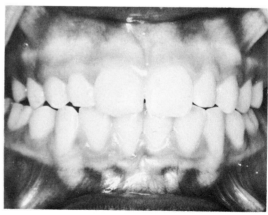

B

Fig. 2.1 A, Anterior dentition of my daughter at the age of 7 years. B, At the age of 11 years. Note spontaneous correction of transient crowding.

The permanent incisors remain lingual throughout their development and if a deciduous incisor fails to shed, the permanent one will normally erupt in the lingual position. It will tend to move in a favourable direction once the deciduous tooth has been shed, but may be locked in crossbite in the case of an upper incisor. These teeth are often rotated before eruption in order to occupy less space. In a crowded mouth this rotation may persist after eruption; typically lateral incisors are disto-lingually and central incisors mesio-lingually rotated. The premolars migrate at an early stage from their lingual position so as to lie between the roots of the deciduous molars before they commence to calcify, and normally remain there until they erupt. The upper first molar develops in the tuberosity of the maxilla with its occlusal surface facing somewhat distally. It moves downwards and forwards as growth takes place until it erupts, its former position being occupied by the second molar and finally the third molar. Similarly the lower molars develop in the ascending ramus of the mandible, where their occlusal surface is tilted mesially. These teeth move forward as growth takes place and are replaced in the ascending ramus by the second and then the third molar. It will be appreciated that the upper molars move forwards and downwards during eruption whereas the path of the lower molars is essentially mesial with little or no vertical movement. In a crowded mouth it is not unusual for a developing lower third molar to overlap the second molar on its buccal side. From the position of the developing molars at a given age, it is possible to infer, to some extent, the degree of inherent crowding.

ERUPTION OF THE PERMANENT
INCISORS (see Fig. 2.3)

In the ideal mouth, the deciduous incisors are spaced throughout their useful life. It was for long believed that the spacing, seen in the deciduous incisor region before the eruption of permanent successors, was the result of a growth mechanism to make sufficient room for the larger permanent teeth. Clinch, Baume and Sillman have shown this to be a fallacy. The deciduous incisors may erupt in contact with each other or spaced, but usually remain unchanged until they are shed. As growth of the maxilla takes place, this may cause a spacing of the roots of the teeth, but the crowns remain in the same relation, so that they appear to tilt towards each other in the later stages of their existence. Increase in inter-canine width, necessary to accommodate permanent incisors, usually occurs as these teeth are erupting. They are frequently crowded when they first erupt, but this crowding may be eliminated as eruption takes place. Once the incisors have fully erupted, it is unusual, but not unknown, for crowding to improve. It is not possible to predict at the age of 7 or 8 whether a crowding in the incisor segment will persist, or as in Figure 2.1, correct itself spontaneously. Broadbent calls this stage of transient crowding the 'ugly duckling' stage. There is a further slight increase in available space as the permanent canines erupt to replace their deciduous predecessors.

In average terms, there is 1–2 mm increase in intercanine width during the time that the deciduous incisors are in the mouth. During the eruption of incisors and permanent canines there is about 3.5 mm increase in the upper arch and 3 mm in the lower. This is achieved to some extent by a labial growth of the appropriate part of the alveolus causing a change in shape of the upper dental arch, and also by the fact that the permanent anterior teeth are more proclined than their deciduous predecessors. It should be borne in mind that few individuals are average and the amount of growth taking place varies quite considerably in different children. If the deciduous incisors are in contact and not spaced, then this should be regarded as essentially a crowded condition. The correlation in size of deciduous and succeeding permanent teeth is not very high, so that this lack of space may be caused by large deciduous incisors which can be replaced by relatively smaller permanent teeth. On average unspaced teeth tend to be associated with slightly more growth in inter-canine width. Nevertheless, we must accept that where the deciduous incisors are in contact there is a probability that the permanent incisors will be crowded. If the deciduous incisors themselves are crowded, then it can be regarded as certain that their permanent successors would be similarly afflicted.

When the permanent incisors do erupt in a crowded state, it is impossible to predict accurately their final alignment but it is wise to be guarded in assessing prognosis.

DEVELOPMENT OF THE DENTAL ARCHES (see Fig. 2.4)

Arch length is usually defined as the length of a perpendicular, drawn from the contact point of the upper central incisors, to a line joining the distal contact points of the second deciduous molars or second premolars. Arch circumference is the length of a line drawn around the teeth, usually passing through the buccal cusps of posterior teeth and incisal edges of the incisors. The arch length changes very little after the eruption of the second deciduous molars. In the maxilla, there is a slight increase in arch length between the ages of 6 and 10 years, as the permanent incisors erupt, while the deciduous molars are still present. This is followed by a decrease as the latter teeth are replaced by the permanent premolars. In the mandible the increase does not occur but there is a slight decrease in arch length between the ages of 10 and 17 years. In both jaws this is of the order of 1–2 mm, although there are marked individual variations. In primitive man, there is substantial wear of the contact points between the teeth and this is responsible for a noticeable decrease in arch length. Begg has suggested that in the Australian Aborigine this may amount to the width of a premolar tooth on each side of the jaws. In civilised man, this wear of the contact points is much less severe, and a substantial decrease in arch length would be associated with crowding.

The arch width, measured again across the lingual margins of the fifth tooth (the second deciduous molar or second premolar), also changes comparatively little once the deciduous dentition is established. Between the ages of 3 and 18 years, there is 2–3 mm increase in width of the maxilla, rather more in boys than in girls, while in the mandible there is about 2.5 mm increase in width in both sexes. The increase in width

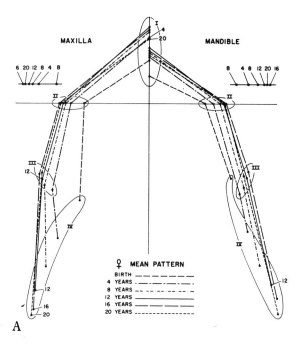

A

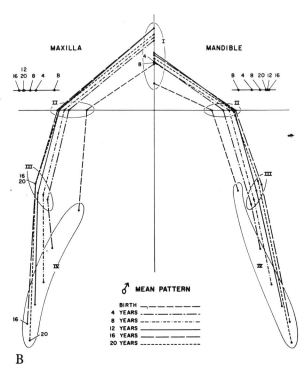

B

Fig. 2.2 Diagrammatic representation of the development of the dental arches. (From Sillman J H 1964 American Journal of Orthodontics 50: 824–42)

between the first permanent molars from the age of 6–18 years is very similar; again rather more in the male than the female. If would seem that there is little change after the age of 11 years, that is, during the period in which orthodontic treatment normally takes place. Here again there is some variation between individuals. This has been illustrated diagrammatically in Figure 2.2, which is taken from the work of Sillman.

The arch circumference changes very little in the maxilla, with an increase of slightly over 1 mm in the male and only half that in the female. In the mandible however, there is a substantial decrease in arch circumference of about 3.5 mm in the male and 4.5 mm in the female. This is perhaps the most outstanding case of individual variation, with obviously a more substantial decrease in arch circumference in crowded mouths.

In general, therefore, there is surprisingly little change in the anterior part of the dental arch once all the deciduous teeth have erupted. There is some change in shape with a corresponding increase in inter-canine widths. The main increase in size occurs posteriorly as space becomes available for the erupting molars. The permanent incisors being substantially larger than their deciduous predecessors, require some increase in inter-canine width, but the premolars are usually smaller than the deciduous molars. Although the permanent canines are larger than the corresponding deciduous teeth, the total length of the permanent canine and two premolars is usually less than that of deciduous canine and molars. This discrepancy in size is sometimes called the 'lee-way space' and is greater in the mandible than in the maxilla. This is one of the reasons why there is greater decrease in arch circumference in the lower jaw. As previously indicated, there is a correlation in the size of deciduous and corresponding permanent teeth, but it is a comparatively low one, and we do sometimes see small deciduous teeth replaced by large permanent ones or vice-versa.

DEVELOPMENT OF THE OCCLUSION
(Fig. 2.3 and 2.4)

At birth the gum pads can hardly be said to have an occlusion, but if they are brought into contact, they usually meet in the region of the future first deciduous molar. There is a space in the future incisor region and it has been suggested that this accommodates the nipple, although it usually closes at 5–6 months, shortly before the deciduous incisors erupt. This space is not present in all newly born infants, and it has been suggested that its absence is related to a deep overbite later in life. Such a relation is certainly not absolute but there may be a correlation in some cases. It would seem possible that in the earlier stage of intrauterine development there is a mandibular protrusion, but certainly this has disappeared by 64 days and by 110 days the growth of the mandible is lagging behind that of the maxilla, so that shortly before birth there is usually a distinct mandibular retrusion. This is not infrequently present at birth, although the mandible usually catches up before the deciduous dentition is complete.

There is a forward growth of the mandibular arch relative to the maxillary dentition which continues at a slow rate throughout infancy and childhood. This is reflected in changes which occur in the occlusion of the deciduous molars. It seems probable that, at least in some cases, when the first deciduous molars erupt the terminal planes of upper and lower molars (that is the posterior margins of the teeth), are in line with each other, and that the normal step, with the terminal plane of the lower molar slightly anterior to that of the upper molar, occurs as the second deciduous molars erupt (Fig. 2.3). While this is uncertain, there can be no doubt that in a substantial proportion of individuals the terminal planes of the second deciduous molars are in line when they first erupt. For normal occlusion to develop, this has to give way to a 'stepped' condition, so that the mesial cusps of the lower first permanent molar are somewhat in advance of those of the corresponding upper tooth. Baume has suggested that this cusp-to-cusp situation occurs in 76 per cent of individuals immediately after eruption of the deciduous molar with a step in the remaining 24 per cent. Clinch and Sillman feel that this is too high a proportion although they do not suggest alternatives.

There is, therefore, in many individuals, a need for a change in relationship of the fifth teeth so

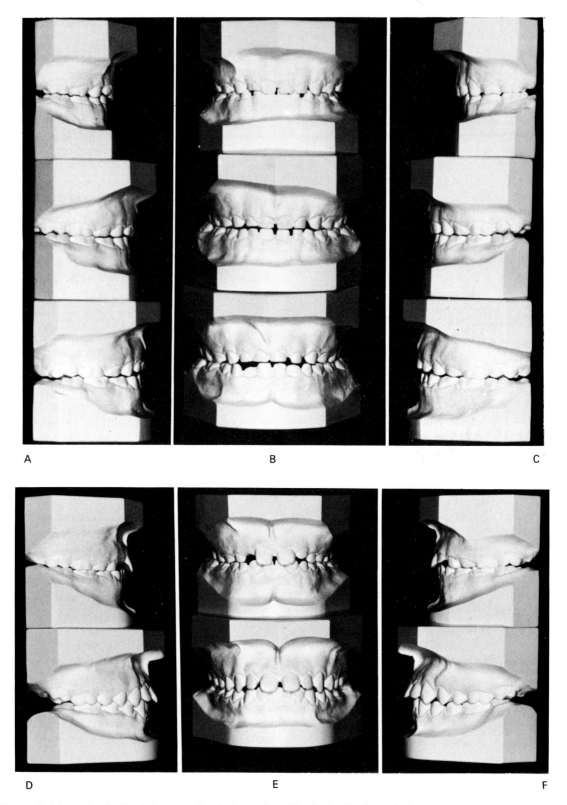

Fig. 2.3 Serial models of a developing normal occlusion, collected by the late Professor S. Friel and reproduced by permission of the Curator, British Society for the Study of Orthodontics.

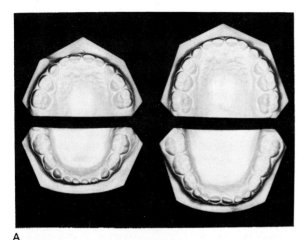

A

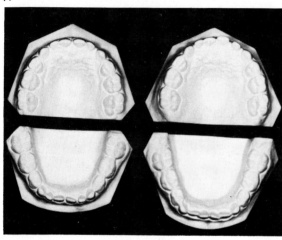

B

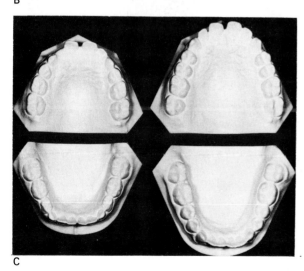

C

Fig. 2.4 Occlusal view of the serial models of the case shown in Fig. 2.3.

as to allow the first molars to come into a normal occlusion. This may occur at one or more of a number of stages as itemised below.

1. The second deciduous molars may erupt with a 'step' between their distal surfaces.

2. The lower arch may move forward as the second deciduous molars are erupting.

3. Very occasionally the whole lower arch apparently moves forward during the stage to the complete deciduous dentition — that is from 2 to 6 years.

4. Frequently, there is a forward movement as the first permanent molars are erupting.

5. The lower molars may move forward as the lower permanent incisors are erupting.

6. Baume has drawn attention to the existence of noticeable space between the upper deciduous lateral incisor and deciduous canine, and between the lower deciduous canine and first molar. These are similar to spaces found in the great apes and their purpose is to accommodate the pointed tip of the opposing deciduous canine tooth. He has suggested that closure of these spaces, especially that in the lower jaw, is the mechanism whereby the relationship of the permanent first molars is corrected. In fact the closure of the space is correlated with a decrease in overbite and a blunting of the pointed tips of the deciduous canines. While it may contribute to an improvement in molar relationship it is certainly not the sole cause.

7. Finally there is some further change in the first molar relationship as the deciduous molars are replaced by permanent premolars, the 'lee-way space' being greater in the lower than in the upper dental arch.

It will be appreciated that this forward movement of the lower dental arch reflects the relative increase in mandibular prognathism compared to that of the maxilla. At the same time there is usually a tendency for the overbite of the deciduous incisors to decrease, becoming edge-to-edge towards the end of their existence. In men living under primitive conditions the permanent incisors normally erupt with a positive overbite but this gradually disappears to produce an edge-to-edge occlusion in the mature individual. This would appear to be partly due to the continuing forward movement of the lower arch, and partly to attritional wear of the incisor teeth. In civilised man it does not occur. The overbite prevents the forward movement of the lower incisors which therefore frequently become crowded in the adolescent period.

This apparent forward movement of the lower dental base and of the attached dentition, is in fact caused, at least to some extent, by the forward and upward rotation of the mandible during growth to which attention has been drawn in the last chapter.

This then has been a description of the development of ideal dental occlusion. It is uncommon for any child to follow this path exactly. Some will develop malocclusions, while others may depart from the ideal path only to recover later and produce an occlusion which may be ideal or at least acceptable.

SUGGESTED READING

Bonnar E M E 1956 Aspects of the transition from deciduous to permanent dentition. Transactions of the British Society for the Study of Orthodontics 41–54

Clinch M 1966 The development of the deciduous and mixed dentitions. Transactions of the British Society for the Study of Orthodontics 83–92

Leighton B C 1971 The value of prophecy in orthodontics. Dental Practitioner 19: 218–23

Sillman H H 1964 Dimensional changes of the dental arches; longitudinal study from birth to 25 years. American Journal of Orthodontics 50: 824–42

3

The aetiology of malocclusion: skeletal and soft tissue factors

It would be idle to pretend that we have a full understanding of the aetiology of malocclusion in modern man. Like most of the ills to which man is heir, his dental occlusion is a result of a mixture of genetic and environmental factors — a mixture of nature and nurture. In the early days of the specialty, under the influence of Edward Angle, the importance of environmental factors was grossly exaggerated. Indeed, Angle himself refused to accept that genetic factors played any part at all. This was surprising. The relationship of the jaws to each other and of the soft tissues which surround them, are reflected in facial appearance and the similarity between close relatives and the very close similarity between identical twins, is evidence of the importance of genetic factors in shaping the jaws.

It is in fact generally accepted that the genes play a large part in producing the face and the dentition of the individual. The face is made up of many independent parts and it is not surprising that the inheritance of the face as a whole is multifactorial. We resemble our close relatives but even identical twins are not exact duplicates. The importance of genetic factors has been investigated by the collection of family histories — usually of Class III malocclusion — while twin studies, especially those of Lundstrom, have shown that for most dimensions of the face and jaws, these factors are paramount. This is not to say that environmental factors can be completely eliminated. It seems likely, however, that such factors play their part at an early stage after, or even before birth.

The incidence and especially the severity of malocclusion varies between different races and is probably highest in people of Western European origin. Although malocclusion has been found in the skulls of individuals who died in the Middle Ages, it has increased, in both incidence and severity, over the last 200 years. In particular, there would appear to have been an increase in crowding of the jaws with a decrease in size of the dental arches. This may in part be due to the mixture of genes which results from an industrial revolution but it is difficult to believe that this is the whole story. Dickson has drawn attention to the increase in variation which occurs in a species, when an unnaturally large proportion of young animals live to maturity, and are able themselves to reproduce — when we lose the benefits accruing from 'survival of the fittest'. In more primitive communities, the majority of children who are born do not themselves live to become parents. In all advanced countries this has been completely reversed over the last 200 years, so that nowadays even the most handicapped may themselves have children. The increased variation which results from this, so far as the dentition is concerned, constitutes a malocclusion. Suggestions that the increased crowding is due to a decreased function, resulting from prepared foods, seems to have been discredited.

In considering the aetiology of malocclusion, it is convenient to look at the subject from the point of view of the skeletal pattern, the soft tissues and the dental pattern. It should be realised that these are not independent of each other and that considerable interaction takes place between them.

SKELETAL PATTERN

The basal part of the jaws, on which the teeth and

alveoli are situated, are related to each other in three planes of space: antero-posterior, vertical and lateral. The mandible is attached to the skull only through its articulation with the squamous part of the temporal bone. This does not articulate directly with the maxilla since the sphenoid bone lies between. It is perhaps surprising that in most individuals the teeth erupt in such a position that upper and lower teeth occlude in a very close approximation to the ideal. Not so surprisingly, quite a small discrepancy in the relationship of the dental bases will produce a malocclusion.

Antero-posterior relationship

We have seen that the mandible is normally related to the maxilla in such a way that the teeth will erupt into normal occlusion or a Class I malocclusion. There will be no antero-posterior discrepancy. If the mandible is placed posteriorly relative to the maxilla, we have a situation which we call a Class II skeletal pattern. The lower posterior teeth will tend to occlude too far distally with the upper cheek teeth, and the incisors will erupt with some increase in overjet. Similarly, if the mandibular base is too far forward, relative to the maxillary base, we will have a Class III skeletal pattern with a corresponding malocclusion of the posterior teeth and a tendency for the lower incisors to erupt labially to the uppers. A number of authors have analysed malocclusions showing a malrelationship of the dental arches and it would appear that this malrelationship can occur for a number of different reasons. The Class II skeletal pattern can be produced by a small mandible relative to a large maxilla. Although this does occur, it is in fact comparatively uncommon and the jaws are normally of comparable size. This can be demonstrated when we come to take impressions of the teeth; it is quite uncommon to find a marked discrepancy in the size of impression tray required for upper and lower impressions. Again, the Class II skeletal pattern may be caused by the maxilla being placed too far anteriorly, either because it is long or because the anterior base of skull, to which it is attached, is unduly long for the rest of the face. Although possible, this is also comparatively uncommon. The most common factor in producing a Class II skeletal pattern

arises because the mandibular joint is placed too far posteriorly to the maxilla, thus carrying a mandible of normal size too far backwards. This process cannot be reversed by treatment. It can be brought about by discrepancies in any or all of a number of areas in the base of skull, a common cause being an unusually large angle between the anterior and posterior bases of skull where they meet at the sella turcica. Nevertheless, it is unusual to find a single discrepancy which has produced malrelationship of the dental arches. Most individuals depart from the mean values in several parts of the skull and these departures may exacerbate each other or one may tend to compensate for another.

Examples of this are shown in Figure 3.1. In this figure, the lateral skull tracings of four children, exhibiting a Class II skeletal pattern are each superimposed on the outline diagram for 12-year-old Swedish boys taken from the work of Björk and previously shown in Chapter 1. In Figure 3.1A the skeletal discrepancy is essentially due to a forward position of the maxilla. This in turn would appear to be due to the abnormally long anterior base of skull. It will be seen that the distance from sella turcica to the base of the nasal bone is increased and this has carried the maxilla forward in an otherwise normally proportioned face. In Figure 3.1B the position of the maxilla is reasonably normal. The temporo-mandibular joint is somewhat posteriorly placed due to an increase in the angle between anterior and posterior bases of skull — the so-called saddle angle. Even so, this does not entirely account for the marked skeletal discrepancy which is exacerbated by the short horizontal ramus of the mandible and in this case there seems genuinely to be a small lower dental base relative to the upper. Figure 3.1C shows a similar condition, although here the mandible is of normal size and the posterior position of its joint is largely responsible for its postnormal relation with the maxilla. The situation in this case is complicated by a downward and backward rotation of the lower face relative to the base of skull and this serves to worsen the skeletal discrepancy. Finally, in Figure 3.1D we see a skeletal discrepancy associated with a combination of several factors. The anterior base of skull is of normal length but the maxilla is situated in a

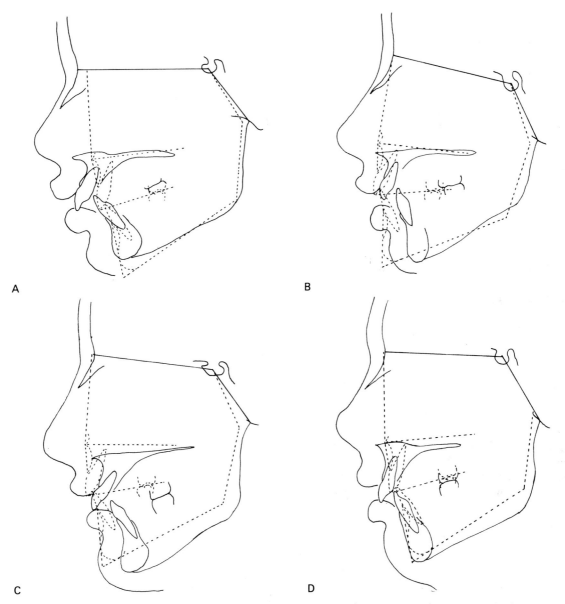

Fig. 3.1 Tracings of four individuals exhibiting a Class II skeletal pattern, each superimposed on Björk's outline for 12-year-old Swedish children. A, The long anterior base of skull has carried the maxilla anteriorly. B, A retroplaced mandible associated with a large saddle angle. The mandible is also small. C, Retroplaced mandibular joint with large saddle angle. The lower face has rotated downwards and backwards. D, Essentially prognathous maxilla.

forward position on this base of skull. The mandibular joint is situated too far posteriorly, but the mandible is longer than average, compensating for this effect, so that the overall skeletal pattern and the malocclusion reflect the position of the maxilla.

Similarly, a Class III skeletal pattern can be brought about by many factors, most of which are the reverse of those already described. In this case however, it is rather more common to find a genuine discrepancy in size between mandibular and maxillary bases. Examples of the skeletal discrepancies in Class III malocclusion, are illustrated in Chapter 12.

The vertical relationship

In discussing the vertical relationship of the dental bases, we are essentially considering a malrelation of the anterior part of the lower facial height and its relationship to the posterior part. If the anterior lower facial height is unduly increased, as seen in Figure 3.2A, the incisor teeth will continue to develop beyond their normal occlusal level but only to a limited extent. Eventually they will 'run out of steam' and if the condition is sufficiently severe, the patient will present with an anterior open bite. In extreme cases we may find that the patient occludes only on the distal part of the most distal molar teeth with the open bite increasing as one passes forward in the mouth. Typically, the lower border of the mandible is steeply inclined in these cases.

Where the lower facial height is abnormally small, as shown in Figure 3.2B, there may well be a tendency to a very deep overbite of a type which is particularly difficult to treat. However, in cases with a small lower facial height, the situation is rather more complex. It would seem that the anterior teeth have a powerful tendency to develop to a certain level but the way in which this actually takes place varies between individuals, depending to a large extent on other aspects of the skeletal and soft tissue pattern. Four examples of this are shown in Figure 3.3. All of these children show very small lower facial heights. In all the cases if the teeth were tilted to a normal angle and any antero-posterior skeletal discrepancy removed, a deep overbite would be present. In practice, however, this is not always the case. In Figure 3.3A a hyperactive lower lip, described in the next section, has retroclined the lower incisors and proclined the upper teeth, so that the overbite is not indeed complete onto the palate. In Figure 3.3B a Class II skeletal pattern has caused the upper incisors to be further labially than the lowers so that although the interincisal angle is normal, there is a deep overbite. In Figure 3.3C a different soft tissue pattern has caused both upper and lower incisors to be retroclined, producing a high inter-incisal angle and an overbite so deep that the upper incisal edges were traumatising the gingival margin labially to the lower incisors. The reverse of this is seen in Figure

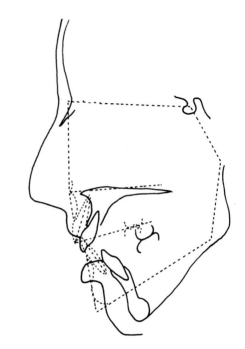

A

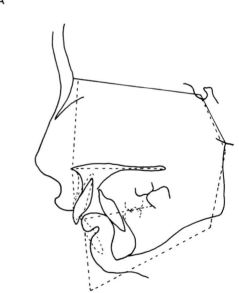

B

Fig. 3.2 Tracings of two individuals, similarly superimposed on Björk's standard outline, with A, an increased anterior lower facial height and B, a decreased height.

3.3D, where both upper and lower incisors are markedly proclined, possibly due to the action of the tongue, and the overbite is actually reduced. Nevertheless, even in this case, if the teeth were tilted lingually, a deep overbite would be present.

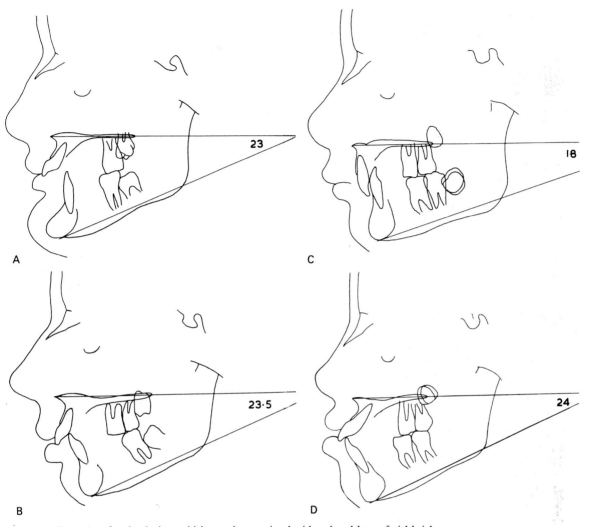

Fig. 3.3 Examples of malocclusions which may be associated with reduced lower facial heights.

In general, those severe discrepancies of vertical incisal relationship which are related to a similar discrepancy in skeletal pattern are particularly resistent to treatment unless natural growth is unusually favourable.

The lateral relationship

An abnormality in the width of the bony dental bases will often be associated with a crossbite. If the maxilla is narrow relative to the mandible, this will produce the conventional buccal crossbite, with the buccal cusps of the lower posterior teeth occluding buccally to those of the upper

posteriors. This can be seen, to some extent in Figure 3.4A, where the upper dental arch is appreciably smaller than the lower. It will be seen that the posterior teeth are at a normal angle to their bases and the crossbite seen in Figure 3.4B reflects the skeletal discrepancy rather than any tilting of the teeth. This patient had a Class III jaw relationship (Fig. 3.4C) and the antero-posterior discrepancy contributed to the lateral one, since a wider part of the lower jaw lay opposite a narrower part of the upper. In Figure 3.4D the models have been placed in a more normal relationship and the postero-anterior view in Figure 3.4E shows that this eliminates some, but

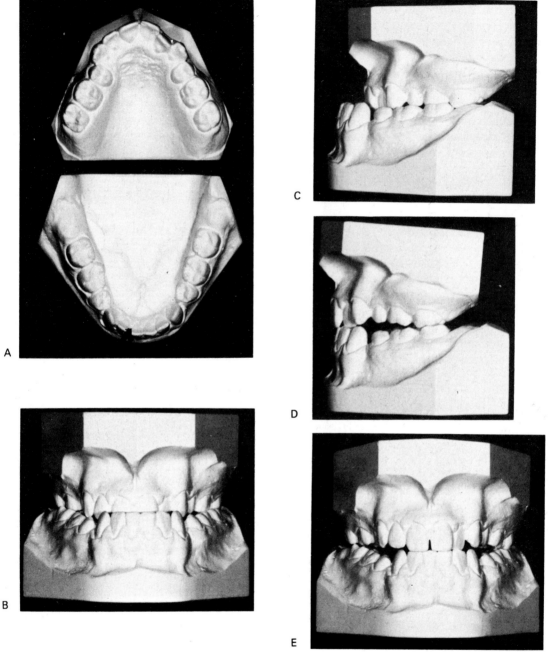

Fig. 3.4 Buccal crossbite of lower posterior teeth, due partly to a discrepancy in width of the skeletal bases. The Class III skeletal pattern also contributes, as illustrated when the models are placed in more normal relation (D and E).

not all of the crossbite. The antero-posterior skeletal discrepancy may therefore contribute to a lateral malocclusion. In a case where the lower arch is a narrow one, a lingual crossbite will be produced (Fig. 3.5). In the latter case the buccal cusps of the lower teeth occlude completely lingually to the upper teeth so that there is no occlusal contact between the occlusal surfaces of the posterior teeth. This is sometimes called 'scissors bite'.

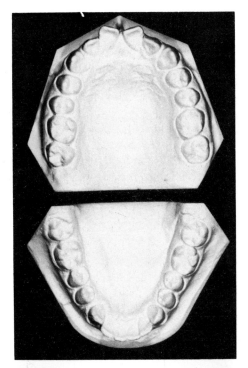

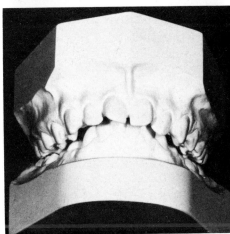

Fig. 3.5 Bilateral lingual crossbite of lower posterior teeth, associated with a discrepancy in width of skeletal bases

A skeletal discrepancy in the lateral direction may be caused by a genuine difference in width of the dental bases. It may also, as we have seen in Figure 3.4, be the result of an antero-posterior skeletal discrepancy where this is extreme. If the mandibular base is postnormal to the upper, we may find that a narrower part of the lower arch corresponds to a given part of the upper, the converse of that which we have seen in connection with a Class III skeletal pattern.

SOFT TISSUES

There is little doubt that the muscles around the mouth can have a profound effect on the occlusion. The teeth lie within the alveolar arch between the tongue on the one side and the lips and cheeks on the other. Since teeth are normally stationary, it is logical to believe that they are in a position of balance between these muscular structures, that is either the forces exerted by the muscles exactly balance or they lie in a position where there is no force. The mandible is slung from the skull and at rest, lies in a second, vertical position of balance between the elevators and depressors of the mandible. We have therefore to consider two groups of muscles: firstly the muscles of expression, supplied by the seventh nerve but also including the tongue, and secondly, the muscles of mastication, supplied by the fifth cranial nerve.

Muscles of expression (including the tongue)

The anterior teeth lie between the tongue and the lips. It is usual to describe the lips as lying in light contact when at rest. In a large proportion of chil-

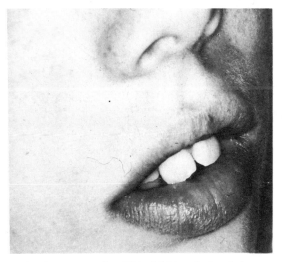

Fig. 3.6 Incompetent lips. This child breathed entirely through his nose.

dren, probably a majority, this is not the case. Many children have their lips apart at rest and have in the past been described as 'mouth-breathers'. This again is a fallacy. The majority of children who is habitually have their lips apart, breathe perfectly normally through the nose (Fig. 3.6). Mouth-breathing is invariably the result of an obstruction in the nasal passages, either complete or partial.

Lips which are held apart at rest are described as incompetent. The degree of incompetence will vary greatly and if it slight, the individual may make an almost unconscious effort to hold them together. A child is described as having competent lips when these are held naturally in contact at rest. This should not be confused with children who hold their lips in contact as a result of slight muscular contraction. Truly competent lips exist only in a minority of children. On the other hand the majority of adults hold their lips together at rest and this change of posture has never been satisfactorily explained, although Vig and Cohen have shown that the lips usually grow more during childhood than do the underlying bones.

There are doubtless many reasons why a child should hold his lips apart at rest, but often this is due to a skeletal discrepancy. If the anterior lower facial height is increased and the lips are of

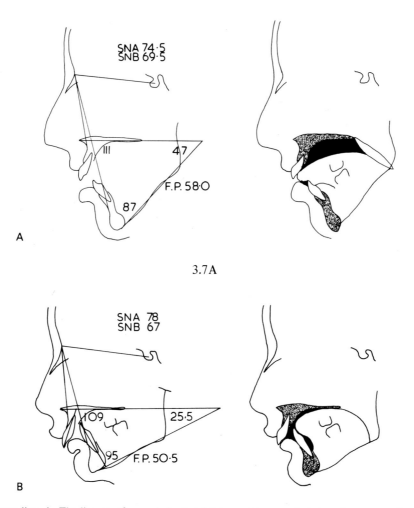

Fig. 3.7 Incompetent lips. A, The lips are of normal size but fail to meet because their insertions are too far apart, vertically. B, The incompetence results from an antero-posterior displacement of their insertions. (These are the same patients as in Fig. 3.2.)

normal length and inserted in their normal places, then logically they will not comfortably meet. This is illustrated in Figure 3.7A which shows the patient already considered in Figure 3.2. Similarly, if there is a gross Class II skeletal pattern, so that the insertion of the lower lip is too far back relative to the upper, again it may be difficult for the individual to hold these lips together without an effort (Fig. 3.7B). It may also be that in some cases the lips themselves are of inadequate size to bridge the gap — the traditional phrase 'short upper lip' may well be a real one.

Even where the lips are held apart at rest, it is necessary that the front of the mouth should be sealed. If this is not so, saliva will escape between the lips and the child will drool! This anterior oral seal will also facilitate normal nasal breathing, although the latter could be achieved by a posterior seal between the dorsum of the tongue and the soft palate. The anterior seal may be produced in a number of ways. If the lips are only slightly incompetent then, as suggested above, the slight effort necessary to hold them together will be made more or less unconsciously. Where the incompetence is due to a Class II skeletal pattern, with a postnormal mandible, then the natural rest position of the mandible may be modified and a habitual rest position adopted, with the mandible displaced downwards and forwards, enabling the individual to bring the lips into contact (Fig. 3.8). The third possibility is that the seal with be produced by a lip–tongue contact. The exact mechanism for this depends on a number of factors and especially the height of the lower lip line relative to the upper incisors. This in turn will be affected at least in part by the vertical relationship of the skeletal bases. If the lip line is high, as shown in Figure 3.7B, the seal will be produced almost entirely by the lower lip resting under the upper incisors in contact with their lingual surface and with the anterior part of the hard palate. If on the other hand the lip line is low (Fig. 3.7A), the seal will be produced mainly by the tongue resting between the incisors, coming into contact with the lower lip. In many cases both lip and tongue contribute to the seal. This lip–tongue contact will have the effect of 'dispersing' the teeth, that is of proclining the upper incisors and possibly retroclining the lowers, thus increasing any natural tendency to an overjet. Its effect is greatest where the seal is produced primarily by the lower lip.

So we may have a situation where a Class II skeletal pattern has taken the lower dentition too far posteriorly relative to the upper, thus producing not only a postnormal occlusion of the posterior teeth but also an increase in overjet. If the lower lip line is relatively low, this overjet will probably reflect the skeletal discrepancy without any proclination of the upper incisor teeth (Fig. 3.7A). If the lower lip is high, the lower lip may be drawn under the upper incisors, thus proclining them and increasing the overjet still further (Fig. 3.7B). Alternatively, a high lower lip line may have the effect of retroclining the upper incisors if it comes to lie on their labial surface,

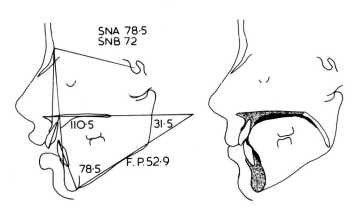

Fig. 3.8 Incompetent lips associated with mild skeletal discrepancy. Lips held together as a result to habitual forward posture of the mandible.

producing a typical Class II Division 2 appearance. As we shall see in later chapters, the height of the lip line has an important bearing on the prognosis for treatment, especially in Class II Division 1 malocclusion. If the upper incisors are resting on the outer surface of the lower lip and they can be retracted so as to rest on the inner surface of the same lip, then the patient is provided with a natural permanent retainer and the result is on the whole more likely to be stable than in the case shown in Figure 3.7A. In this latter case, the lip is not effecting the upper incisor position and will not do so following treatment.

The role of the tongue is more controversial. It has long been realised that if an individual has an anterior open bite or an incomplete overbite, the tongue protrudes through the gap so formed, in swallowing, speech and indeed often at rest. It seemed logical to assume that this 'tongue thrust' was the cause of the incomplete overbite. In fact in the majority of instances the reverse would seem to be the case: the incomplete overbite has to be occluded by the tongue in order to produce a seal, as described above. Ballard has suggested that the position labio-lingually of the incisor teeth is determined primarily by the lips and that the tongue acts in a secondary capacity, rather like a plunger adapting the teeth into the mould produced by the lips. If the lips are full and flaccid the teeth will be proclined until resisted by the lips, producing a bimaxillary proclination. Where the lip tone is high, the tongue can only take them as far as the lips will allow, producing a typical bimaxillary retroclination. The former is usually associated with a reduced overbite or even anterior open bite, while the latter is usually associated with a deep overbite of the Class II Division 2 type.

Bimaxillary proclination is sometimes associated with a tongue which is apparently unduly large. It is a common clinical finding that an anterior open bite of this type will resolve during childhood and that a bimaxillary proclination will become less marked. It was assumed that this was because the tongue grew less than the surrounding oral tissues although Cohen has recently shown this to be fallacious. In fact the tongue becomes relatively larger during childhood in most individuals. It is also comes to lie lower down in the oral cavity due to the increased height of the lower face during growth and this lower position is probably the reason for the uprighting of the anterior teeth where this occurs.

It would seem that the above description is something of an over-simplification. Several authors have investigated the resting pressure of lips or cheeks and the tongue on the teeth (see Gould & Picton, 1962 and Proffit, 1978) and there has been a general consensus that the resting pressure of the tongue is greater than that of the cheeks and lips. The missing factor is probably provided by the 'chain' of interdental periodontal fibres, holding the teeth in contact. If these fibres are destroyed, in periodontal disease, the teeth often tend to migrate. Nevertheless, this additional factor does not invalidate the importance of basic muscular balance.

It was formerly believed that the main effect of the lips and tongue in positioning the anterior teeth took place during such activities as swallowing, speech and facial expression. It has become more fashionable in recent years to assume that the main effect of the soft tissues takes place at rest. This is indeed probably the major factor but it seems unwise to ignore function altogether. The frequency with which a person swallows varies very widely, both between individuals and between the different times of the day. The average frequency of about once per minute is therefore rather meaningless. It may well be that a lip to tongue contact in swallowing has an important reinforcing effect in proclining upper incisors especially where the lip is too low to affect the incisors at rest, but is drawn in during swallowing.

Soft tissue patterns are infinitely variable but it seems possible to recognise two types of case in which the function of the soft tissues is of considerable importance, although both of these are quite rare in an extreme form. In the first type the lower lip appears to be hyperactive, particularly during facial expression. This lower lip has been described as 'strap-like' or 'sling-like'. An example of this is shown in Figure 3.9. Its effect will depend on the height of the lip relative to the dentition. Where the lip line is low it will effect primarily the lower incisor region, either retroclining these teeth or indeed, causing the anterior alveolus to grow upwards and lingually so that the whole of the lower incisor segment is moved bodily in a lingual direction. This will result in a very marked chin. In the girl shown in Figure 3.9A, it will be seen that both these effects have been produced. Such a hyperactive lower lip is resisted by the tongue, which may protrude into contact with the lip to produce an incomplete overbite, even in patients with a small lower facial height. The height of the lower lip again enters into the picture. If it is high the lower lip will contract lingually to the upper incisors and will cause incisor proclination. If however the lower lip contracts on the labial side of the upper incisors, it will cause a marked retroclination of these teeth, producing a very severe Class II Division 2 incisor relationship. The girl shown in Figure 3.9A had the upper incisors resting on the lower lip although, because of the severe skeletal discrepancy, these teeth were not unduly proclined. Treatment in this case was prolonged and difficult but eventually the overjet was reduced to the patient's satisfaction. Figure 3.9C shows her as an adult with the hyperactive lower lip still very noticeable but with the upper incisors inside this lip and well aligned (Fig. 3.9E). Orthodontic treatment has effectively turned her from a Class II Division 1 malocclusion into a Class II Division 2 type.

The second type of abnormal soft tissue behaviour is the so-called endogenous tongue thrust. Although the majority of tongue thrusts are probably secondary to the position of the teeth and have only, at most, a minor effect in any resulting open bite, it would seem that a small proportion of patients exhibit some lack of finer control of their tongue. In these cases the tongue protrudes very actively between the anterior teeth during swallowing and speech, and probably lies in this position even at rest. It is often associated with a speech defect, producing a sigmatism (an abnormality in pronunciation of the letter 's') but pronunciation of other consonants may be affected. Such an endogenous tongue thrust, if powerful enough, will produce a bimaxillary proclination, an anterior open bite, or an incomplete overbite. Such a case is shown in Figure 3.10. This boy shows a typical lack of facial

expression — the reverse of that shown in Figure 3.9. He exhibited an increased overjet with a very incomplete overbite. Treatment was conventional, leading gradually to an upper removable appliance with a labial bow to move the upper incisors palatally. In fact after a very short time they failed to move further and indeed when the force on the incisors was increased, these teeth became markedly loose. There was no doubt therefore that the appliance was being worn but presumably its effect was being resisted by the action of the tongue. The second tracing shows the final position of the teeth very little changed from the original.

This type of endogenous tongue thrust is excessively rare and it is very difficult to differentiate it from the normal secondary type of tongue thrust. Indeed, although two types of abnormal muscle activity have been described, it should not be felt that patients fall neatly into these two categories. Variation is little short of infinite in both type and severity. Thus a patient with a slight tendency towards an endogenous tongue thrust may be capable of controlling this if the teeth are moved into a normal position, although with a more severe abnormality we may encounter the resistance shown in Figure 3.10.

If the anterior teeth lie in a position of balance between lips and tongue, presumably the posterior teeth lie in a similar position between the cheeks and tongue. This may be the reason why expansion buccally of the cheek teeth is almost invariably followed by relapse. It is more difficult to assess whether abnormalities here can affect the occlusion. It has been suggested that a low tongue position, possibly but not necessarily associated with an increased lower facial height, may be the cause of a crossbite of the posterior teeth, since the pressure of the buccinator muscle is not balanced by that of the tongue. It has been suggested that any factor which causes the individual to maintain a lowered position of the mandible will remove the tongue from the upper arch and this produces a muscular imbalance, a narrower upper arch and probably a crossbite. In this category may be included mouth-breathing and digit-sucking, both of which are discussed in the next chapter and an example of the latter is shown in Figure 3.15. It has also been suggested

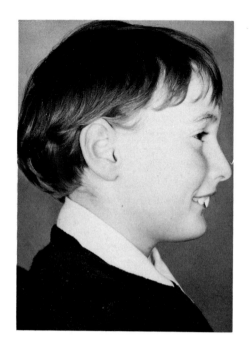
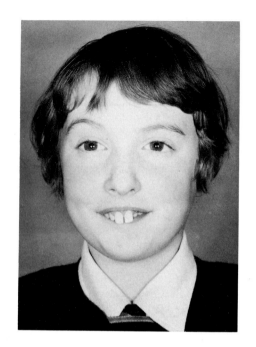

A

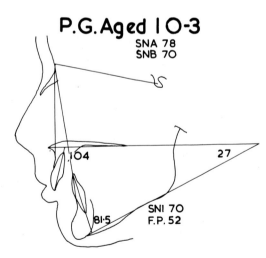

P.G. Aged 10·3

SNA 78
SNB 70

164   27

81·5   SNI 70
              F.P. 52

B

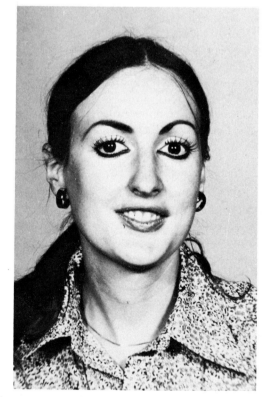

C

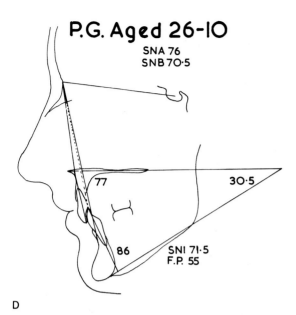

P.G. Aged 26-10

SNA 76
SNB 70·5

77   30·5

86   SNI 71·5
          F.P. 55

D

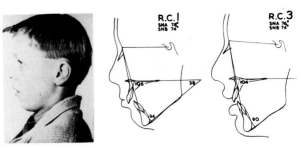

Fig. 3.10 Patient with 'endogenous' tongue thrust. Attempts to reduce the overjet were unsuccessful and resulted in excessive mobility of the teeth.

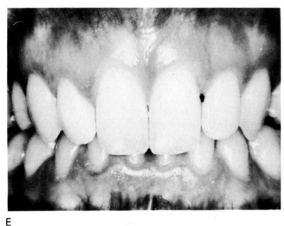

E

Fig. 3.9 A, Photographs of patient at age 10 years. Note hyperactive contraction of the lower lip in smiling. B, Lateral skull tracing, showing retroclination of lower incisors and retroplacement of alveolus. C, Photograph and D, tracing at age 27 years: 12 years after end of treatment. Hyperactive lip activity still present but E, patient now has Class II Division 2 malocclusion.

that a high tongue position may be the cause of a narrow lower arch and reverse crossbite, although this would seem to be a confusion of cause and effect.

Muscles of mastication

The muscles of mastication, derived from the first branchial arch, are responsible for opening and closing the mouth and for producing lateral jaw movements. They also hold the mandible in its natural rest position. During the period of the Second World War, Thompson and Brodie came to the conclusion that this rest position was an essential part of the individual's make-up and was unalterable. They suggested that the mandible came to rest as a result of muscle tone with the tonic contraction of the elevators of the mandible exactly balanced by that of the depressors. These ideas have since been modified in two respects. Firstly, it has come to be realised that the rest position of the mandible is essentially part of the individual's posture and although the elasticity of the muscles may play a small part, its position is essentially determined by feed-back mechanisms. These probably come from the position of the tongue, lips, cheeks and teeth relative to each other and possibly to some extent from the joint itself. Secondly it has been appreciated that the rest position is less immutable than was originally thought. It can be modified to some extent by the position of the head and by the age of the patient and presence or absence of teeth. In an orthodontic context the most interesting modification is that seen in certain cases of Class II Division 1 malocclusion. Where the overjet is only moderately increased (Fig. 3.8) this is frequently associated with incompetent lips which are essentially due to the Class II skeletal pattern, which carries the insertion of the lower lip too far back relative to the upper. The patient may be able to overcome this and hold the lips in contact by modifying his rest position and holding the mandible in a forward posture. This will mean that the condyle of the mandible will lie on the eminentia articularis, and the movement from rest to occlusion will involve an upward and backward translation of the condylar head, compared with the normal rotation seen in most individuals. The space between the posterior teeth — the free-way space or interocclusal clearance — is usually greater in these cases. It will be seen in Figure 3.8 that this allows the individual to bring the lips into contact and to produce an anterior oral seal, although the extent of 'forward posture' which the individual can maintain is quite limited. Ricketts showed, many years ago, that following treatment of this type of patient with reduction of the overjet, the forward posture of the mandible would disappear and the condylar head would return to the fossa in both rest and occlusion. Perhaps the individual could keep his lips in contact without the forward posture because the upper incisor teeth were no longer in the way. A similar situation occurs in most patients with Class II Division 2 malocclusion (Fig. 3.11). These individuals usually have no difficulty in keeping their lips in contact and the downward and forward displacement may be necessary to bring the incisor teeth into a more comfortable and functional relationship and possibly also to correct the 'over-competence' of the lips.

The situation in Class III malocclusion is rather different. This concerns those patients in whom the lower incisors occlude labially to the upper incisors with a deep overbite. These individuals can often achieve an edge-to-edge relationship of the incisor teeth and the details of this will be dealt with in a later chapter. One feature is that they cannot assume their natural endogenous rest position since the incisor teeth would get in the way, and in these cases, the habitual rest position occurs with the incisors in an edge-to-edge position. Again this often involves an increase in the free-way space.

As already indicated, it is therefore suggested that the individual has an inherent or endogenous rest position to which he will often return following successful orthodontic treatment. From this rest position, it is possible to adopt an alternative, habitual rest position which is dictated by a feedback mechanism from the lips and incisor teeth. This may present yet another method of producing an anterior oral seal in cases with incompetent lips.

MANDIBULAR ROTATION

We have already seen in Chapter 1 that during growth the mandible does not maintain a constant relation to the rest of the skull. Figure 1.9 showed lateral skull tracings of two children, in one of whom the mandible rotated forward and upward during growth, while in the other, the mandible rotated downwards and backwards. It would seem that in fact a slight forward and upward rotation is the normal condition, and in good occlusion the mandible essentially rotates about the point where the lower incisal edge occludes on the cingulum of the upper incisor. In the case shown in Figure 3.12A, however, the point of rotation lies further back in the region of the premolars or molars, so

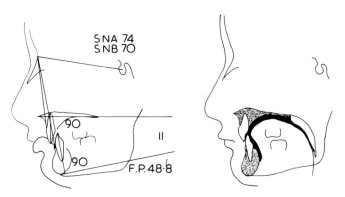

Fig. 3.11 Tracings of patient with severe Class II Division 2 malocclusion. A, In occlusion: note the 'over-competent' lips. B, In the habitual rest position.

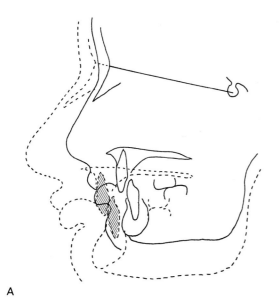

A

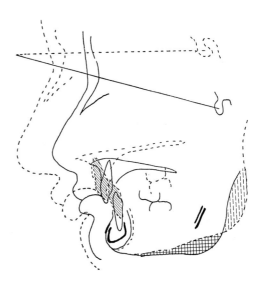

B

Fig. 3.12 Patients showing extreme mandibular rotation, previously shown in Fig. 1.9. A, Patient, also shown in Fig. 3.11, traced at ages 9 and 16 years, showing apparent normal growth. B, Superimposed on Björk structures to show extreme forward rotation. C, Patient showing extreme backwards rotation.

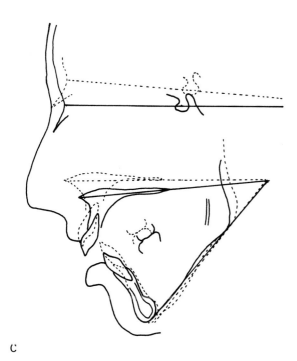

c

that as the rotation occurs the lower incisors tend to move upwards producing a deep anterior overbite of a type which is often difficult to treat. Björk seems to imply that this is to some extent due to a high inter-incisal angle and an unfavourable relation of the incisors to each other. If the incisors were in normal relationship, the rotation

would take place about these teeth and it is only where the inter-incisal angle is high, so that the lower incisors can slide over the uppers, that rotation takes place about a point further back in the arch. This explanation may well be an oversimplification. The case shown in Figure 3.12C the rotation downwards and backwards about a point in the premolar or molar region, is associated with a reduced overbite or even an anterior open bite.

The reason for these two extreme forms of rotation is controversial. It has been suggested that a forward rotation is due to greater vertical growth of the vertical ramus of the mandible than of the combined alveolar regions. This is undoubtedly a fact, but it would seem more probable that the verticle growth of the alveoli is secondary to the position of the mandible. Møller, using electromyography on young adults, noted that the muscle force of the elevators of the mandible was greater in 'forward rotators' than in 'backward rotator'. This was confirmed by J. P. Moss and also, using strain gauges attached to the teeth, by Profit et al. (1983). The last author found, however, that when the same experiment was carried out on children, there was no appreciable difference between the two types of rotation. He suggests that the difference in adults is due to the greater mechanical advantage in the forward type of rotation. Further investigation is clearly desirable.

MANDIBULAR DISPLACEMENT ON CLOSING

In most individuals the mandible will close from the rest position, by a hinge action in the temporomandibular joint. Where there is a forward habitual rest position, this will be associated with some degree of posterior translation of the condylar head. In a proportion of patients, the mandible does not remain in centric jaw relationship during closure to the inter-cuspal position. This is because one or more teeth meet in an uncomfortable relationship if the normal path of closure is followed. Such a tooth is sometimes described as having an initial or premature contact. When the tooth first erupts the individual finds closure on this tooth uncomfortable or even painful and the mandible is therefore displaced to the minimum extent which will allow a comfortable closure. An intercuspal position is gradually developed in this displaced position unless treatment is instituted to correct the initial contact. Such a displaced inter-cuspal position is sometimes called a 'bite of comfort' or 'bite of convenience'.

The most obvious example of this occurs on a Class III skeletal base. In such a case the incisor teeth erupt into an edge-to-edge relationship. This is not comfortable and since the mandible cannot retrude further, it is protruded so as to allow the posterior teeth to come into contact. This is demonstrated in Figure 3.13 and it will be seen in this patient, as is usually the case, that the condition is associated with a deep overbite. It is interesting that where the deep overbite is present, as the mandible continues to close the condyles are able to move posteriorly, due to angulation of the incisor teeth, until in the occlusal position the condyle is often fully retruded into its correct position in the fossa. Such as case is illustrated diagrammatically in Figure 3.14. The original

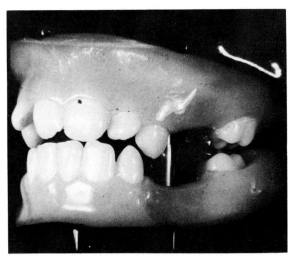

A

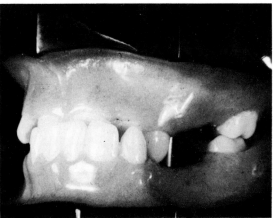

B

Fig. 3.13 Acrylic models of patient with Class III skeletal pattern and deep overbite. A, On initial contact with incisors edge-to edge. B, In occlusion

tracing with the solid outline shows the condition in the patient before orthodontic treatment. The dotted outline has in fact been produced diagrammatically. A second piece of tracing paper was superimposed on the first and the outline of the mandible traced a second time on this piece. A drawing pin was then inserted in the region of the condyle so that the second tracing could rotate on the first and as it was swung downwards and backwards it came into the edge-to-edge occlusion which was in fact present in the mouth. To achieve this diagramatically, it was necessary for

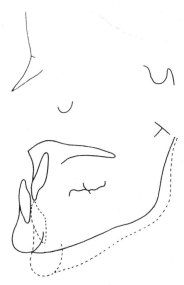

Fig. 3.14 Tracing of patient with Class III incisor relation and deep overbite. This patient could achieve an edge-to-edge incisor relation. The dotted outline has been produced by 'rotating' the mandible backwards around the mandibular joint region.

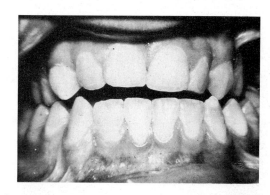

A

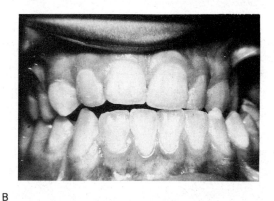

B

Fig. 3.15 Patient with a narrow upper arch. A, On initial contact the condition is symmetrical but the posterior teeth meet cusp-to-cusp. B, In occlusion the mandible is displaced to the patient's left, producing an apparent unilateral crossbite. The patient also sucked the right thumb, which may be the cause of the narrow upper arch.

the lower incisors to pass 'through' the upper incisors. Clearly this does not happen in nature and in order for the patient to close from the edge-to-edge relationship to the occlusal position, the mandible has to be protruded to disengage the incisors but as it closes up the condyle returns to its position in the depth of the fossa, so that in this position there is in fact no displacement of the mandible. This feature seems to be confined to those cases with a deep overbite. In an individual with a Class III incisor relationship and a shallow overbite, who can achieve an edge-to-edge occlusion, the condyles are displaced forward on the eminentia articularis in occlusion.

Mandibular displacement can however occur in many other cases. If the upper dental arch is narrow relative to the lower, the posterior teeth may erupt so that the upper buccal cusps, instead of overhanging the lower buccal cusps, meet cusp-to-cusp (Fig. 3.15). Similarly, the lingual cusps will also meet head-on. Such a position is uncomfortable and the individual will displace the mandible to one side, in this case the patient's left, producing an apparent unilateral crossbite (Fig. 3.15B). This will also produce an apparent facial asymmetry which can be very satisfactorily

corrected by bilateral expansion of the upper arch. Indeed mandibular displacements may occur with only one, or a small number, of teeth forming the initial contact, as shown in Figure 3.16 where a single instanding incisor has caused the patient to displace the mandible forward shortly after its eruption, into an inter-cuspal position which is not in centric jaw relationship. The remaining teeth have erupted into a good occlusion in this position so that, in the adult patient illustrated, correction will be quite difficult, since not only must the instanding incisor be corrected, but also the occlusion of most of the remaining teeth. Similarly, isolated premolars in crossbite can cause a lateral displacement. In fact where any tooth appears to be in crossbite, the patient should be carefully

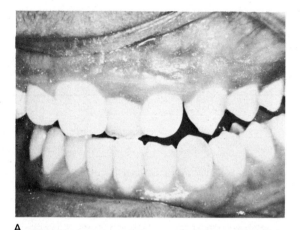

A

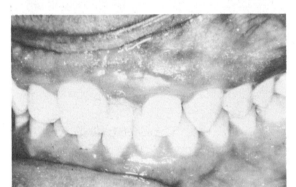

B

Fig. 3.16 Adult patient with instanding /1. A, Initial contact. B, Occlusal position with mandible displaced anteriorly.

examined to see if there is a displacement of the mandible on closing.

Although the mandibular displacement originally occurs because of the discomfort in closing in centric jaw relationship, the individual quickly learns to avoid the uncomfortable tooth. Closure therefore takes place directly into the inter-cuspal position without any need to feel the way. Indeed, if one is attempting to diagnose such a displacement, it is extremely difficult to persuade the individual to close in centric jaw relationship, since he knows that in this position teeth will meet in an uncomfortable or even painful relationship. Nevertheless, if the discomfort is eliminated, even

by fitting an orthodontic appliance which caps the posterior teeth, the individual will return to the centric path of closure within a matter of minutes. As already indicated, it is desirable to treat any mandibular displacement as early as possible to prevent the rest of the dentition developing in the displaced position, as has occurred in Figure 3.16B.

SUGGESTED READING

Ballard C F 1963 Variations of posture and behaviour of the lips and tongue which determine the position of the labial segments; the implications in orthodontics, prosthetics and speech. Transactions of the European Orthodontic Society: 67–93

Björk A 1947 The face in profile. Svensk Tandlakare Tidskrift 40: Suppl. 8B

Björk A, Skieller V 1972 Facial development and tooth eruption. American Journal of Orthodontics 62: 339–383

Cohen A M 1977 Reorientation of the mandible and tongue during growth. British Journal of Orthodontics 4: 175–80

Dickson G C 1969 The natural history of malocclusion. Transactions of the British Society for the Study of Orthodontics 55: 148–64

Gould M S E, Picton D C A 1962 A method of measuring forces acting on the teeth from the lips, cheeks and tongue. British Dental Journal 112: 235–42

Lundstrom A 1949 An investigation of 202 pairs of twins regarding fundamental factors in the aetiology of malocclusion. Dental Record 69: 251–64

Lundstrom A 1984 Nature versus nurture in dento-facial variation. European Journal of Orthodontics 6: 77–91

Proffit W R 1978 Equilibrium theory revisited: factors influencing the position of the teeth. Angle Orthodontist 48: 175–86

Proffit W R, Fields H W, Nixon W L 1983 Occlusal forces in normal and long-faced adults. Journal of Dental Research 62: 566–70

Proffit W R, Fields H W, Nixon W L 1983 Occlusal forces in normal and long-faced children. Journal of Dental Research 62: 571–4

Proffit W R 1986 On the aetiology of malocclusion: The Northcroft Lecture 1985. British Journal of Orthodontics 13: 1–12

Richardson A 1970 Dento-alveolar factors in anterior open bite and deep overbite. Dental Practitioner 21: 53–7

Ricketts R M 1952 A study of changes in temporomandibular relationships in the treatment of Class II malocclusion. (Angle). American Journal of Orthodontics 38: 918–33

Schudy F F 1968 The control of vertical overbite in clinical orthodontics. Angle Orthodontist 38: 19–39

Subtelny J D, Subtelny J D 1973 Oral habits — studies in form function and therapy. Angle Orthodontist 43: 347–83

Vig P S, Cohen A M 1979 Vertical growth of the lips: a serial cephalometric study. American Journal of Orthodontics 75: 405–15

4

The aetiology of malocclusion: local factors

Ideally, the size and number of the teeth is such that they will exactly fill the space available in the alveolar part of the jaws with neither spacing nor crowding. Departure from this ideal in one form or another, is the main cause of malocclusion to arise from the teeth themselves. It will be seen from Figure 4.1 that the sizes of both teeth and jaws vary considerably and there seems to be comparatively little relationship between the size of the teeth and of the jaws. The correlation between these two sizes is often referred to as the tooth/tissue ratio, although this is usually a purely descriptive term and not at present the subject of accurate measurements. Other causes of malocclusion involve variations in the size of individual teeth or groups of teeth and variations in their number, shape and position.

ABNORMALITIES OF TOOTH/TISSUE RATIO

It will be recalled that phylogenetically the teeth and jaws are of very different origins. The teeth

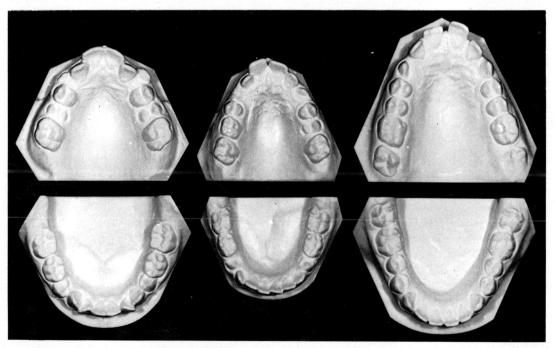

Fig. 4.1 Study models of three children in the early permanent dentition. Note the variation in size of both teeth and dental arches.

are ectodermal in origin from the scales of primitive fish, while the jaws are mesodermal in origin and come originally from the gill arches. It is not therefore surprising that they tend to be inherited separately, and that we can have a patient with small teeth in large jaws or large teeth in small jaws. It would seem that the sizes of both structures are largely genetically controlled and in the case of the teeth, their final size is determined at an early stage. No change is possible in their size once the whole of the occlusal surfaces of their crowns is calcified.

It would seem that in a modern Anglo-Saxon population the incidence of crowding is noticeably greater than that of spacing (although of course many cases of spaced teeth do not come to the orthodontist). The reason for this factor has never been satisfactorily explained and it would seem that it is largely a development of the last 200 years. In medieval times although some crowding of the teeth did occur, it was less common and usually less severe. In other races crowding of the teeth is certainly less common than in those of Western European ancestry. Happily, dental crowding is one of the few inherited diseases which can be satisfactorily and permanently cured — teeth can be extracted!

ABNORMALITIES IN THE NUMBER OF TEETH

Congenital absence of teeth

This may vary from the absence of a single tooth to complete anodontia. Where anodontia is more or less complete, it is sometimes associated with dysplasia of other ectodermal structures; nails, hair and sweat glands may be deficient. By definition, anodontia implies a complete absence of teeth and anything less complete may be called hypodontia or oligodontia. The most frequently absent teeth are third molars, upper lateral incisors, lower central incisors and second premolars. However, any tooth in the head may occasionally fail to develop either alone or in company with others.

The absence of third molars does not seriously affect the occlusion but it may influence orthodontic treatment when the decision has to be made whether or not to extract other permanent teeth, especially other molars. The absence of a second premolar is more often found in the lower jaw. In such cases the second deciduous molar is often retained well beyond its usual time for shedding, and occasionally it may be decided to retain this deciduous tooth as long as possible. The only effect of this is to retain the lower first permanent molar in a slightly post-normal position relative to the upper tooth, since the deciduous molar is usually wider than a corresponding premolar. If the deciduous molar is carious, depressed or for some other reason a poor risk, it should be removed and the space either retained for an ultimate bridge or closed mechanically. If the lower arch is crowded, the space should normally be closed, and the absence of a lower second premolar may obviate the need for the extraction of this or another tooth.

The absence of the upper lateral incisors will have one of three effects on the dentition. The space may remain open and local in which case it may be filled by a suitable prosthetic replacement. Secondly, it may close completely, in which case the upper canines may well be disguised to simulate the lateral incisors and the condition accepted, although extractions in the lower arch may be necessary to balance the condition. Thirdly, and most commonly, the condition may close partially with spacing between the two central incisors and sometimes between the canine and first premolar (Fig. 4.2). In an otherwise normal occlusion this is unsightly, and orthodontic treatment may be necessary to localise the spacing so that a prosthetic replacement for the missing tooth or teeth may be inserted. If such a condition is associated with a generalised crowding it may be possible to close the space mechanically, often in conjunction with extractions in the lower arch only.

The absence of a lower incisor (Fig. 4.3), is easily overlooked since the space is usually closed and the remaining teeth well aligned. It may be that the condition is acceptable but if the permanent canines are in a normal relationship, crowding may occur in the upper incisor region due to the difficulty of occluding four upper incisors over three lower ones.

In general, the effect of the absence of any tooth

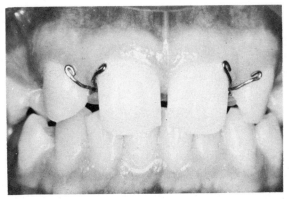

A

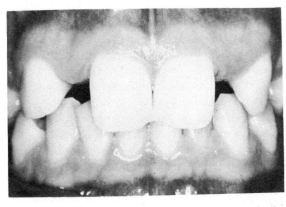

B

Fig. 4.2 A, Patient with congenitally absent 2/2 in an uncrowded mouth. Spacing exists on each side of 3/3 and also between 1/1. A removable appliance is *in situ*. B, Following localisation of the spacing to permit fitting of a prosthesis.

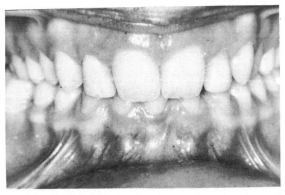

Fig. 4.3 Patient with congenital absence of one lower central incisor. This can easily be overlooked.

will depend on the overall degree of crowding. If overcrowding is not present then there will be more or less local space and some local tooth movement may be required. On the other hand, it is undesirable to condemn a child to the permanent wearing of any form of prosthesis, and if there is any suggestion of crowding of the teeth, it may well be possible to close the space, this usually being associated with compensating extractions in the opposing arch.

Premature loss of deciduous teeth

The early loss of the deciduous incisors and canines is not common. As they are usually spaced in a normal occlusion, their loss is often without effect on the permanent teeth, unless this loss is the result of trauma. In the latter case the developing permanent teeth may be displaced, dilacerated or both. This may be checked radiographically at the time of the accident, but no treatment is indicated, and it should be borne in mind that quite severely displaced permanent incisors may in fact find their way back into the mouth in the normal or into a treatable position. Deciduous canines are occasionally lost early due to resorption of their roots by the adjacent permanent lateral incisor. This occurs in very crowded mouths and the resultant malocclusion is the cause rather than the effect of the early loss of the deciduous tooth.

The effect of the loss of the deciduous molars is more serious, although even this has been somewhat exaggerated in the past. If the deciduous molars are lost early, one of three things may happen. The space may close to a greater or lessor extent. It may remain unchanged, or the space may partially close and then re-open when the premolars erupt. The actual result will depend on a number of factors:

1. The inherent tooth/tissue ratio. In general the space will tend to close where the mouth is inherently crowded and the result is essentially a localising effect, producing crowding in the canine and premolar region, but possibly reducing crowding of the posterior molars. Occasionally, in border-line cases, the space may close somewhat and then re-open, although this may involve the

crowding of other teeth such as the canine or incisors.

2. Other things being equal, the loss of space will be greater following the extraction of an upper deciduous molar rather than a lower one, and following the loss of a second deciduous molar, rather than a first. The unilateral loss of a first deciduous molar, especially in the lower arch, may cause a displacement of the centre line of the incisors, although here again it is probable that the effect has been exaggerated; a displaced centre-line may, in some cases, correct itself spontaneously.

3. The effect of the loss of deciduous molars is particularly severe if this occurs before the first permanent molars erupt. For this reason, a special effort should be made to retain the deciduous tooth until the first molar has erupted, even if it cannot be saved for its full life-time.

4. There is no evidence that the early loss of deciduous molars has any effect on the size of the jaws and dental bases.

Loss of permanent teeth

Any of the permanent teeth may be lost for a variety of reasons, but the most frequent are the incisors, which are usually lost as a result of trauma, and the first molars, which may be extracted as a result of caries.

Following the loss of a permanent incisor — usually a central incisor — there is a tendency for the space to close to some extent. This is particularly true where there is an inherent tendency to crowding. Here again, there are two possible lines of treatment: either the space may be retained at its full width, so that a prosthesis may ultimately be fitted, or the space may be closed mechanically, with parallel movement of the adjacent teeth maintaining the original centre-line. In the latter case, the lateral incisor on the affected side may be disguised to simulate a central incisor by means of a crown. Alternatively, it may be built up to simulate a central incisor using composite resin as shown in Figure 4.4. This requires considerable restorative skill and should only be carried out where the root of the lateral incisor is adequate to support the larger size of crown, and the long-term prognosis for such a tooth is uncertain. In suitable cases the space may be closed without any

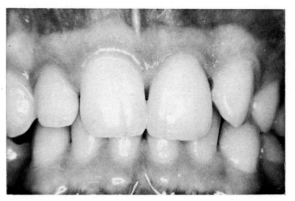

Fig. 4.4 /1 was lost due to trauma and /2 moved into its place. This tooth now carries an over-sized jacket crown.

alteration in the shape of the lateral incisor. A well-known film star of yesteryear had a successful career with only one central incisor. In such a case, the permanent canine may be disguised to simulate a lateral incisor.

The effect of the early loss of permanent first molars parallels to a considerable extent that resulting from the early loss of deciduous molars. The following factors are important: (1) if the mouth is inherently crowded the space will tend to close spontaneously to a greater or lesser extent. On the other hand, in the absence of crowding, the space will not close although adjacent teeth may drift into the space with a production of spacing elsewhere in the dental arch. (2) The effect is somewhat different in the two dental arches. Space closure is usually more complete in the upper arch and is produced very largely by mesial migration of the second molar. Salzmann has suggested that if the upper first molar has a width of 10 mm the space, in a typical case, will be closed by 9 mm mesial drift of the second molar and only 1 mm distal drift of the second premolar. The upper premolars drift distally to a maximum of 2 mm and remain essentially in contact during this. This may cause a slight relief of crowding of a canine but the effect on the labial segment is minimal. The second molar will probably rotate mesio-lingually and the premolars may rotate disto-lingually, but the teeth do not usually tilt appreciably.

In the lower arch, again to quote Salzmann, if the first molar has a width of 11 mm it is likely

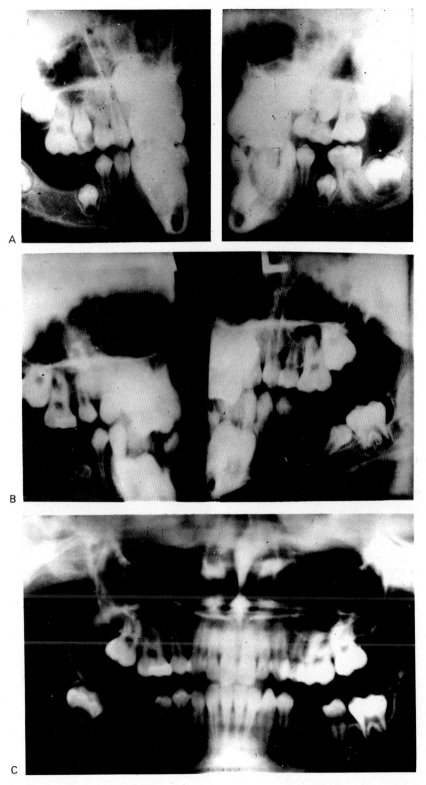

Fig. 4.5 A, 6̄/ has been extracted and /6̄ is grossly carious and unsaveable. B, Following extraction of /6̄, /5̄ has migrated distally and impacted against /7̄. C, Spontaneous uprighting of /5̄.

that the second molar will drift mesially 5 mm and the second premolar drift distally 4 mm. That is, the teeth drift to an almost equal extent, and there is frequently some residual spacing. It is not unusual to find a space occurring between the two lower premolars, and where the dental base is long with an uncrowded mouth, this space may be the width of a premolar tooth. This is particularly liable to happen if the first molar is extracted before the age of 9. Figure 4.5 shows how this occurs. It might be thought that the retention of a deciduous molar would prevent the distal drifting of the second premolar but this is not necessarily the case. The distal root of the deciduous molar may be resorbed with the second premolar erupting distally to it (Fig. 4.6).

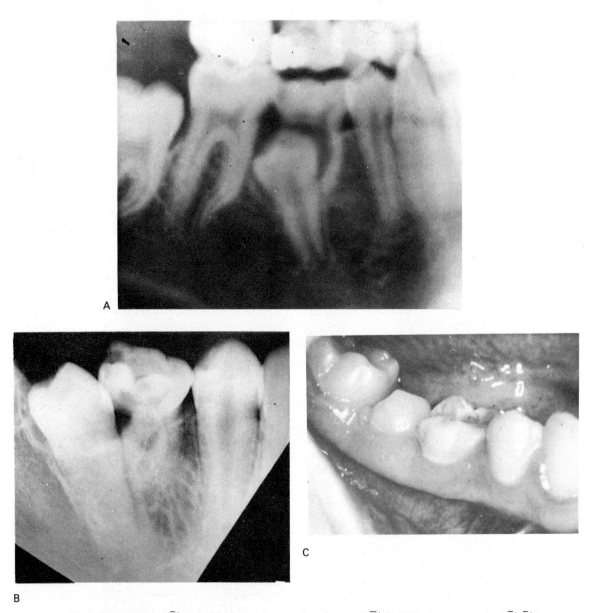

Fig. 4.6 A, Slight displacement of $\overline{5}/$ has caused unequal resorption of roots of $\overline{E}/$. B, Following extraction of $\overline{6}/$, $\overline{5}/$ has erupted distally to retained $\overline{E}/$. C, Intra-oral view.

While the second molar and second premolar may rotate, a more serious sequel in the lower jaw is the tilting of these two teeth toward each other which usually occurs. On the other hand, the distal drifting of the lower premolars may well relieve the crowding of the lower labial segment to some extent. It may also allow the lower incisors to drop lingually, but this is usually quite minor in extent and certainly never causes a major malocclusion. (3) The result will be effected by the age at which the first permanent molars are extracted. If it is hoped that the space will close satisfactorily, then the first molar should be extracted at about the age of 10 or 11 years, more precisely when the lateral incisors and first premolars have erupted but not the second premolars, canines or second molars. Very early loss runs the risk of the distal migration of the lower second premolar. At the other extreme, if the first molars are extracted after the second molars are in occlusion, it is very unusual for a satisfactory alignment with space closure to occur without appliance therapy. On the other hand, if it is proposed to carry out orthodontic treatment of a malocclusion in the anterior part of the mouth, then extraction should if possible be delayed until the second molars are in occlusion. Any mesial migration will then be slower and can be controlled with suitable appliances. (4) If it becomes necessary to extract the first permanent molars, then some consideration should be given to the necessity for balancing these extractions. If a lower first molar is lost and the upper tooth retained, then the lower second molar will probably tilt mesially, with over-eruption of the upper first molar. There will be some residual spacing while the traumatic effects on the lower second molar may ultimately cause the loss of this tooth or may even give rise to temporo-mandibular joint dysfunction. If the upper molar only is lost, the result is less serious. Especially if this takes place before the second molar has erupted, this latter tooth will often come forward to occlude satisfactorily with the lower first molar. The upper third molar may then erupt to occlude with the lower second molar. It should be borne in mind that the usual reason for a first molar to be lost is the result of caries, and on the whole lower first molars are more caries-prone than the upper teeth. The lower

molar should therefore only be retained if its prognosis is perfect. If it is proposed to carry out orthodontic treatment, then the loss of a lower first molar may be 'balanced' by the extraction of an upper premolar or vice-versa since the closure of the space can be controlled with suitable appliances.

It has been suggested that extractions of first molars on one side of the mouth should be balanced by extracting the corresponding teeth on the opposite side. This seems unnecessary if the contralateral teeth are in good condition (although caries is often symmetrical), and if extractions are indicated to relieve crowding, more convenient teeth such as premolars, may be extracted on the opposite side. Any effect on the centre-line of the teeth is likely to be minimal following the loss of a permanent molar.

Some 40 years ago, Wilkinson suggested that the symmetrical extraction of all four first permanent molars was the panacea for all dental ills. This is certainly not the case. With careful selection and timing, an acceptable result may be achieved even without orthodontic treatment but this is exceptional and often the result is not so good as would at first sight appear (Fig. 4.7). It is often noticeable, as here, that the best results in the lower arch occur in those cases where, prior to extraction, $\overline{5/5}$ are completely impacted and without space.

Retention of the deciduous teeth

The deciduous teeth are normally shed a short time before the eruption of the corresponding permanent teeth. If this permanent tooth is absent or seriously displaced resorption of the roots of the deciduous tooth may not take place and it may be retained for many years beyond its normal term. Occasionally a deciduous tooth fails to resorb despite the presence of its permanent successor. This is usually because the deciduous tooth is non-vital and infected. In this case the permanent tooth will erupt in an ectopic position. This is usually self-correcting if the deciduous tooth is extracted but in a case such as that shown in Figure 4.8A the central incisor may be displaced so as to occlude lingually to the lower incisors where it is locked by the occlusion. Similarly a

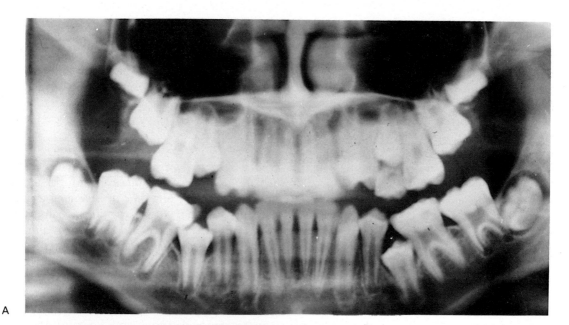

A

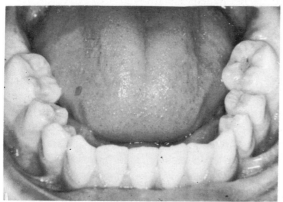

B

Fig. 4.7 A, Before extraction of first molars. Note impaction of lower second premolars. B, Intra-oral view 2 years later; no orthodontic treatment in the lower arch. C, Radiograph taken at the same time. Although this might be considered a 'good' result, there is considerable mesial tipping of $\overline{7|7}$.

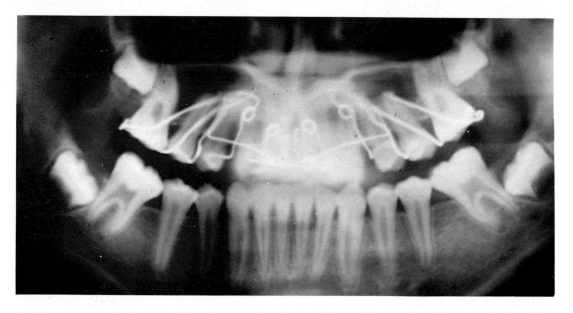

displaced premolar may be held by the occlusion and fail to correct itself when the deciduous molar is lost (Fig. 4.8B).

Retention of deciduous teeth is usually, therefore, a local matter. The age at which these teeth are shed is very variable between individuals but occasionally a patient is encountered in whom all or most of the deciduous molars remain firm even though the permanent teeth are lying close beneath them and apparently ready to erupt. If the deciduous molars are retained beyond the fourteenth birthday it is usually desirable to have these teeth extracted provided that the premolars are close beneath them. If the premolars are

deeply placed, new bone may form over their crowns following loss of deciduous molars and this may delay the eruption of the permanent teeth.

Delayed eruption of permanent teeth

This may be general or local. As indicated above, the dates of eruption of all teeth vary very widely, especially premolars, canines and second molars. They tend to be later where there is a tendency to crowding. Undue importance should not be attached to moderately delayed eruption of teeth, where the pattern of eruption is otherwise normal and radiographic investigation shows all teeth to be present and in a good position. The eruption of teeth may be generally delayed and the teeth themselves gravely misplaced in certain endocrine dysfunctions and osteodystrophies.

Eruption may be delayed locally due to impaction, misplacement, the retention of deciduous teeth or the presence of supernumeraries. If one or two teeth are unduly late in erupting, compared with other teeth in the arch and particularly with a fellow on the opposite side, then a full investigation should be made to locate the position of the unerupted tooth to make sure that there is no reason for its delayed eruption.

Supernumerary teeth

Supernumerary teeth may be found in any part of the mouth and in most locations they bear some resemblance to normal teeth of that region. They are particularly liable to occur at the ends of tooth series. Thus a fourth molar is occasionally seen and this is particularly common in people of West African descent. Such teeth may interfere with the eruption of the lower third molar.

They may also occur in the upper jaw, as seen in Figure 4.9A, where there is also a supernumerary denticle on the buccal side of $/\underline{6}$ and the crowns of supernumerary premolars adjacent to the roots of the lower permanent premolars. These are typical of supernumerary premolars. Their proximity to the roots of the permanent teeth makes their removal hazardous. They do not usually interfere with the occlusion and their roots frequently do not form and the teeth remain stationary. They should be kept under observation

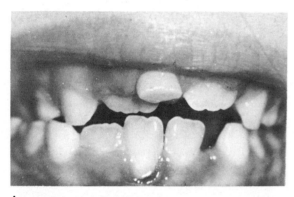

A

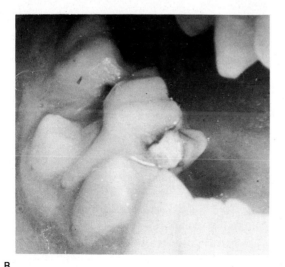

B

Fig. 4.8 A, Retained non-vital deciduous incisor causing lingual displacement of $\underline{1}/$, which may become locked in crossbite. B, Retained $\overline{E}/$ similarly displacing $\overline{5}/$.

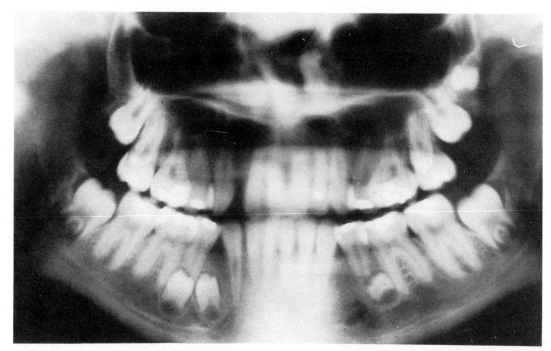

A

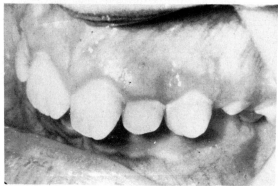

B

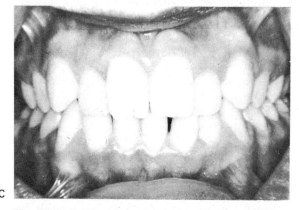

C

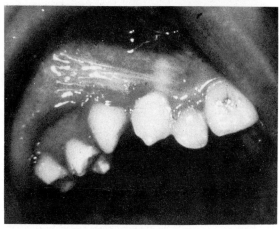

D

Fig. 4.9 A, Radiograph showing supernumerary upper left fourth molar, denticle on buccal side of /6 and supernumerary lower premolars. B, Supplemental upper lateral incisor. C, Additional lower incisor in well-aligned arch. This can be easily overlooked. D, Supplemental 3/ in case of oro-facio-digital syndrome.

and only removed if they show signs of migration or of cyst formation.

I have never personally seen a supernumerary canine, although Professor Milan Markovich tells me they can occur in oro-facio-digital syndrome, and kindly provided me with the transparency which forms Figure 4.9D. More commonly, but still very rarely, a small odontome, usually of the compound composite type, forms close to the crown of the upper canine and prevents its eruption. Supplemental incisors are not uncommon and are usually seen in the upper lateral or lower incisor regions (Fig. 4.9B, C). Supplemental upper central incisors are seen only in patients

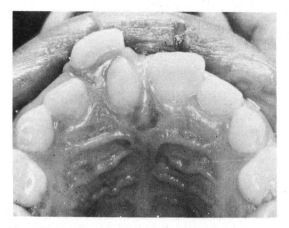

Fig. 4.10 'Mesiodens' associated with displacement of upper **central** incisor. Unusually, the supernumerary tooth has **erupted**.

teeth do not usually resemble their neighbours. Such a tooth is often referred to as a mesiodens, although in fact it is never in the mid-line but always to one side or other of the suture. There seem to be two distinct types of supernumerary found in this region. The type shown in Figure 4.10 is usually described as 'peg-shaped' and may occasionally be seen erupted as here but more usually is lying unerupted and often pointing posteriorly or even upwards towards the nose (Fig. 4.11). It is associated with displacement of

with clefts of the lip. Supplemental teeth usually present no problems, provided they are noticed, but it is very easy to overlook the presence of an additional lower incisor.

The supernumerary teeth which cause the greatest problems in orthodontics are those lying close to the mid-line in the upper arch. These

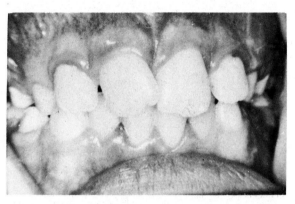

A

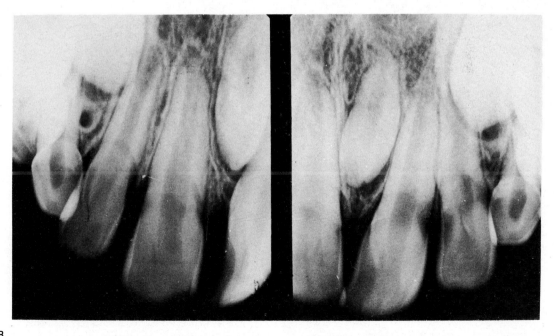

B

Fig. 4.11 A, Intra-oral view. Note imbrication of 1/1 and distal displacement of root apices. B, Intra-oral radiographs showing 'mesiodens' lying between the central incisors.

the immediately adjacent teeth but its extraction is not followed by the self-correction of these displaced permanent teeth. It is necessary to move them mechanically, and even then they show a tendency to go back to their original position. The second type of mesiodens is a more tuberculate tooth and may be incisiform in shape, although not resembling any particular permanent tooth. Its effect is to prevent the eruption of the permanent central incisor and the typical picture is of a child attending with all the incisors present except for one central incisor in the upper arch. There is no history of extraction and on X-ray examination, the supernumerary tooth is seen lying usually on the lingual side of the permanent tooth. Both these types of supernumerary may sometimes be bilateral. The latter type will be dealt with in more detail in Chapter 9.

ABNORMALITIES IN THE FORM AND POSITION OF TEETH

Teeth of abnormal shape and size

These include gemination and fusion, macrodontism and microdontism (Fig. 4.12A, B) supernumerary cusps and dilacerated incisors. They give rise to very localised malocclusions, unilaterally or bilaterally. The prognosis for dividing geminated or fused teeth is poor, even if they have separated pulp chambers, and the best solution usually involves their extraction. Dilacerated teeth can be moved in the normal fashion (contrary to the old wives' tale). If the dilaceration is very severe it may not be possible to align the crown, since to do so would place the root in an impossible position, as in the case shown in Figure 4.12C. In such a case, also, the truncated root would not

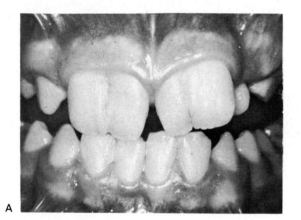

A

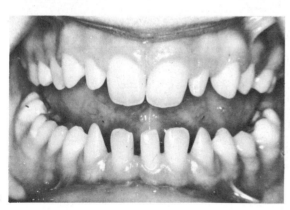

B

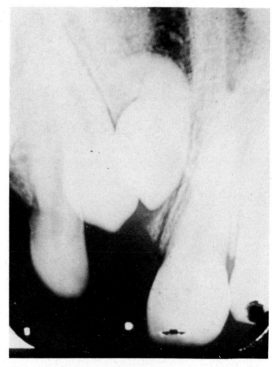

C

Fig. 4.12 A, Geminated macrodont incisors. 2/2 were present, as normal teeth but palatally displaced. B, Microdont incisors. C, Dilacerated 1/.

support the functioning crown. A mild dilaceration is no impediment to tooth movement.

Total displacement and transposition

The classical picture of transposition is for the upper permanent canine to erupt in the labial sulcus, between the two premolars (Fig. 4.13A). It may be possible to bring it forward into its correct place, using banded appliances, or alternatively to move the first premolar mesially into the canine position, and to accommodate the canine in the arch between the premolars. Very occasionally the canine may lie in the line of the arch, between the premolars (Fig. 4.13B).

A rather common transposition is that where a permanent lower lateral incisor erupts distally to the canine (Fig. 4.13C). The incisor is usually very distally inclined, with its labial surface facing anteriorly, giving the impression that it is the result of an abnormal direction of eruption, rather than a true transposition. Again each case should be treated on its merits.

Traumatic displacement of teeth

Teeth may be displaced following a blow on the jaw. This applies particularly in the incisor region where a newly erupted incisor may be driven back into the bone by a blow or an unerupted tooth

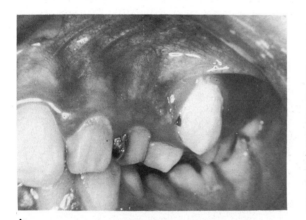

A

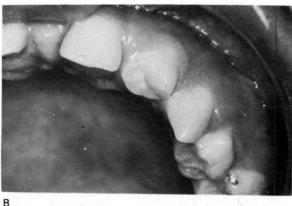

B

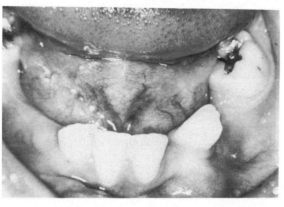

C

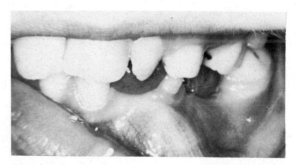

Fig. 4.13 A, Transposed /3, lying in buccal sulcus between /45. B Transposed /3 in line of the arch. C, Distally displaced /2, with its crown lying distally to /3, although its root apex is more normally placed.

may be displaced by damage to is deciduous predecessor. If the displaced tooth is not damaged, it will have a strong tendency to return to its original position and may erupt normally. It is certainly worth observing it for some time since, in any case, no treatment is indicated. Not infrequently however, it becomes dilacerated to a greater or lessor extent and may fail to erupt for this reason. An example is shown in Figure 4.12C, to which reference has already been made.

Impaction of teeth

Late erupting teeth may become impacted due to a lack of space in the arch. This can usually be relieved by appropriate extractions but the position and angulation of the impacted tooth should be carefully considered before doing so. Teeth have a natural tendency to upright them-

selves, and a second premolar, which is distally impacted against a first molar, will usually free itself if the first premolar is extracted to make room for it to come into the arch. If the first molar is extracted the premolar may, as we have already seen, migrate distally. A rather different problem arises where the impacted tooth is, at least for the time being, the most posterior in the dental arch. This obviously occurs in the case of third permanent molars but may sometimes be seen involving upper first or lower second molars. An upper first molar can occasionally erupt and become impacted with its mesial marginal ridge beneath the contact point of the second deciduous molar. Having just broken the gum, it then fails to continue to erupt. Some authorities recommend that the condition be left alone but in this case food lodgement tends to cause caries and gingivitis in this region. Alternatively an effort may be made to disimpact

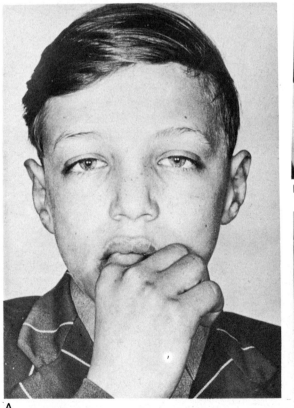

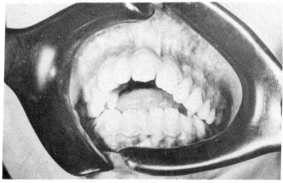

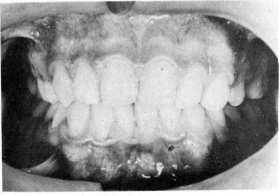

Fig. 4.14 The effects of prolonged sucking of the knuckle of the right index finger in a boy of 14 years. A, The boy demonstrating the habit. B, The intra-oral result thereof. C, The same case following orthodontic treatment.

the tooth or the second deciduous molar may be extracted. Unfortunately, even when this is carried out the tooth does not always erupt and it would seem that there may be a localised failure of alveolar growth. An impacted lower second molar may be successfully treated by mechanical appliances as described by Vig and by Reynolds with or without the extraction of the third molar.

OTHER LOCAL CAUSES OF MALOCCLUSION

Habits

Any force acting on a tooth will cause it to move provided the force is great enough and is applied for sufficient time each day. The tooth or teeth in question will then move until the effect of this force is balanced by that of the opposing soft tissues. The best known example of this is undoubtedly finger-and thumb-sucking but others of varying degrees of probability have been described. Digit-sucking in infancy is extremely common and probably takes place in about half of all babies. The reason for it is not known, apart from the importance which sucking obviously plays in a baby's life. The habit does not seem to be associated with the type or duration of feeding or with parental deprivation. It usually commences within the first year of life and usually continues at least into the fourth year. Occasionally it goes on very much longer and the boy shown in Figure 4.14 was still sucking the knuckle of the right hand at the age of 14 years and this is by no means a record. The most common of a number of variants is for the individual to suck the thumb holding it in a vertical position with the nail towards the lower teeth. One or two fingers may be sucked in a similar position or the knuckle may be involved as in the case shown. Either hand may be affected and it is not necessarily associated with handedness (that is right-handed people do not necessarily suck the right thumb). The typical effect is shown in Figure 4.15B although in an extreme form. The incisors are proclined and this is usually asymmetrical with greater proclination present on the side of the digit involved. The lower incisors may be tilted lingually to a slight extent but this is not invariable. The overbite is always incomplete and frequently reduced. The condition is essential local, although if it is persistent in a somewhat crowded mouth, the upper posterior teeth may come forward, maintaining contact with the canines. Extractions may then be necessary to allow the anterior teeth to be corrected. There is some controversy concerning the effect of digit-sucking in the production of a narrow upper arch and crossbite. There appears sometimes to be a coincidence of the two conditions, as in Figure 3.15 but, as shown here, this is not invariable. Thus Bowden (1966) found no increased tendency to crossbite in 116 digit-sucking children. Leighton (1969) found that such a crossbite was eliminated if the habit ceased before establishment of the permanent dentition, while Larsson (1972, 1975) found a higher incidence of crossbite in 4-year-old finger-suckers but not in 9-year-olds, who were still sucking. Other authors' findings are equally contradictory but it would seem that a crossbite, unilateral or bilateral, is an uncommon feature of digit-sucking and may be self-correcting. Once the habit is discontinued, the incisor teeth show a strong tendency to correct themselves. Bowden has shown that in the mixed dentition the overjet will correct itself within about 12 months, although the overbite will take considerably longer to re-establish. It would seem that self-correction is probably more rapid, the younger the patient. Appliances will probably be required if the condition were encountered in the complete permanent dentition but even so, the teeth usually move well and the result is stable (Fig. 4.12C).

Abnormal fraenum labii

At birth the fraenum labii superioris is attached to the incisive papilla. As growth proceeds and the teeth erupt, the attachment of the fraenum to the gum normally 'recedes' to a point about mid-way between the alveolar border and the reflection of the mucosa. The main factor in causing this seems to be the apposition of the central incisor teeth. Where the deciduous incisors are spaced, as is usually the case, the fraenum remains attached to the incisive papilla. When the permanent incisors erupt they may also be spaced due to inherent smallness, to absence of lateral incisors or because

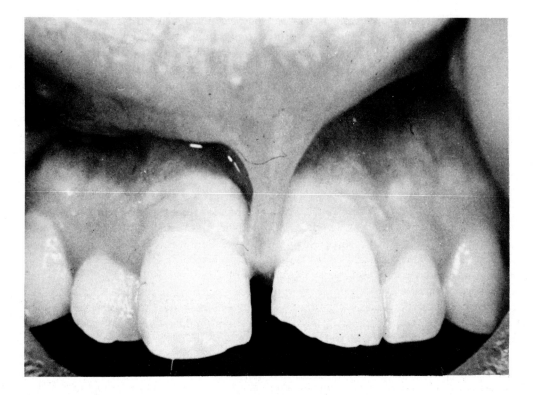

A

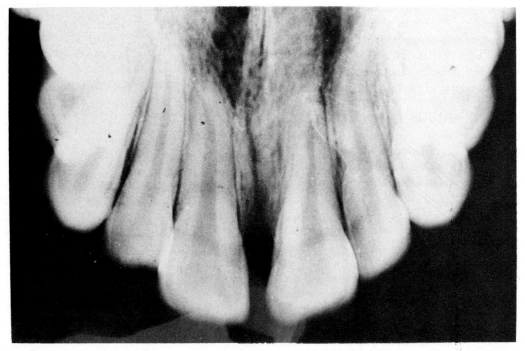

B

Fig. 4.15 Superior labial fraenum which is probably the case of the median diastema. A, Intra-oral view. B, Radiograph.

in a narrow maxilla their apices are crowded together and the crowns consequently tilted apart. A transient spacing is not uncommon during normal development (Fig. 2.1A). In these cases the fraenum will remain attached to the incisive papilla and is not necessarily the cause of the diastema. The operation of fraenectomy or removal of the fraenum between the incisor teeth has long been practised and the majority of such operations were completely unnecessary.

On the other hand, a rather different type of fraenum is very occasionally seen and one such is illustrated in Figure 4.15. This may occur in a mouth which is otherwise crowded and appears to be the primary cause of the diastema. Such a fraenum is thick and 'fleshy' and runs quite horizontally from the crest of the alveolus to the vermilion margin of the lip. In the radiograph the alveolar bone between the incisors exhibits a notch, like an inverted V (Fig. 4.15B), and this indicates the position of the fibrous tissue in the line of the suture. If the fraenum appears to be of this type, it should be removed, the operation involving not only removal of the fraenum itself but the complete dissecting out of the soft tissue in the line of the alveolus. The best time for this is probably just before the permanent canines erupt. It should be emphasised that this type of abnormal fraenum is excessively rare and even when it has been removed, it is unwise to promise a perfect result.

MOUTH-BREATHING

In the heyday of Dr Angle it was necessary to find an environmental cause for all cases of malocclusion. Prominent upper incisors were often associated with an open-lip posture, believed, usually incorrectly, to be a sign of oral respiration (see next chapter), so 'mouth-breathing' was regarded as a common cause of Class II Division 1 malocclusion. This belief was eventually discredited, with the opposite extreme prevailing — that there was no connection between oral respiration and malocclusion.

Linder-Aronson, from an examination of a large number of children attending an ENT clinic, found a rather typical pattern associated with an inability to breathe through the nose (see Linder-Aronson, 1979). A case is shown in Figure 4.17. The facial appearance is somewhat typical; there is an increase in both upper and lower facial heights, with a narrow upper arch and a tendency to posterior crossbite, and to an anterior open bite. Upper and lower incisors are retroclined. Following restoration of normal respiration, Linder-Aronson found a tendency for the dental abnormalities to be self-correcting.

PATHOLOGICAL CAUSES OF MALOCCLUSION

Malocclusion and displacement of the teeth can be caused by a wide variety of pathological conditions

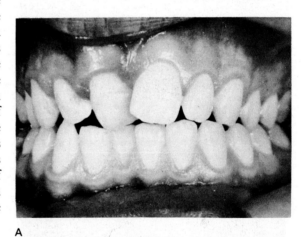

A

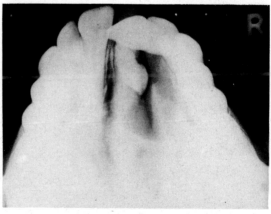

B

Fig. 4.16 A, Gross displacement of the roots of 1/1, with consequent imbrication of the crown. B, Radiograph to show dentigenous cyst in conjunction with supernumerary tooth.

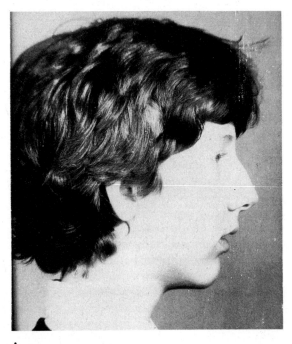
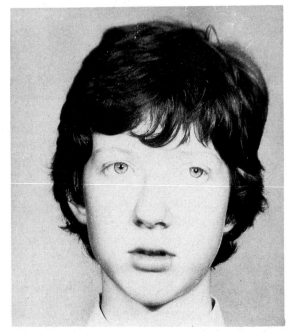

A

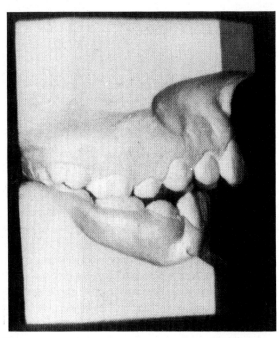
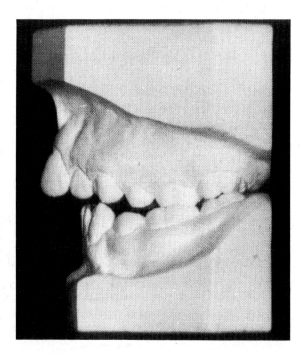

B

Fig. 4.17 Patient was unable to breathe through her nose. A, Full-face and profile photographs. B, Study models; note narrow upper arch with tendency to open the bite. C, Lateral skull radiograph; note enlarged adenoids. D, Tracing; note that incisors are retroclined.

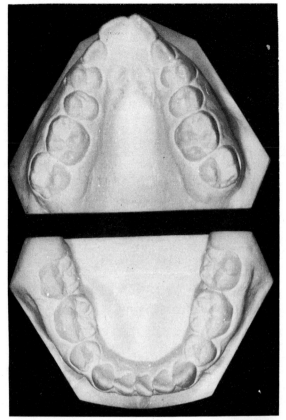

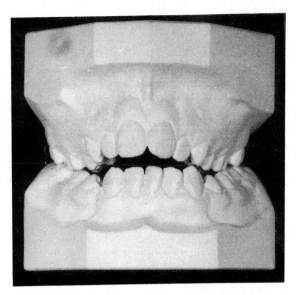

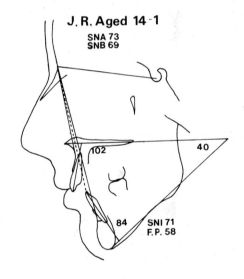

J. R. Aged 14·1

SNA 73
SNB 69

102

40

84

SNI 71
F. P. 58

D

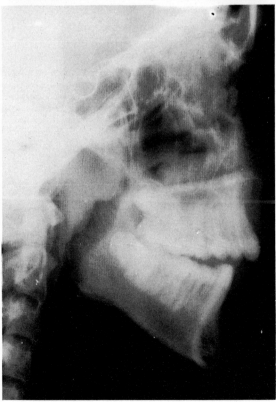

C

of which it sometimes forms an important diagnostic sign. In examining a patient with his X-rays, the orthodontist should always look beyond the malocclusion and indeed beyond the teeth and be on the watch for any abnormality. Most conditions are rare and frequently self-evident but the possibility should not be forgotten that the malocclusion may be due to a fracture of the jaw (treated or untreated) the presence of a cyst (Fig. 4.16), neoplasm or inflammatory condition. These should be considered particularly where the malocclusion is of unexpectedly recent onset.

SUGGESTED READING

Bergström K, Jensen R, Martensson B 1973 The effect of superior labial frenectomy in cases with midline diastema. American Journal of Orthodontics 63: 633–8

Bowden B D 1966 A longitudinal study of digital and dummy sucking. Australian Dental Journal 11: 184–90

Bowden B D 1966 The effects of digital and dummy sucking on arch widths, overbite and overjet: a longitudinal study. Australian Dental Journal 11: 396–404

Bowden B D 1966 A longitudinal study of the effects of digit and dummy sucking. American Journal of Orthodontics 52: 887–901

Broadway R T, Gould D G 1960 Surgical requirements of the orthodontists. British Dental Journal 108: 187–90

Clinch L M 1959 A longitudinal study of the results of premature extraction of deciduous teeth between 3–4 and 13–14 years of age. Dental Practitioner 9: 109–26

Di Biase D D 1969 Midline supernumeraries and eruption of the maxillary central incisor. Transactions of the British Society for the Study of Orthodontics 55: 83–8

Hallett G E M, Burke P H 1962 Symmetrical extraction of first permanent molars. Factors controlling results in the lower arch. Transactions of the British Society for the Study of Orthodontics: 238–55

Howard R D 1978 Impacted tooth position. Unexpected improvements. British Journal of Orthodontics 5: 87–92

Larsson E 1972 Dummy and finger-sucking habits with special attention to their significance for growth and occlusion. 4. Effect on growth and occlusion. Swedish Dental Journal 65: 605–34

Larsson E 1975 Dummy and finger-sucking in 4 year olds. Swedish Dental Journal 68: 219–24

Leighton B C 1969 The early signs of malocclusion. Transactions of the European Orthodontic Society 353–68

Linder-Aronson S 1979 Respiratory function in relation to facial morphology and the dentition. British Journal of Orthodontics 6: 59–71

Popovich F, Thompson G W, Main P A 1977 The maxillary incisal diastema and its relationship to the superior labial frenum and intermaxillary suture. Angle Orthodontist 47: 265–71

Reynolds L M 1976 Uprighting lower molar teeth. British Journal of Orthodontics 3: 45–52

Ronnerman A 1965 Early extraction of deciduous molars and canines. Transactions of the European Orthodontic Society: 153–67

Salzmann J A 1938 Study of orthodontic and facial changes and effects on dentition attending loss of first molars in five hundred adolescents. Journal of the American Dental Association 15: 892–905

Thilander B, Jakobson S O, Skagius S 1963 Orthodontic sequelae of extraction of first permanent molars. Odontologisk Tidskrift 71: 381–412

Vig K W L 1976 Some methods of uprighting second molars — II. British Journal of Orthodontics 3: 39–44

5

Orthodontic diagnosis

In no branch of dentistry does diagnosis play a more important part than it does in orthodontics. A treatment procedure which involves the slavish following of a 'philosophy' associated with a particular appliance may be successful in a proportion of cases but sooner or later important factors will be overlooked and mistakes made. Any diagnosis depends on the careful collection of a case history and in order to do this successfully it is important to follow a standardised routine. That which follows has been employed for many years, and while it is not the only routine which is possible, it is suggested that the reader should use it initially, until he finds something better.

Before commencing the diagnosis, the operator should have with him records of varying importance.

1. Study models of the present condition of the mouth are so important as to be almost essential. They enable the operator to examine the dentition closely, not only from the labial and buccal surfaces but also, if he wishes, from the lingual surface. It is traditional in orthodontics that these models should be prepared to a high standard and their bases trimmed according to conventional patterns (Fig. 5.1). Although the trimming of the bases is not essential, it helps to inculcate a feeling of neatness and order in both the operator and his assistants. Angle is believed to have said that he would judge the competence of an orthodontist by the standard of his study models and while this is not absolutely true, there is a grain of truth in it. These models should of course be retained throughout treatment for not only are they an aid to diagnosis but they are also invaluable for following the progress of the treatment under-

taken, and finally to check for any indication of relapse.

2. Appropriate radiographs of the mouth are essential. I shall return to this matter later.

3. Cephalometric lateral skull radiographs are a valuable tool both in diagnosis and in following the progress of treatment. They are not essential and very many patients have been treated successfully without their help. In the past of course many broken limbs have been successfully repaired without radiological help, although this would be now considered to be essential, and it may be that in the future we shall regard cephalometric radiographs as equally essential. Again I shall return to this topic in the next chapter.

EXAMINATION OF THE PATIENT

As the patient is brought to the chair, a general observation should be made of his body posture and behaviour and especially of his facial expression and the activities of his facial muscles. Note the patient's height and general appearance and attempt to correlate this with his chronological age — is he tall or small for his age and what is his (or more particularly her) relation to puberty? A girl who has reached menarche, or a boy whose voice has broken, is likely to have passed the pubertal growth spurt.

It is always advisable to obtain a brief medical history. This need not take long and there are comparatively few conditions which would effect orthodontic treatment. In many cases, it would be a matter of asking whether the patient has had any serious illnesses, whether he is currently receiving

61

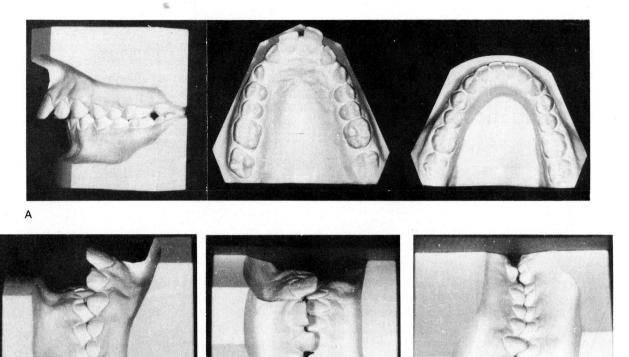

A

B

Fig. 5.1 A, Study models, trimmed with the occlusal plane parallel to the base of the model. B, When the teeth are in the intercuspal position, the backs and sides of the models bases should lie in the same plane, so that the models will stand on the flat.

any treatment from the doctor and whether he is currently taking any pills or medicines.

ORTHODONTIC EXAMINATION

Skeletal pattern

Having seated the patient in the dental chair, the relationship of the dental bases to each other should be assessed in all three planes of space.

Antero-posterior

In order to assess the antero-posterior relationship of the dental bases, the patient should be asked to sit upright in the hair and to look at a point on a level with his eyes — that is to look straight ahead. Traditionally in this position, the Frankfort plane should be approximately parallel to the floor, but this is not always the case and it is less important than having the patient in a natural head position. The first finger of the right hand is then used to palpate the alveolar outline in the midline of the upper jaw as high in the reflection of the mucosa as possible. The second finger similarly palpates the alveolar outline at the mucosal reflection of the lower jaw. By feeling the relative position of these two fingers (Fig. 5.2A), it is possible to assess the relationship of the alveolar bone overlying the apices of the incisors in the two

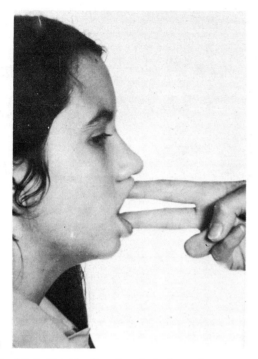
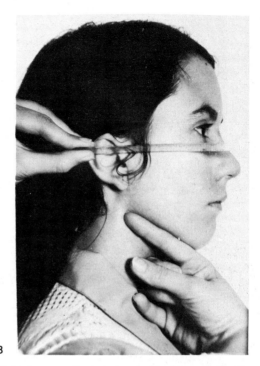

Fig. 5.2 A, The 'two finger' method of assessing antero-posterior skeletal pattern. B, Assessing the Frankfort-mandibular planes angle.

jaws. For a Class I skeletal pattern, the first finger should be slightly anterior to the second finger. If it is more than slightly anterior, then the skeletal pattern may be regarded as Class II, while if the first finger is posterior to the second finger, the skeletal pattern is Class III. Although somewhat subjective, this is probably the most efficient method of assessing the skeletal pattern in this dimension.

The vertical relationship

The vertical relationship of the dental arches should now be assessed. A clinical assessment of the angle between the Frankfort and mandibular planes should be made (Fig. 5.2B), classifying the angulation of the lower border of the mandible as normal, high or low. This should be supplemented by a clinical assessment of the lower facial height; that is, the distance from the lower border of mandibular symphysis to the lower border of the nose should be compared with the height of the face as a whole, and also with one's recollection of a normal face. Put more simply, has the indi-

vidual got a long face and particularly, a long lower face or an abnormally short one (Fig. 5.3).

Lateral

Finally, the width of the dental bases in the molar and premolar regions should be compared between the two arches. This is of prime importance where there is a crossbite of the posterior teeth and in such a case, one attempts to assess whether it is due to a discrepancy in the width of the dental bases or whether it is produced by a tilting, buccally or lingually, of the appropriate parts of the dentition.

Soft tissue patterns

The muscles of facial expression

At rest. The lips should be examined without disturbing the patient, firstly to assess whether or not they are competent. Competent lips are held together without any contraction, conscious or unconscious, of the muscles surrounding them. As

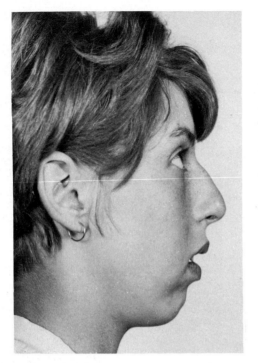
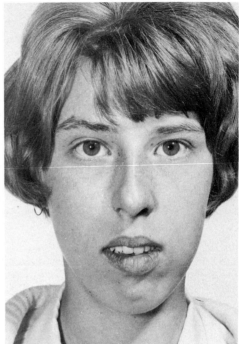

A

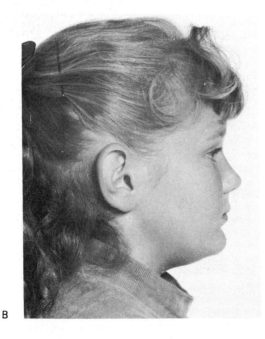
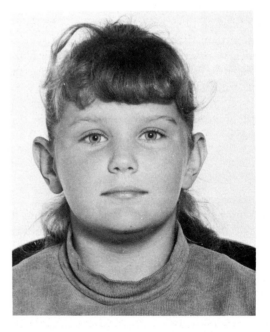

B

Fig. 5.3 A, Photographs of girl with high Frankfort-mandibular plane angle and increased lower facial height. B, The opposite condition: a low Frankfort-mandibular plane angle and lower facial height.

indicated in Chapter 3, incompetent lips may in fact be held together by a light contraction of the circumoral muscles if this can be easily achieved. While this is an interesting academic point, it is of little clinical importance. Where the lips are apart at rest, they are incompetent unless the individual is forced to breathe through the mouth. In patients with the lips apart the next test would therefore be to check that the individual is breathing normally through the nose. As indicated in Figure 5.4, this can be achieved by the use of a small hand mirror or by holding a small wisp of cotton wool in front first of the nose and then of the mouth. It is reiterated that the vast majority of children with their lips apart at rest are breathing prefectly normally through their nose. If however, they are breathing through their mouth, this will usually be found to be associated with a nasal obstruction and, assuming the child does not have a cold, it might be advisable to refer this for further investigation by the appropriate specialist.

Now, with the lips fully relaxed, assess the height of the lower lip relative to the upper incisors. If there is an increased overjet, the position of the upper incisal edges relative to the lower lip should be noted, that is, resting on the lower lip, biting into the lower lip or inside the lower lip. In cases of very deep overbite, it is also advisable to relate the height of the lower lip to the upper incisor teeth.

The position of the tongue should be assessed as best as possible, especially if there is an incomplete overbite. it should be particularly noted whether the tongue is in contact with the lower lip at rest.

From the above examination, assess the manner in which the anterior oral seal is produced. Is this a result of holding the lips together, of trapping the lower lip beneath the upper incisors or of holding the tongue in contact with the lower lip?

In function. It is important to assess the behaviour of the tongue and lips during such normal functions as speech, swallowing and facial expression. This is best done when the patient is relaxed and not consciously 'performing'. Although notes of the facial behaviour should be made at this stage, they should be the result of the observation throughout the period during which the

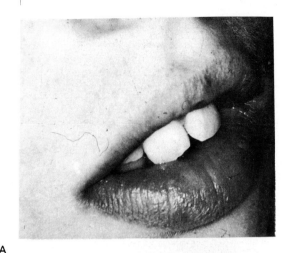

A

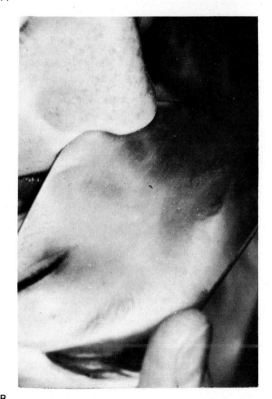

B

Fig. 5.4 A, Patient with incompetent lips. B, A small mirror or polished spatula held beneath nose will indicate if nasal respiration is present. The same test may be repeated in front of the oral cavity.

patient is in the chair. Special note should be made of hyperactivity of the lower lip during such activities as smiling and other forms of facial expression, and also of any abnormal tongue

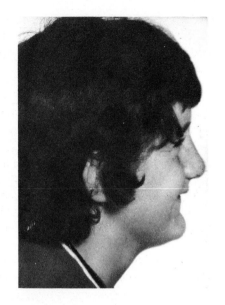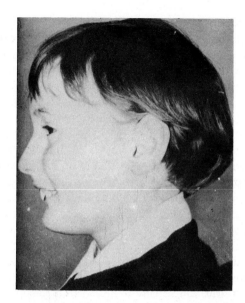

A

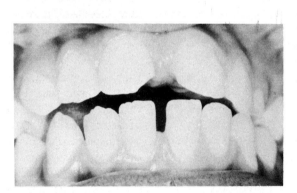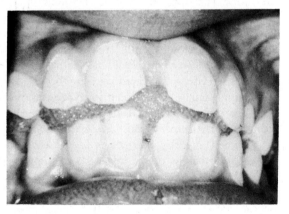

B

Fig. 5.5 A, Hyperactive contraction of the lower lip. The girl on the right has a Class II Division 1 and the boy on the left a Class II Division 2 malocclusion. B, 'Endogenous' tongue thrust, producing anterior open bite.

activity (Fig. 5.5). The patient will usually swallow following a prolonged intra-oral examination and the operator should be ready to observe this at that time.

Posture and path of closure of the mandible

Rest position. For this examination, the patient should again be sitting comfortably with the head unsupported and looking approximately straight ahead. An effort should be made to ensure that

the patient is relaxed and this may be achieved by talking to him reassuringly. When satisfied that the patient is indeed in this relaxed state he should be told that you are proposing to part his lips so as to look at the position of his teeth but that you do not wish him to move his lower jaw in any way. Without this warning (and often with it!) the patient will tend to move into the intercuspal position as soon as his lips are touched. The lips are then parted and a relationship of the upper incisors to the lowers noted. In particular the degree of overbite in this position should be noted. The patient should then be asked to close the posterior teeth together and movement of the mandible during this closing is again noted. The rest position which you have observed may be either the true or a habitual rest position. In the former case, the mandible will close through 2 or 3 mm around a hinge axis located in the condyles. If a habitual rest position is present, there will be a horizontal translation of the mandible usually upwards and backwards in closing. The degree of interocclusal clearance (freeway space) can be approximately assessed. If there is any doubt that the patient was relaxed when this examination was carried out, it should be repeated at a later stage. A further guide to the rest position may be obtained by merely looking at the extra-oral appearance of the patient at rest and then asking him to close his teeth together (without touching him) and observing the amount and direction of movement of the chin point.

Mandibular displacements. The above examination assumes that the patient is closing in the true centric jaw relationship. This may not necessarily be the case. The patient should therefore be examined for any mandibular displacement in closing, and special attention should be given to this where any tooth or group of teeth are in crossbite.

For this examination, the patient should be asked to relax the lower jaw completely and to allow you to close the teeth together. The chin is grasped lightly by the operator, with the fingers on the patient's left side and the thumb on the right (for a right-handed operator). An effort is then made to move the mandible up and down. The patient will usually resist this initially and some perseverance is necessary to achieve the relaxed movement required. It is often helpful to tell the patient that the teeth may meet in an unusual way, but to assure him that you will not allow him to hurt himself. The patient frequently has a recollection of pain when closing in centric jaw relationship due to the premature contact on the appropriate tooth, and he may be unwilling to do this. When the mandible is fully relaxed, it is moved upwards on a hinge axis until the teeth come into contact and a note made whether this is in a position of maximum intercuspation or whether other teeth are contacting prematurely.

Study models are very helpful in this context, especially if the teeth responsible for the initial contact are instanding, or if the lingual cusps of teeth are the culprits.

Speech

Speech again is best assessed during the whole of the examination, but if there is any reason to suspect an abnormality, the patient may be asked to read from a suitable book or to recite suitable phrases. The most common and relevant abnormality is in pronunciation of the letter 'S' (a sigmatism). This may be assessed by asking the patient to count from 60 upwards. A really young patient who may be unable to do so, can be asked to recite the words 'sing a song of sixpence'.

Habits

Although habits, such as finger and thumb-sucking may be considered at this stage, it is not advisable to ask the patient whether he sucks his finger or thumb. it is better during the whole of the examination, to look out for the stigmata of these habits and at a later stage to challenge the patient with a phrase such as 'You suck your right thumb don't you?' Patients are frequently, and parents occasionally, so self-conscious about these habits that they will deny them unless it is made clear that you have little doubt of their existence.

The extra-oral appearance of a persistent digit-sucker is somewhat typical. The upper lip appears full and almost as if it is swollen as a result of trauma. A little experience will make its recognition easy, and the operator may then look for the other stigmata of the condition.

INTRA-ORAL EXAMINATION

Having assessed the skeletal and soft tissue pattern, now turn to a detailed examination of the teeth themselves, although the operator will probably have already made a cursory examination. The first stage is to list all the teeth present in the mouth. This might appear self-evident but it is comparatively easy to overlook a supplemental lower incisor or one which is congenitally missing where the space has closed naturally, as illustrated in the preceding chapter (Figs. 4.3 and 4.9C). Other supplemental teeth, also, can sometimes be overlooked, while deciduous and permanent teeth can be confused in some cases. Having listed those teeth which are erupted, it is then important to account for both the presence and position of all unerupted teeth. This is achieved radiologically and there are a number of possible techniques.

1. The type of half plate radiographs sometimes referred to as 'bi-molar' has been described, together with a suitable positioning device, by Gould (1968). This can be produced by simple apparatus and in skilled hands will show all the posterior teeth and even sometimes lateral incisors. It is comparatively economical, both in materials and X-ray dosage, and very reliable.

2. Panoramic X-rays. These are of two types. The orbiting panoramic radiograph (for example the orthopantomogram) is essentially a tomographic X-ray with tube and film moving in opposite directions. It gives a very clear picture but can fail to show a tooth which is appreciably displaced from the line of the dental arches (Fig. 5.6). It is not usually satisfactory for incisor teeth and with all these techniques, it is usually advisable to take a standard occlusal X-ray of the upper anterior teeth and where necessary the lower teeth. The static panoramic radiograph is taken by placing the tube inside the patient's mouth and gives a more reliable picture but is not well tolerated by children because of the bulk of the equipment.

These radiographs will confirm the presence or otherwise of all the teeth but further views may be necessary if there is any suggestion that one or more teeth are displaced from their normal unerupted position. This applies particularly where the teeth are late in erupting or where there is a lack of resorption of their deciduous predecessors. Permanent canines are particularly prone to displacement and will be dealt with in detail in Chapter 9.

Having accounted for all the teeth, a thorough examination of these teeth is desirable. A note should be made of any carious cavities present and also of any very large restorations. Caries should normally be treated before orthodontic treatment is commenced, the only exception being where it is proposed to extract the carious tooth. Similarly, the periodontal condition and oral hygiene should be assessed and orthodontic treatment should not be commenced until the latter is of a high standard.

DENTAL EXAMINATION

This is carried out by considering the segments of teeth individually, firstly with the mouth open and secondly, in the intercuspal position.

Incisors

First examine the lower incisors, making a note of the presence of crowding or spacing and of any rotations which may be present. Also note the angle which the long axis of the lower incisors makes to their base as represented by the lower border of the mandible.

Next carry out a similar examination of the upper incisors for crowding, spacing and rotations and this time their angulation is referred to the Frankfort horizontal plane.

Now ask the patient to close the teeth together. Most patients will close naturally into the occlusal or intercuspal position but a few children, especially the younger ones, become nervous and will close anywhere except in their true occlusal position. There are various techniques for encouraging the patient to occlude normally, of which the most satisfactory is probably to place a small piece of paper on the occlusal surface of the posterior teeth and ask the patient to bite this. The occlusion so produced can be checked against the study models where the intercuspal position will usually be self-evident.

Having achieved occlusion, the overjet is then measured by means of a suitable small ruler, as demonstrated in Fig. 5.7, and noted down in millimetres. It is necessary for this part of the examination to acquire a ruler on which the graduations starts from the end of the ruler itself. Metal has the advantage of being easily sterilised. The overbite is then noted and this can also be measured or alternatively merely described in general terms. Finally, the upper and lower centre lines between the central incisors should be

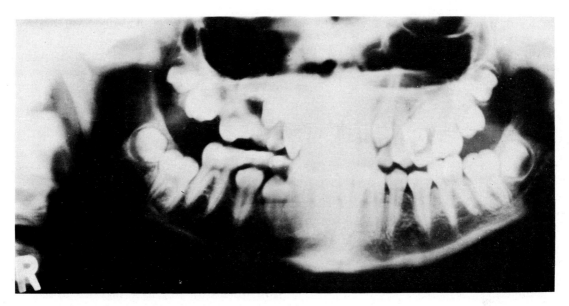

A

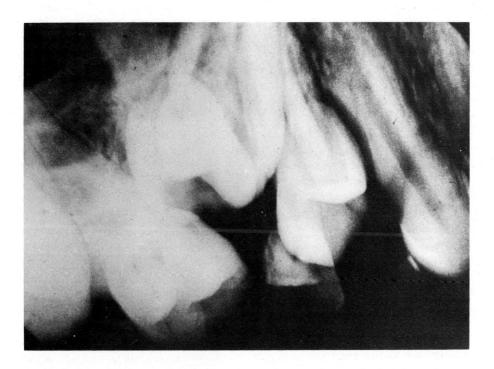

B

Fig. 5.6 A, Orthopantomogram radiograph. Note the displacement, of 64/ and the deeply impacted tooth lying between them. Note also unsatisfactory respresentation of incisors. B, Intra-oral radiograph of 64/region showing two impacted teeth, a submerged E/ and unerupted 5/.

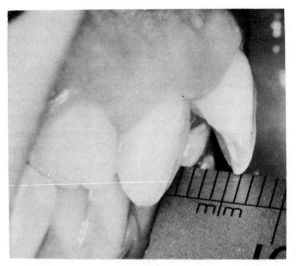

Fig. 5.7 Measuring the overjet.

checked against each other and also against the centre of the respective jaws. Any mandibular displacement should again be noted, and the offending tooth or teeth identified.

Buccal segments

The buccal segments include the canines, premolars and molars, so that the canine teeth tend to fall for some purposes, in both segments. Here again they are first examined with the mouth open and then with the teeth in occlusion.

A note is made of the presence and position of any crowding or spacing, together with the displacement or impaction of any teeth. This is reasonably self-evident in the region mesial to the first molars but an assessment should be made of crowding distal to these teeth. The upper molar teeth normally develop in the tuberosity above and behind their mesial neighbour. The lower molars similarly develop distal to their neighbour in the ascending ramus of the mandible. The operator should therefore examine the region of the tuberosity, both in the mouth and in radiographs, and calculate whether there is sufficient space available for eruption of the second and third molars. Clearly a situation which is normal at the age of 6 will not be normal at the age of 18. The dental arches grow primarily in length in order to make space for the developing molars and if, in a child of 11 or 12 years, the second and third molars are

lying in echelon above and behind the first molar, as in Figure 5.8, this is indicative of a lack of space. The condition is often referred to as 'stacking' of the molars. A similar assessment may be made in the region distal to the lower first molars.

From the assessment of the ante-molar and post-molar crowding, note the length of the dental bases relative to the size of the teeth. This is of importance in considering the need for and site of extractions.

Next examine the angulation of the teeth in the buccal segments. If it is proposed to extract the first premolars, then if the canines are mesially inclined, as in Figure 5.9A it is comparatively simple to tilt them distally into the space created by the extraction. If they are upright or, worse still, distally inclined, as in Figure 5.9B then their retraction will be more difficult if distal tilting is not to become extreme, and fixed appliance therapy will be necessary. Distally inclined molars, a common feature where the dental bases are short, will come forward readily. If space is at a premium, precautions may be necessary to discourage this. If all the cheek teeth, including

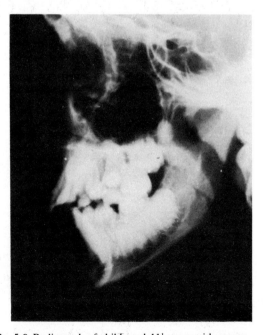

Fig. 5.8 Radiograph of child aged 11½ years with severe crowding. Note 'stacking' of posterior upper molars with lower molars developing in the vertical ramus.

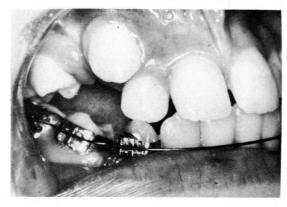

A

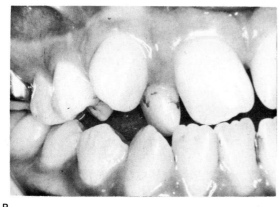

B

Fig. 5.9 A, Mesially inclined upper canine, which will respond well to mechanical retraction. B, Distally inclined canine would present considerable difficulty in retraction.

the molars, are mesially inclined, then they will probably respond well to distal movement, with or without extraction of the second molars.

Now ask the patient once more to close the teeth together and examine the occlusion of the cheek teeth, both mesio-distally and bucco-lingually.

The mesio-distal relationship can be described by means of Angle's classification. In ideal occlusion, the mesio-buccal cusp of the lower first permanent molar occludes between the buccal cusp of the second upper premolar and the mesio-buccal cusps of the first upper molar (Fig. 5.10A). This relationship is also present in Class I malocclusion. Class II malocclusion is present when the mesio-buccal cusps of the lower first molar occludes between the two buccal cusps of the

upper first permanent molar (Fig. 5.10B). In describing the antero-posterior relationship of the teeth, it is conventional to describe the displacement of the lower teeth relative to the upper, so that a Class II malocclusion may also be called a postnormal occlusion or occasionally referred to as distocclusion. Similarly, if the mesio-buccal cusp of the lower first molar occludes between the buccal cusps of the two upper premolars, this is referred to as Class III malocclusion, prenormal occlusion or mesiocclusion (Fig. 5.10C). In practice, we do not always find an accurate cusp-in-groove relationship of the posterior teeth and strictly speaking, according to the Angle classification, the dividing line between the classes is the cusp-to-cusp relationship. It is often convenient to refer to an occlusion, as for example 'slightly post-normal' when the relationship is on the Class I side of cusp-to-cusp but still not in an ideal position.

In assessing the mesio-distal relationship of the teeth, it is usual to describe it not only for the first molars but also for the canines so that we may write that a patient has an occlusion which is 'Class I on the molars but class II on the canines' (Fig. 5.10A). Cases may well arise where, for example, the first molars have been lost and the canines have not yet erupted, where we would describe the relationship by means of the premolars.

Having described the mesio-distal relationship of the cheek teeth, we now look at the bucco-lingual relationship indicating if the patient has a crossbite, either lingual or buccal, or a tendency in that direction.

Where a crossbite of one or more teeth is present, it is particularly important to examine the patient carefully as he moves into occlusion and to note whether the mandible is displaced from the true centric jaw relationship in that position.

This completes the purely dental examination but there are certain other details which should be noted.

1. The opportunity should be taken to collect details of a family history of a similar malocclusion. This may be obtained from the patient but in the case of children, a more certain source is the parent. Such a history, although not always reliable, is sometimes helpful.

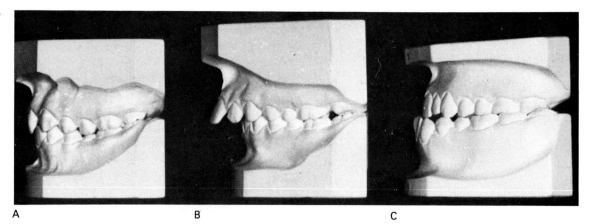

Fig. 5.10 Relationship of posterior teeth in Angle's classification: A, Class I. B, Class II. C, Class III.

2. The patient and/or parent should then be asked the reason for their attendance. This may appear to be a statement of the obvious, but it is not uncommon to find that the patient is present because the dentist told them to come, and they have no idea of the reason for this. In such a case the operator should find out whether the patient and the parent are worried by the malocclusion and whether they are anxious to have it corrected. In many cases the malocclusion will have little effect on the health apart from the psychological one.

3. Arising out of this, an attempt should be made to assess the likely degree of co-operation, and the operator should ensure that the patient fully understands the nature of orthodontic treatment, the likely duration and frequency of attendance required, and the need to wear the appropriate type of appliance. A photograph of a patient wearing a fixed banded appliance is useful to show patients, to ensure that they understand what is involved. Appliances should always be of the simplest type possible to achieve the required result but patients should not be allowed to dictate their own treatment. The patient who refuses to wear bands is the one most likely to complain if the result is less than perfect.

Diagnosis

From the information collected, we now make our diagnosis which is essentially a resumé of the case history, together with a consideration of the inter-relationship between the various factors and their effects on treatment and prognosis. For example, the two patients whose study models are illustrated in Figure 5.11 both have large overjets. In the case shown on the left the upper incisors are very proclined with a very mild Class II skeletal pattern, while in the patient shown on the right, the incisors are at their normal angulation and the overjet almost exactly mirrors the skeletal discrepancy. Other things being equal, the malocclusion on the right will be more difficult to treat and the prognosis more limited. If in addition the patient does not know why she has been referred and is unwilling to wear banded appliances, it is probably better to abandon the exercise altogether!

THE CLASSIFICATION OF MALOCCLUSION

Mankind is infinitely variable, yet man always wishes to classify. This is nowhere more true than in facial form and variations of the occlusion. Classification can be a useful method of describing different types of malocclusion but it should not be assumed that all patients falling into a given class are identical or warrant the same form of treatment.

Angle's classification (Fig. 5.10)

Some reference has already been made to this but classification will here be described in detail. It

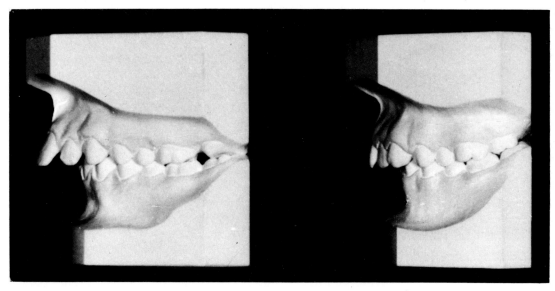

Fig. 5.11 Models of two patients with increased overjets. *Left* on Class I skeletal pattern, *Right* on Class II base.

was invented by Edward H. Angle and is essentially a classification of antero-posterior relationship of the dentition. For the purist, since it is a classification of malocclusion, normal occlusion does not enter into the picture and should simply be described as normal occlusion and not as Class I occlusion.

Class I malocclusion comprises those in which the first permanent molars are, as already described, in normal relationship to each other. The malocclusion is therefore an essentially dental one, with a normal relationship of the arches in the antero-posterior dimension, although this may be associated with an increased or reduced overbite and/or a crossbite. Generally speaking it involves the condition of crowding or spacing, rotation of teeth and local abnormalities. Any of these conditions may of course be found superimposed on a malrelationship of the dental arches: that is a Class II or Class III malocclusion.

Class II malocclusion is found in those cases where the lower first molar is in postnormal relationship to the upper. It is divided into two divisions. Division 1 comprises those cases where there is an increase in overjet, usually, but not necessarily, with proclined upper incisor teeth (Fig. 5.12A). Division 2 comprises those cases in which the upper incisors are retroclined, usually

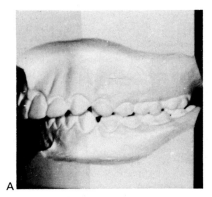

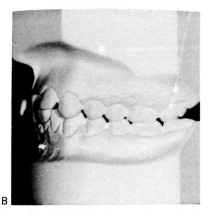

Fig. 5.12 A, Class II Division 1 malocclusion. B, Class II Division 2 malocclusion. These are 'typical' cases.

with an increase in overbite. Not infrequently the lateral incisors are proclined giving the very typical appearance (Fig. 5.12B), although this is not a necessary part of the condition.

Sub-division is a rather archaic term and is used by Angle where the buccal segment on one side of the mouth is in Class I relationship and on the other in Class II relationship. This would be described as 'Class II sub-division'. There is not a series of sub-divisions, and the term is rather a quaint one.

Class III malocclusion comprises those cases where the lower first permanent molars are in prenormal occlusion. This is frequently found in association with an anterior crossbite, where the upper incisors are occluding inside the lower incisors.

The British Standard Classification of incisor relationships

Although Angle's classification is strictly based on the relationship of the posterior teeth, it is becoming increasingly common to use these classes to describe the incisor relationships without giving regard to the relationship of the molars. This has been regularised by the use in British Standard number 4492 of a classification of incisor relationship. This reads as follows:

'Class I — The lower incisor edges occlude with or lie immediately below the cingulum plateau (middle part of the palatal surface) of the upper central incisors.

Class II — The lower incisor edges lie posterior to the cingulum plateau of the upper incisors.

Division 1 — The upper central incisors are proclined or of average inclination and there is an increase in overjet.

Division 2 — The upper central incisors are retroclined. The overjet is usually minimal but may be increased.

Class III — The lower incisor edges lie anterior to the cingulum plateau of the upper incisors. The overjet is reduced or reversed.'

It will be re-emphasised that while both these classifications, together with the skeletal classification already described, are useful as adjuncts in describing a malocclusion, they should not be regarded as more than this. In the ensuing chapters, we shall consider various types of malocclusion on the basis of Angle's classification, but it should not be assumed from this that all the cases falling into one class are necessarily similar.

SUGGESTED READING

British Standards Institution 1983 BS4492, British Standard Glossary of Terms Relating to Dentistry. London, British Standards Institution.

Gould D G 1968 A head positioner for oblique lateral jaw radiography. Dental Practitioner and Dental Record 18: 397–8

6

Cephalometric radiology

The cephalostat was developed in the period after the First World War by B. Holly Broadbent at Western Reserve University in Cleveland Ohio. It evolved from a radiographic craniostat (that is a device for holding dried skulls in a predetermined position in order to radiograph them) which had been designed by Wingate Todd. The finance for the development and its early use was provided by Mrs Charles Bolton and her name is commemorated not only in the Bolton study but also in a point and a plane within the head.

It is certainly possible to undertake orthodontic diagnosis and treatment without the use of cephalometric radiographs. It is also possible to treat fractures of long bones without the use of radiography. Both types of treatment were undertaken for many years before appropriate equipment was invented. Nevertheless, lateral skull radiographs give considerable information, of use both in diagnosis and in the monitoring of treatment, which is not available elsewhere. The necessary equipment may be readily purchased, although expensive, and lateral skull radiographs are being used increasingly, not only in hospitals, but also in private practice. Broadbent originally intended that the lateral skull radiograph should be partnered by a postero-anterior radiograph, thus enabling any point to be located in three dimensions. As we shall see in Chapter 9, this technique is very useful in locating buried teeth, but apart from this, the use of postero-anterior radiographs has proved disappointing. In taking the lateral radiograph, it is usual to ask the patient to close his teeth into occlusion in the intercuspal position. It is always necessary to check that this has been achieved by examination of the radiograph immediately after development. It is occasionally useful to take a second radiograph in the habitual rest position although, again, this has been found less useful than was originally hoped, and such an examination is reserved for cases where it is of particular importance.

Figure 6.1 shows a patient in the cephalostat. The ear posts are tightened into the external auditory meatuses sufficiently to steady the head. They should not be painful and over-tightening, in an effort to stabilise the position of the head, is coun-

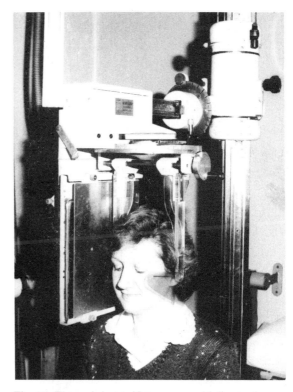

Fig. 6.1 The cephalostat. Note perspex with line to show Frankfort plane.

terproductive. The patient can of course rotate his head vertically about the ear posts and some guidance is necessary to ensure the radiographs are all taken with the head in approximately the same position. A pointer may be added to the apparatus with its tip at the same level as the upper border of the ear posts. This can then be aligned with the lower border of the left bony orbit, located by the palpation, thus ensuring that the Frankfort plane is horizontal. Such a pointer is somewhat frightening and possibly dangerous, and an alternative method is to have a wall mirror in front of the patient, in which the patient is asked to look at his own eyes. This should bring the head into the natural head position.

It is obviously convenient to have the radiographic picture occupying a similar part of the film but the main reason for having standardised head position arises when we also take a posteroanterior view of the same patient. Unfortunately, nature has not endowed us with holes in the front and back of the head and the postero-anterior view is therefore less standardised than the lateral view. It is reasonably accurate in the lateral plane but in the vertical plane, information should as far as possible, be taken from the lateral skull radiograph.

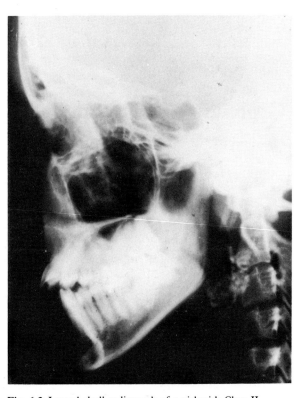

Fig. 6.2 Lateral skull radiograph of a girl with Class II Division 1 malocclusion and high mandibular angle. Note especially calcified lymph nodes at angle of mandible and also apical resorption of upper incisors.

CEPHALOMETRIC DIAGNOSIS

The radiograph

There is a tendency to regard the lateral skull radiograph as being the raw material from which a tracing is prepared. Although tracing and subsequent analysis can be of considerable use, and will be dealt with in the next section, before this is considered the radiograph itself should be closely examined with the following points in mind.

1. The whole radiograph should be scanned and normal structures identified. Any abnormal or pathological condition should also be noted and if appropriate, further advice or treatment sought. The radiograph shown in Figure 6.2 reveals a calcified mass in the region of the angle of the mandible which was identified as a harmless calcified lymph node. It also shows that the roots of the upper central incisors are abnormally short.

This latter fact caused us to take full mouth radiographs which revealed that there had been excessive resorption of the roots of a considerable number of teeth. This is obviously something one would wish to know before commencing extensive orthodontic treatment. The lateral skull radiograph is particularly useful for monitoring any resorption of central incisors, since the film is not appreciably distorted and one can actually measure the length of the tooth before and after orthodontic treatment.

2. The amount of crowding present anterior to the first molar can readily be assessed by clinical examination of the patient or models, but crowding posterior to the first molar is often concealed, since the appropriate teeth are unerupted. This has already been mentioned in the previous chapter. Figure 6.3 shows radiographs of two girls both aged 11 years who will be referred to frequently during this chapter. The

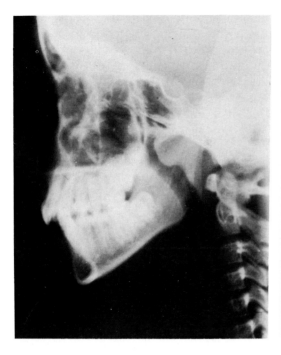
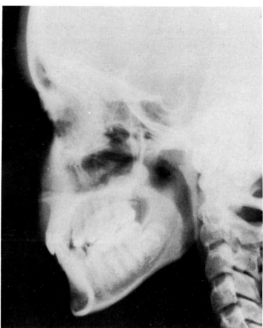
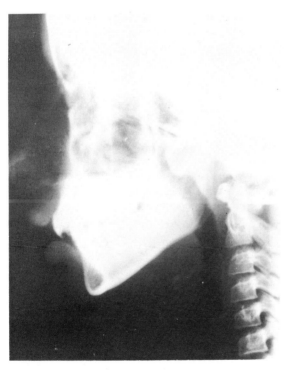
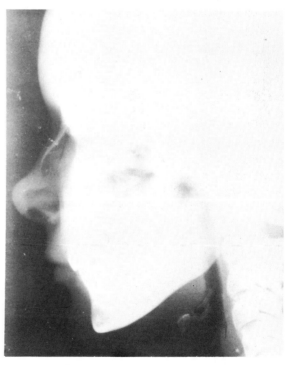

Fig. 6.3 Lateral skull radiographs of *left* Anne and *right* Sheila. Anne has a Class II Division 1 malocclusion with gross crowding. Sheila approximates to the ideal. The upper part of the illustration has been printed to show the hard structures and the lower part, from the same negative, to show the soft parts.

girl on the left, Anne, had a malocclusion with crowding anterior to the molars but it will be observed that there is a gross lack of space for the developing second molars which are 'stacked' above and behind the first molar, with the third molar commencing calcification even further back. In the lower jaw the second molar is developing in the vertical ramus of the mandible, although there is at present no sign of the developing third molars. The girl on the right, Sheila, had a normal occlusion and has been selected as being a close approximation to the ideal. Her third molars are developing in a position only slightly more crowded than that of the second molars in the girl on the left. Anne received orthodontic treatment involving the extraction of four premolars and even so, the third molars remained deeply impacted. In the case of Sheila, they erupted uneventfully.

3. With careful positioning of an aluminium wedge, it is possible to get a clear picture of the soft tissue outline of the face. This is seen particularly well in Figure 6.3 in the lower picture. Although it is not possible to see both hard and soft structures in a photographic print, these may be seen clearly in the original radiograph, the lips and nose being especially clear on the right hand side. Even if this refinement is not available, the soft tissues may be seen by projecting a sufficiently bright light through the radiograph from an unshaded electric bulb or a dental operating lamp. In a good radiograph it may also be possible to see the outline of the tongue and soft palate, as again see in Sheila in Figure 6.3. Anne also shows some adenoidal enlargement although this is comparatively mild. The relation of the lips to the incisor teeth may be assessed from the lateral skull radiograph in the vertical plane and, occasionally usefully, in the horizontal plane. The significance of this relationship has already been mentioned in previous chapters.

4. The radiograph may be used to identify and to some extent localise the position of unerupted teeth. Figure 6.3 indicates that no third molars have so far developed in the lower jaw for Anne (although they may of course still appear) and also that Sheila has two lower third molars, since the outline of both may be clearly seen. In the upper jaw, the situation is less clear cut, since the two

outlines are fairly accurately superimposed. It is not possible from a single radiograph to position an unerupted tooth accurately. Very exact positioning may however be achieved with the use of a corresponding postero-anterior radiograph, as described in Chapter 9.

5. It is also possible from the radiograph to assess the angulation of teeth and degree of overjet and overbite, although these are probably better assessed from the tracing.

Cephalometric analysis

Although to Broadbent goes the credit for the development of the cephalostat and the collection of much useful data, it was not until 1948 that Downes suggested that the skeletal and dental picture could be analysed by comparing measurements on the tracing of the lateral skull radiograph with known standards. Since then a considerable number of such analyses have been developed, to some of which reference will be made in the list of suggested reading at the end of this chapter.

Cephalometric analysis is normally made on a tracing of the lateral skull radiograph. This is done either on tracing paper or acetate film. The latter is probably more dimensionally stable but is also somewhat more expensive. The paper is placed on top of the radiograph and illuminated from below. The X-ray viewer should be masked so that extraneous light does not escape around the outline of the film. It is also useful to have a piece of card or black paper with a hole approximately 3 inches in diameter. This can be placed over the film and allows the identification of faint structures which would otherwise be difficult to position. It is an additional help if the room can be darkened. The outline should be traced either with a very hard pencil (4H) or with a very fine ink stylus. The tracing is then removed from the radiograph and the appropriate lines drawn, again with the fine stylus or hard pencil. It is customary for measurements to be made either in the form of angles, measured with a protractor, or of proportions or ratios. Direct linear measurements are not popular, since heads vary in size and some enlargement is inevitable in producing the radiograph.

In the analysis of cephalometric radiographs, it

is necessary to have data with which to compare the figures measured in the individual under consideration. A particularly thorough review of the available analyses up to the year 1957 is given by Krogman and Sassouni (1957), but this book, which was published privately, is not always readily available. Many of the published analyses go into great detail with a large number of measurements, and this gives rise to a very real tendency for the orthodontist to believe that a complete diagnosis may be made from cephalometric radiographs alone. Lateral skull radiographs are one very useful tool in the completion of a diagnosis but they are only an aid, to be taken with other radiographs, study models and photographs and most important, the clinical examination of the patient himself.

Two points should be borne in mind. Firstly, the measurements made from tracings of a radiograph are by no means exact. Table 6.1 lists the 'error of the method' as assessed by a number of investigators for those measurements used in the 'Eastman' analysis. Table 6.1A shows the error as calculated by seven graduate students as part of

their M.Sc. theses, while Table 6.1B is taken from sources in the literature. The former is noticeably more accurate than the latter, probably due to the use of an electronic digitiser as described later in this chapter. The error of the method is a statistical device, somewhat similar to a standard deviation. Thus if the error of the method for the angle SNA is 0.60°, this means that in approximately ⅔ of individuals, one's tracing will be within 0.60° of the correct value. In 95 per cent of individuals it will be within a range of twice this figure and in virtually all the individuals it will be within a range of three times this figure. The figures in Table 6.1 are for duplicate tracings of the same radiograph and take no account of the error arising in taking the film itself. To estimate this would involve unjustifiable radiographic exposure, but estimates have been made by Björk, Backlund and recently by Perera. It would seem that errors from this source are negligible except in the case of porion. This is usually defined as the uppermost point on the shadow of the ear-post of the machine and Steiner has drawn attention to the variation which can arise in positioning this in the external auditory meatus. Both ends of the Frankfort plane are, for different reasons, of low accuracy and it is recommended that this should not be used as a plane of reference. Secondly, because of this inaccuracy and because of the wide range found in any study, there is no point in giving a standard value to two places of decimals. Table 6.2 shows the figures reported by various investigators in samples of varying sizes and ages. In some cases the samples were selected, usually as having excellent dental occlusion, whereas in others they were random samples. All are for Caucasian children. Nevertheless, the mean figures and the standard deviations are reasonably

Table 6.1 'Error of the method' in making measurements of lateral skull radiographs

A. Postgraduate students — E.D.H.

	A*	B*	C*	D*	E	F*	G
SNA	0.34	0.43	1.33	0.40	0.27		
SNB	0.35	0.25	1.02		0.28		
ANB	0.25	0.36	0.60		0.20		
SNI	0.36	0.25					
M/M			0.85	0.69	0.39	0.67	0.54
SN/Max.		0.78		0.56			
F.P.		0.30		0.26	0.40		0.25
1 — Max. P.	0.97	0.96			1.28	0.88	
1̄ — Mdb. P.	1.16	1.16			1.02	1.31	

*Using the digitiser.

B. Other publications

	Björk 1947	Backlund 1963	Mills 1964	Mills 1966	Perera 1977	Johannsen 1972	Graveley & Benzies 1974
SNA	0.60		0.84	0.89	1.21	0.55	0.78–1.31
SNB	0.62		0.54	0.72	0.91	0.46	0.54–1.12
ANB				0.41		0.43	0.57–1.03
SNI			0.58	0.75		0.39	
M/M	0.99	1.05	1.20	0.80	0.67	0.89	0.83–1.37
F.P.						0.26	
1 — Max. P.	1.39	1.53	2.20	1.32	0.97		2.11–2.23
1̄ — Mdb. P.	1.48	1.31	1.81	2.06	1.90		1.64–1.81

Table 6.2 Means and standard deviations of lateral skull parameters as calculated by various authors. The bottom line gives the standard figures

	No. in Sample	Age	SNA	SNB	ANB	SNI	1 — Max. P.	1 — Mdb. P.	M.M.P.A.	SN/Mx. P.A.	F.P.
Harkness & Brown 1972	216	12	80.96 (3.25)	77.62 (3.18)	3.37 (2.19)		108.15 (6.6)	94.51 (6.08)	25.85 (5.17)		54.81 (1.55)
	23	9	80.28 (2.82)	77.37 (3.17)	2.91 (2.07)		109.56 (4.69)	93.89 (4.84)	28.52 (3.16)		
Mills 1973	24	14	81.06 (2.87)	77.67 (3.26)	3.35 (2.23)		112.10 (5.76)	94.04 (4.85)	26.71 (4.08)		54.60 (2.18)
	34	11.19	80.80 (2.7)	77.51 (3.0)	3.29 (2.0)				27.88 (3.4)		54.65 (2.15)
Johannsen 1972	34	16.54	81.49 (3.08)	78.50 (3.11)	2.99 (2.05)				26.79 (4.24)		55.01 (2.07)
Björk &	243	12	81.3 (3.3)	77.8 (3.4)	3.4 (2.3)	80.37 (3.45)	110.5 (6.0)	92.1 (6.7)	28† (6†)	8.0 (3.0†)	
Palling 1954	243	20	82.0 (3.7)	79.3 (3.7)	2.7 (2.6)	81.07 (3.62)	111.2 (6.4)	90.5 (7.2)			
Ballard 1956	250	—	81.0 (3.5)	77.5 (—)	3.5 (—)		109 (6)	92.5 (6.5)	28.0 (—)	8.0	
Weinberg & Kronman 1966	30	11.6									54.86 (1.97)
Goldman 1959	50	Adult	81.22 (3.11)	79.79 (3.21)	1.42 (2.17)						54.5 (2.26)
Coben 1955	47	8									54.2 (2.18)
Riedel 1952	52	Adult	82.01 (3.89)	79.97 (3.60)	2.04 (1.81)			93.09 (6.78)			
	24	7–11	80.79 (3.85)	78.02 (3.06)	2.77 (2.33)			93.52 (5.78)			
Backlund 1963	142	10–11					109.9 (5.4)	91.1 (6.4)	28.7 (5.2)		56.0*
	138	10–11					109.8 (5.4)	89.7 (6.4)	28.1 (5.2)		55.0*
Kerr 1979	18	10	8.17 (4.2)	78.2 (3.7)	3.5*		104.8 (5.4)		28.2*	5.9 (2.7)	
	17	10	81.7 (4.2)	78.2 (3.7)	3.5*		109.5 (6.6)		27.3*	7.5 (2.3)	
	18	15	81.6 (4.2)	78.4 (4.2)	3.2*		108.4 (7.4)		26.5*	7.7 (3.5)	
	17	15	81.5 (2.4)	79.0 (2.9)	2.5*		110.7 (7.4)		25.7*	7.8 (2.9)	
Eastman Standard			81.0 (3.0)	78 (3)	2	= SNA	109 (6)	93 (6)	27 (4)	8.0 (3.0)	55 (2)

† Quoted from Ballard 1956
* Calculated from the author's mean figures

close to each other and on the final line I have suggested values which may be used in practical analysis. For each measurement the first column indicates the standard value and the second column the range, on either side of this, which may be regarded as reasonably normal. This latter figure is of course, a 'rounded' standard deviation. It is suggested that the measurements given in this Table, illustrated in Figure 6.4, should provide the basic cephalometric analysis of Caucasian individuals. Table 6.3 gives similar figures for children of Negroid and Chinese races. These have mostly been taken from the American literature. Most of the black population of the United Kingdom came originally from the West Indies, where there is some racial mixture, and figures for cephalometric analysis are less reliable. Children from the Indian sub-continent are, of course,

Table 6.3 Suggested standard cephalometric standard figures for patients of African and Chinese origin.

	African	Chinese
SNA	85	83
SNB	80	80
ANB	5	3
M/M Angle	28	28
$\underline{1}$ to Max. Pl.	118	113
$\overline{\underline{1}}$ to Mand. Pl	98	96

mostly Caucasian. These have been used for some years at the Eastman Dental Hospital, London and serve to give a useful picture of the lateral skull appearance without the wood being obscured by the trees. For specific purposes, other measurements may be required and average values for a wide range of such measurements may be obtained from the articles quoted at the end of this chapter. For the moment it will suffice to consider the measurements suggested in some detail.

THE SKELETAL PATTERN

SNA, SNB, and ANB

The points A and B may be taken to delimit the area of bone around the apices of the teeth, where basal and alveolar bone meet. The angles SNA and SNB will therefore indicate the prognathism of upper and lower dental bases if we assume that the anterior cranial base, as indicated by SN, is reliable for this purpose. In practice this is not the case and this fact should always be kept in the back of one's mind if the figures conflict with one's clinical assessment. The difference between these angles, the angle ANB, is used to give an assessment of the antero-posterior dental base relationship. Thus Figure 6.4 shows tracings of the radiographs of the two girls. Anne, shown on the left, has an angle SNA of 78.5° indicating that her maxillary base is somewhat retrognathous relative to the upper face. The angle SNB at 72° shows a distinct retrusion giving her a somewhat receding chin. The difference between these angles, that is the angle ANB, is 6.5° higher than the standard value of 3° and well outside the normal range. Sheila on the right, has an angle SNA of 82° which is only one degree higher than the standard value, while SNB at 78.0° is coinci-

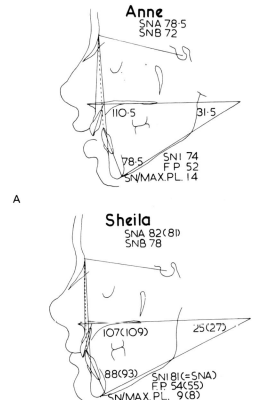

Fig. 6.4 Lateral skull tracings of the girls. A, Anne and B, Sheila. The latter approaches closely the standard figures, which are given in parentheses after the actual measurements.

dent with the standard. Indeed, this tracing was chosen as being very close to the ideal values.

The use of this angle ANB to indicate the skeletal discrepancy, is however only moderately satisfactory for reasons first mentioned by Ballard (1951) and indicated in Figure 6.5. Figure 6.5A is a tracing of Sheila as in Figure 6.4B, with the angle ANB at 4° well within the normal range. Figure 6.5B has been produced by extending the line SN anteriorly to produce an artificial Nasion, N'. If the angles SN'A and SN'B are now measured it will be seen that the angle SN'A has decreased by 4°, while the angle AN'B is 2° less than in Figure 6.5A. In Figure 6.5C, on the other hand, the Nasion has been moved posteriorly to the position N''. This increases the angle SN''A by 4° from the original figure, and the angle AN''B by 1.5°. It would seem therefore that the significance of the angle ANB varies according to the size of the angle SNA. As a rough and ready rule of thumb some correction may be made to the standard values. For every one degree that the angle SNA falls below the standard value of 81°, one should subtract half a degree from the standard angle ANB of 3°. Alternatively, and probably more conveniently, add half a degree to the angle ANB of the patient under consideration, and then compare the 'adjusted' figure with the standard value of 3°. Thus, in Anne's case (Fig. 6.4A) the angle SNA is 2.5° below the datum and one should therefore add half this value to ANB, which thus becomes 7.75° — more severely Class II than initially appeared to be the case. This crude correction works reasonably well for all

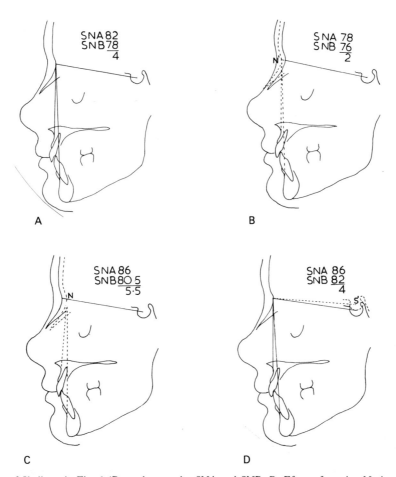

A

B

C

D

Fig. 6.5 A, Tracing of Sheila as in Fig. 6.4B, to show angles SNA and SNB. B, Effect of moving Nasion anteriorly without changing the rest of the skull. C, Effect of moving Nasion posteriorly. D, Effect of raising the point S.

malocclusions but it should be remembered in Class III skeletal patterns, that the mathematical sign enters into the calculation. For example, if the angle ANB were −3.0° and we subtract from this 2° then the final figure will be −5°. In Class III skeletal patterns as the angle SNA decreases, the true discrepancy between SNA and SNB increases, although of course it is a negative one. Indeed this adjustment, although not completely invalid, is less satisfactory if SNB is greater than SNA.

Unfortunately, this correction is not fool-proof. Figure 6.5D again shows the tracing for Sheila with a solid outline showing the true picture. The dotted outline shows a modification to increase the angle SNA to 86° again, as in Figure 6.5C but in this case, the effect has been produced by raising

the centre of the sella turcica to S'. Although this alters the angles S'NA and S'NB it does so by equal amounts and does not effect the angle ANB. In practice, where the angle SNA departs from the datum value, this is usually due to a variation in the relative prognathism of point A compared with Nasion but the discrepancy in the base of skull does sometimes happen and undue reliance should not be placed upon the use of the angle ANB. As already indicated, it is a guide not a god!

There is another case in which the angles SNA and SNB can be deceptive. It is illustrated in Figure 6.6. On the left are the study models of a patient, trimmed in the usual fashion with the base and upper surface of the model parallel to the occlusal plane. This patient would appear to have a Class III dental base relationship albeit a mild

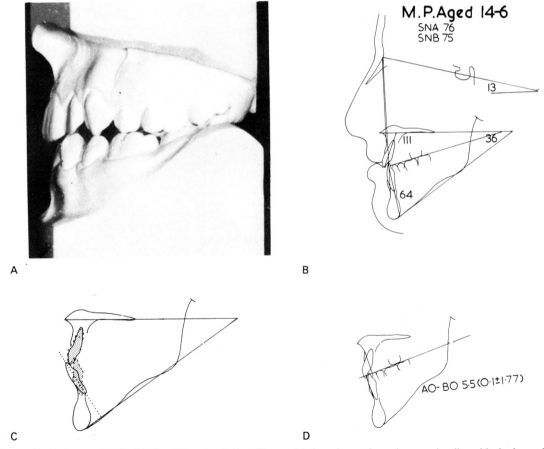

Fig. 6.6 A, Study models of mild Class III malocclusion. The models have been trimmed conventionally, with the base of the model parallel to the occlusal plane. B, Lateral skull tracing. The angle ANB would indicate a Class I skeletal pattern. C, Conversion tracing to assess dental base relationships. D, 'Wits' analysis

one. The tracing on the right shows that in the antero-posterior plane the skeletal pattern is within the realms of normal with the angle ANB of 1° for the angle of 76° for SNA. This would appear at first sight to be a contradiction but the solution lies in the fact that the whole denture is somewhat tilted relative to the base of skull, with its anterior end downwards and its posterior end upwards. This usually arises where the lower border of the mandible is steeply inclined. The upper border and with it the occlusal surface tends to be similarly tilted. Such patients usually have a long lower facial height. The maxilla may also be somewhat tilted in the same direction so that the jaws themselves are rotated upon the skull base. In describing the antero-posterior skeletal relationships in this patient, some qualification is necessary. The mandible is not prognathous and from the point of view of facial appearance, it will be wrong to describe the patient as having a Class III skeletal pattern. Nevertheless, if we are considering only the dentition, then the lower dental base is certainly anterior to the upper dental base and there will clearly be problems in correcting the occlusion. This type of case shows the unwisdom of blindly following angular measurements without giving the matter thought.

It should also be borne in mind that for a given antero-posterior discrepancy in points A and B, the angle ANB will be greater in a short than in a long face. In practice this does not seem to be a serious factor.

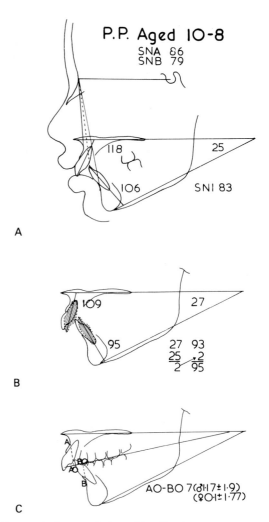

Fig. 6.7 A, Tracing of a boy with a Class II Division 1 malocclusion. B, To show production to 'conversion tracing'. C, 'Wits' analysis

Other methods of assessing skeletal pattern

Since the use of the angle ANB is not always satisfactory, various other methods have been developed to assess the skeletal pattern from the lateral skull radiograph. Two will be mentioned here.

1. 'The conversion tracing' (Fig. 6.7B). This is a method of assessing the relationship of upper to lower dental bases without the intervention of the base of skull. The underlying assumption is that tilting of the teeth is brought about by the effect of soft tissues, including digits, while the bodily displacement of teeth is essentially the result of skeletal discrepancy and probably largely unchangeable. To produce a conversion tracing,

first trace the maxillary and mandibular outlines, together with the attached incisor teeth. These incisors are then traced a second time onto small pieces of tracing paper. A mark is made on the upper incisor at a point $\frac{1}{3}$ of the way down the root from the apex in the direction of the crown. The second tracing is superimposed on the same point and is then tilted lingually until it takes up the standard angle of 109° to the maxillary plane. Its outline is drawn in this new position. A similar technique is followed with the lower central incisor but some modifications are necessary.

Again, a point is selected ⅓ of the way up the root and the second tracing superimposed at this point. It is then tilted until it takes up the standard angle to the maxillary plane. This may of course be done by measuring the angle between its long axis and the maxillary plane but it is more usual to measure the angle of the long axis to the mandibular plane. If the mandibular plane is used, this angle has to be adjusted by reference to the maxillo-mandibular planes angle. For every one degree which this is greater than the mean figure, the mean angle of the lower incisor to the lower border of the mandible should be decreased by one degree and correspondingly, if the maxillo-mandibular planes angle is low, the lower incisal angle should be increased. In this way the lower incisor is placed at its 'standard' angle to the maxillary plane. Thus, is Figure 6.7B, since the maxillo-mandibular planes angle at 25° is 2° less than the standard angle of 27°, the lower incisor outline is corrected to 95°, or 2° greater than the overall standard. When this has been done, it will frequently be found that the two outlines overlap in a completely unrealistic way and the outline of the lower incisor should then be moved downwards along its long axis until its incisal edge just touches the opposing structure. The dental base relationship pattern is then assessed by measuring the overjet, as has been done in Figure 6.7B.

This is a somewhat tedious procedure but produces in most cases an accurate representation of the relationship of the dental bases. It eliminates any reference to the base of skull and therefore in the case in Figure 6.6C, the more realistic diagnosis of a Class III skeletal pattern is produced. The main shortcoming is in the arbitrary selection of the point one third of the way up the root, about which the teeth are tilted. This is most likely to give rise to a misinterpretation in Class II Division 2 malocclusions where it would seem that the teeth in fact tilt lingually virtually about the lingual alveolar crest.

2. 'Wits' analysis. This technique arose because of the difficulties in using the ANB angle described above. It was evolved by Jacobson at Witwatersrand University in South Africa which explains its name. In this technique, a line is drawn along the occlusal plane of the teeth. This is selected somewhat arbitarily to follow the line of the occlusal surfaces of the posterior teeth, a line which is sometimes called the functional occlusal plane. Perpendiculars are then dropped to this plane from point A and point B, meeting the plane at AO and BO. The distance between the points AO and BO is measured and compared with average figures, any difference indicating a skeletal discrepancy. Thus, in Figure 6.7C, the distance of 7 mm is substantially greater than the standard for boys of 1.17 mm. It is a simple technique which again eliminates reference to the base of skull and will indicate the relative positions of the dental bases but neither this nor the conversion tracing would give any indication of prognathism or retrognathism of the jaw bases. Its main disadvantage lies in the difficulty of accurately drawing in the functional occlusal plane. The average figures given are derived from a rather small sample of young adults.

Vertical relation of the jaws

In assessing the skeletal pattern, we should realise that the jaw bases are related to each other in all three planes of space. The lateral skull radiograph will of course only describe two of these but the second, the vertical plane, is of considerable importance. As with the antero-posterior relation, a clinical assessment should always be used in association with cephalometric findings and on the whole it pays to rely on the clinical assessment rather than the cephalometric finding. There are three ways in which the vertical relationship may be assessed.

1. The angle between the lower border of the mandible and the maxillary plane. Any increase above the standard figure for this angle would tend to indicate a steep lower border of the mandible, with the anterior facial height greater than the posterior facial height. Similarly, any decrease in this angle would indicate a small anterior lower facial height relative to the posterior. This is of course only relative and the abnormality may arise either in the anterior or the posterior region, (although the former seems more common), or conceivably at either end of the maxillary plane. Alternatively, some authors prefer to use the Frankfort plane, which has the

disadvantage of being difficult to identify with sufficient accuracy, or the line SN in the anterior base of skull. The latter has its uses but it does not relate one jaw to the other, it relates the lower jaw to the base of skull. For most purposes, the first of these measurements is the most useful.

2. The lower facial height itself may be measured and it is the anterior facial height which is particularly useful. A line is dropped from the lowest border of the symphysis menti (the menton) to touch the maxillary plane at right angles and the length of this line is measured in millimetres. It has the obvious disadvantage that people vary in size, both absolutely and because of variations in age and it is not usually very satisfactory.

3. The facial proportion. This is achieved by making the measurement for the lower face already described and making a similar measurement for the upper face, by dropping a perpendicular from Nasion to the maxillary plane and measuring its length. The lower facial height is then calculated as a proportion of the two heights added together. This is fairly satisfactory and any departure from the average is usually significant. On the other hand there are people who have large or small anterior lower facial heights and correspondingly large or small upper anterior facial heights! It is therefore advisable as indicated above, to use more than one measurement and to compare them with clinical assessment.

TOOTH POSITION

In this context we would normally read the angle of the long axis of upper and lower incisors to their relative bases. It is customary to trace the most prominent incisor and this should be borne in mind if it is not a typical one. The reason for doing this is that it is usually the one most easily seen. This information is particularly valuable in prognosticating as will be described in the next section.

In treating an abnormal overjet, either increased or reversed, the object is usually to bring the upper incisors into a normal relationship with the lowers, without appreciably disturbing the position of the latter. An antero-posterior skeletal discrepancy will increase the difficulty of achieving this. A compensating proclination or retroclination of the lower incisors may make it easier to achieve a normal incisor relationship. Thus (Fig. 6.7A), the patient has an increased overjet and at first sight the ANB angle of 7° would seem somewhat daunting, as would the other assessment of dental base discrepancy. Since the angle SNA at 86° is 5° higher than the standard the 'compensated' figure for ANB is $4\frac{1}{2}°$; rather more reasonable. Furthermore, the lower incisors are proclined to 106°, carrying the incisal edge forward to a more reasonable position.

This effect may be assessed by measuring the angle SNI. If this angle is equal to the angle SNA, then the dentition may be treated as if the skeletal pattern were Class I, even though the facial appearance may deny it. In Figure 6.7C the angle SNI is 3° below SNA, so we have some degree of discrepancy and will either have to move the apices of the upper incisors palatally, or accept a retroclined position of these teeth.

This tilting of the lower incisors may, and often does, serve to compensate for a skeletal discrepancy, but on occasion it may have the reverse effect.

A popular alternative to the use of SNI, serving the same purpose, is to measure the distance of the incisal edge of the lower incisor, either from a line joining nasion to point B or one from point A to pogonion (APo line). The latter line was first used by Downs, although he measured the upper incisor distance and not the lower. Ricketts believes that in an ideal face the lower incisal tip will lie 1 mm anterior to this line ± 2 mm. This allows a range which will include most individuals. Raleigh Williams believes that ideally the lower incisal edge should lie on the APo line.

Although point A may be modified by orthodontic treatment and Po by natural growth, either this line or the NB line is in practice satisfactory for assessing the position of the lower incisor. Unfortunately, Angle's belief that all individuals have the potential for ideal occlusion dies hard, and gives rise to the belief among some orthodontists that so long as one places the lower incisors on the APo line, all will be well. This owes more to necromancy than science, and will often lead to disappointing relapse.

Prognosis

In a limited proportion of cases, it is helpful to use lateral skull radiographs to assess the prognosis for correction of the abnormality. These are usually cases of gross Class II or Class III malocclusion. It has been mentioned in an earlier chapter that there is at present considerable interest in predicting growth in children by means of lateral skull radiographs. This will show the average changes to be expected in a child but of course children are not all average. It does not accurately predict the child whose growth departs radically from the mean figure and although this is a small proportion, it is an important one. In the interests of simplicity, it is preferable where a prognosis tracing is carried out, to assume that no growth takes place. To some extent, this is assuming the worst although of course a few cases will in fact grow unfavourably. Figure 6.8A shows the outline of the jaws and incisor teeth of a severe Class II skeletal pattern. It will be seen that the overjet is almost entirely due to this skeletal discrepancy with the upper incisors already below the average angle to the maxillary plane. The easy way to treat an overjet is to tilt the teeth lingually which can be achieved by simple appliances. The effect of doing this is shown in Figure 6.8B where the solid outline of the upper incisor assumes that it has been tilted about the traditional point close to the root apex. This is probably somewhat more favourable than would in fact be achieved, but even so the position of the central incisor is clearly unacceptable. Its appearance would be grossly unattractive even if it were stable but in practice it would probably relapse. The ideal solution would be to move the tooth bodily in a lingual direction, and even perhaps to move the apex slightly more than the crown. The result of doing this is shown in Figure 6.8C. The appearance of the incisor is much better, but the whole tooth has been moved through the lingual plate of bone of the maxilla. This is not a practical proposition. Although it would seem that the alveolar crest will to some extent follow the tooth, the lingual plate of bone on the level of the apex does so to a very

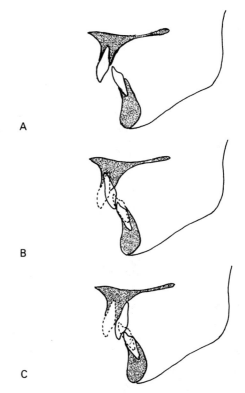

Fig. 6.8 A, Tracing from radiograph of Class II Division 1 malocclusion. B, Prognosis tracing assuming lingual tilting of upper incisors. C, Prognosis tracing assuming only bodily movement thereof.

limited extent, and movement of the root apex into contact with the periosteum may give rise to resorption of the root. It is not therefore possible to move the tooth to this extent. It is necessary to achieve a compromise between the two conditions shown in Figure 6.8B and C and to accept some degree of lingual tilting of the upper incisors in the final condition. As a general rule of thumb, incisors may be tilted lingually until they take an angle of approximately 95° to the maxillary plane. Other things being equal, this will probably be stable and not aesthetically unacceptable.

In order to achieve either of the results shown in Figure 6.8, or the desirable intermediate position, it will be necessary to move the lower incisors vertically downwards. If they were left in their original position, shown by the dotted outline, they would interfere with the lingual movement of the upper incisors and by using our prognostic tracing, we can judge the amount of 'depression' of the lower incisors. The question of overbite reduction will be dealt with in detail in a later chapter but this prognostic tracing gives an idea of the amount of such reduction which is necessary.

Monitoring of progress

Lateral skull radiographs are of considerable value in assessing the changes which have taken place as a result of a combination of orthodontic treatment and natural growth. This may be carried out during treatment if one is in doubt about precisely what tooth movements are taking place, and is particularly valuable at the end of treatment. A great deal can be learnt by comparing tracings of patients at the beginning and end of treatment and if possible some time thereafter. As always, a word of caution is necessary, and undue deduction should not be made from very small changes which may well be the result of inaccuracies.

These assessments may be made by comparing measurements on two successive tracings, either linear, or more usually angular, although a more striking picture can be shown by the superimposition of radiographs. For this purpose both radiographs are traced, preferably with an ink stylus and sometimes usefully in different colours. One tracing is then superimposed on the other and it is possible to see what changes have taken place. This sounds very simple and straightforward, until one considers the sentence 'one tracing is superimposed upon the other . . .'. The question immediately arises as to which points or lines should be used for superimposition. Differing pictures will be given according to the area chosen and it has been said that it is possible to show almost anything by choosing the area of superimposition suitably. The cranium grows considerably less than the face, and the anterior base of skull in particular grows remarkably little after the age of 7 years. This area is therefore frequently chosen for superimposition, the most common structure being the line SN.

Figure 6.9 shows the initial radiograph of Anne and on it has been superimposed a radiograph taken 7 years later, some years after the completion of all treatment. In Figure 6.9A the tracings have been superimposed on the line SN.

Since this line increases in length with normal growth the actual point registered is the point N. It would appear from this the maxilla has grown downwards and backwards, while the maxillary plane has rotated in a clockwise direction. Superimpositions of this type are often used to demonstrate the 'orthopaedic' posterior movement of the maxilla by means of heavy extra-oral forces (although no such forces were used in this case). The mandible has grown substantially with the symphysis coming downwards and forwards thus making some improvement in the skeletal pattern. Turning to Figure 6.9B the radiographs have been superimposed on the same line but this time registered on the centre of sella turcica. The maxilla now appears to have grown downwards and forwards still with a substantial tilting of the maxillary plane. The forward growth of the mandibular symphysis is very much more marked. In Figure 6.9C the radiographs have been superimposed on De Coster's line. This line is simply the uppermost outline of the anterior cranial base and its use depends on the fact that after about the age of 7 years there is apparently no growth in this area. The growth of the anterior base of skull takes place by surface deposition on the frontal and nasal bones and since the fronto-nasal suture is not usually parallel to the line SN the nasion may apparently move upwards or downwards during this growth. The centre of sella turcica similarly moves backwards during growth, and may be displaced upwards or downwards. Figure 6.9C would seem to reduce the amount of tilting in the maxillary outline which now grows almost vertically downwards. The line SN, however, has tilted downwards anteriorly, presumably because of the new situation of the anterior end of the fronto-nasal suture, that is Nasion. These three diagrams show three somewhat different pictures of facial growth and none of them is right and none wrong. Each shows the pattern of growth relative to the structures on which the tracings have been superimposed. Figure 6.9A is the closest approximation to what we see when we look at the patient. While we cannot see the nasion, we can see the skin overlying it and the picture shown here represents the changes in the face which would be visible to the naked eye. We cannot normally see the sella

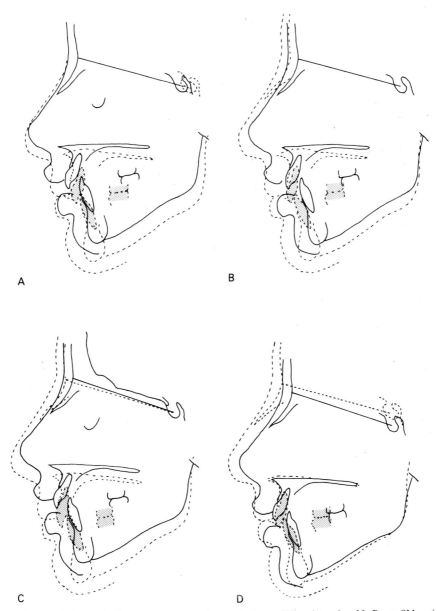

Fig. 6.9 Tracing of Anne, before and after treatment, superimposed: A, on SN registered at N, B, on SN registered at S, C, on the upper outline of the sphenoid bone (De Coster's line), D, on the maxillary outline.

turcica but superimposition on this structure perhaps gives a clearer picture of the way in which the skull grows outwards from its approximate centre. Superimposition on De Coster's line has a great deal to recommend it. It is in fact a structure which is not growing. Unfortunately, it is very difficult to identify accurately and what we gain in realism we probably lose in accuracy.

It will be seen in Figure 6.9A that the apex of the upper central incisor has apparently moved downwards and backwards although this is not confirmed in Figure 6.9B. If we wish to know how individual teeth have moved through the bone, then it is necessary to superimpose the radiographs on the bone concerned as we have done in Figure 6.9D. This shows that in fact the upper

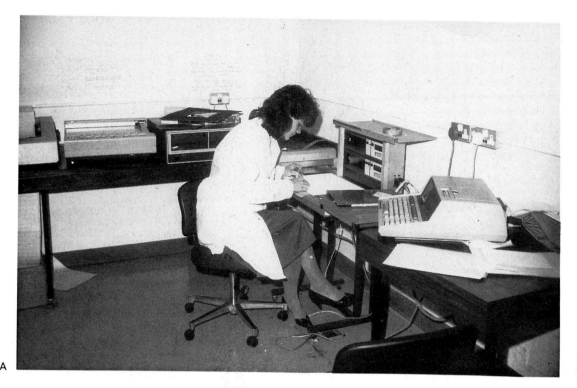

A

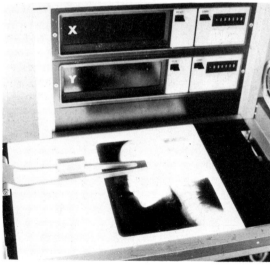

B

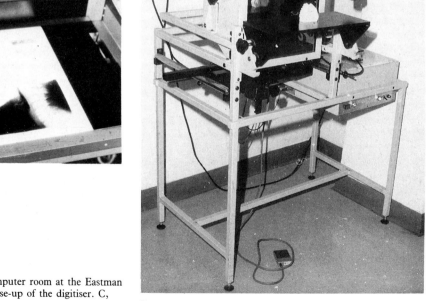

C

Fig. 6.10 A, A corner of the computer room at the Eastman Dental Hospital, London. B, Close-up of the digitiser. C, The reflex metrograph.

incisor has been retroclined by tilting about a point within its root with the apex moving somewhat labially.

These four superimpositions are by no means exhaustive. In Figure 6.9D, the outlines of the maxilla have been superimposed on the anterior vault of the palate which is believed to be a structure where there is minimal surface deposition or resorption. Nevertheless, the maxilla has increased in size and some orthodontists prefer to superimpose on the tip of the anterior nasal spine. If it is desired to show changes of the dentition within the mandible, then the radiographs should be superimposed on the mandible. If Björk's structures are used we will see the actual movement through the bone, whereas if the mandible is superimposed on its lower border, we will get a clearer idea of the situation as it actually faces us.

It is repeated that superimposition of lateral skull radiographs can be very useful provided it is appreciated that these show movements of structures relative to those points on which the radiographs are superimposed. In practice of course, it is not necessary to draw each superimposition and much can be gained by making numerous superimpositions of the two tracings, although they need only be drawn out if required for teaching or publication.

The digitiser

In recent years a piece of electronic equipment has been designed known as a digitiser which enables readings made from lateral skull radiographs or tracings thereof to be passed directly into a computer. A digitiser is now a standard computer accessory or 'peripheral' but the majority of these are not suitable for orthodontic purposes. Figure 6.10 shows an orthodontic digitiser. It consists essentially of an X-ray viewing box on which the radiograph may be mounted and over which it is possible to move a piece of perspex inscribed with fine lines intersecting at right angles. The intersection is placed over the point which it is required to digitise. A button or trigger is then pressed and this has the effect of locating this point within the computer in the form of Cartesian (X,Y) co-ordinates. This refers the point to axes, the location of which is usually completely arbitrary. The process is repeated for the other points which are required and when all such points have been fed into the computer the machine will then calculate such measurements and angles as the operator wishes. Moreover, the readings may be stored within the machinery of the computer and various statistical calculations made on single or more probably a series of radiographs of the same or different patients. In any case the findings will be printed out on paper for permanent record.

Alternatively, the information may be stored on tape or, more usually, on discs, either flexible ('floppy disks') or on hard discs, the latter storing a very large amount of information. With suitable 'peripherals' the computer can draw an outline similar to a tracing, superimpose this as commanded on another tracing, often with a different colour of ink, and even simulate the results of orthognathic surgery, as described in Chapter 16. A recent development is the 'reflex metrograph' with which it is possible to digitise three-dimensional objects such as study models (Fig. 6.10C).

Equipment of this type is, of course, expensive and requires a skilled amateur or professional programmer, since the appropriate programs are not available commercially. Prices of equipment ('hardware') are constantly reducing and, with more standardisation of programming languages, suitable programs may soon become available to the practitioner.

It would seem that the digitising of records has a part to play, more especially in research. With care and the minimising of human error, it can be extremely accurate and can involve considerable saving in time. For most purposes it is not necessary to trace the radiographs, although if the digitising is carried out directly from the film, certain points located on a curve, such as gonion and gnathion, can be difficult to identify accurately. Furthermore, the figures alone are sometimes difficult to visualise without the tracings.

SUGGESTED READING

Broadbent B H 1931 A new X-ray technique and its application to orthodontics. Angle Orthodontist 1: 45–66

Broadbent B H 1936 The face of the normal child. Angle Orthodontist 7: 183–208

Broadbent B H 1937 Bolton standards and technique in orthodontic practice. Angle Orthodontist 7: 209–33

Downs W B 1948 Variations of facial relationships; their significance in treatment and prognosis. American Journal of Orthodontics 34: 812–40

Greenberg L Z, Johnston L E 1975 Computerized prediction: The accuracy of a current long-range forecast. American Journal of Orthodontics 67: 243–52

Jacobson A 1975 The 'WITS' appraisal of jaw disharmony. American Journal of Orthodontics 67: 125–38

Johnston L E 1975 A simplified approach to prediction. American Journal of Orthodontics 67: 253–7

Krogman W M, Sassouni V 1957 A syllabus of roentgenographic cephalometry. Center for Research in Child Growth (published privately in duplicated form), Philadelphia

Mills J R E 1970 The application and importance of cephalometry in orthodontic treatment. The Orthodontist 32–47

Ricketts R M 1973 The application of computers to orthodontics — diagnosis, prognosis and treatment planning. Transactions of Third International Orthodontic Congress, 169–184

Riedel R A 1952 The relation of maxillary structures to cranium in malocclusion and in normal occlusion. Angle Orthodontist 22: 142–5

Schulhof A B, Bagha L 1975 A statistical evaluation of the Ricketts and Johnston growth-forecasting methods. American Journal of Orthodontics 67: 258–76

Steiner C C 1953 Cephalometrics for you and me. American Journal of Orthodontics 39: 729–55

Wylie W L 1947 The assessment of anteroposterior dysplasia. Angle Orthodontist 17: 97–109

Wylie W L, Johnson E L 1952 Rapid evaluation of facial dysplasia in the vertical plane. Angle Orthodontist 22: 165–82

7

Principles of appliance therapy

The purpose of this chapter, as its title suggests, is to consider the basic principles underlying the different types of orthodontic appliance. It is not intended to deal in detail with individual techniques, and for this the reader is referred to the suggested reading at the end of the chapter. As in all sections of the book an effort has been made to keep these suggestions to a length which a postgraduate student might have time to read, but here several longer standard textbooks have also been included for those wishing to pursue techniques further.

It is a feature of orthodontic treatment that a number of techniques, often called 'philosophies', have grown up which involve following *ex cathedra* pronouncements of the appropriate god. This chapter is written in the hope that the reader will understand some of the theory underlying the use of these techniques, and use them selectively, picking the best features of each technique, and employing them in the type of malocclusion for which they are most suited.

Much of this chapter concerns the edgewise technique, but I am reminded of a comment by the late Rudolf Hotz: when a colleague stated that he was an 'edgewise man' Hotz said that he preferred to remove the edge and become a wise man.

ORTHODONTIC WIRE

Orthodontic spring wire is used in a variety of forms and it is desirable that any orthodontist should understand its properties before considering its use in the design and construction of appliances.

Although stainless steel is widely used, other alloys with varying advantages and disadvantages may be employed, especially in fixed appliance techniques.

Stainless steel

There are at least three types of stainless steel and the one which is used in orthodontic spring wire is known as austenitic steel. Austenite is an alloy of iron and carbon with the iron in the 'gamma' form. In ordinary carbon steel this form exists only above the temperature of 723°C. It is maintained in stainless steel at room temperature by the addition of stabilisers, particularly nickel. The type of stainless steel used in orthodontics is also sometimes called 18 : 8 because it contains approximately 18 per cent of chromium and 8 per cent of nickel, although this varies somewhat in modern alloys. With any stainless steel the carbon content is reduced to a minimum; not more than 0.2 per cent. There are usually small proportions of titanium and/or niobium.

Stainless steel in this form has a number of useful properties, and one or two which are less useful.

1. In the first place it is, of course, stainless. The stainless properties are due to the presence of chromium, which when exposed to the air oxidises. This thin film of transparent oxide is very tough and protects the underlying metal from further attack. It also prevents wetting of the surface by solder, and makes soldering difficult unless special fluxes are used to penetrate the oxide film.

2. Unlike carbon steel, stainless steel cannot be hardened by tempering. It is, however, very

susceptible to work-hardening. Wire is made by drawing a cast ingot of steel through a die so as to produce a longer, narrower bar. This is repeated through a series of dies of gradually decreasing diameter, until wire of the appropriate size is produced. Each time the wire is drawn through the die the crystals of steel become elongated, parallel to the direction of drawing, and this parallel arrangement of elongated crystals makes it difficult for them to slip over each other if the wire is deflected at right angles to its length. The wire acquires a false 'temper'. For most orthodontic purposes a hard wire is desirable but if the wire becomes very work-hardened it becomes brittle and unsuitable for orthodontic use. The hardest workable wire is desirable for most purposes and especially for archwires for fixed appliances. Moreover working of the wire, as in the construction of clasps and springs, further increases its brittleness, and excessive bending, especially in correcting misplaced bends, should be avoided. The hardness of stainless steel causes severe wear of pliers, which are sometimes coated with tungsten carbide to increase their life.

3. If the wire is heated above the temperature of recrystallisation, about 800°C, the strained crystals are no longer present, the work-hardening disappears and the metal becomes soft. This is carried out between each drawing operation except the last. In the case of soft wire, such as ligature wire, heating is the final operation. If a piece of soft wire is required, it can be produced by heating a piece of hard wire to red heat, and allowing it to cool. This can be a disadvantage, and in welding or soldering stainless steel, care must be taken to minimise the effect of the inevitable softening which will occur locally when the metal is heated.

4. This softening of the wire only takes place if the wire is heated above 800°C. It is, however, possible to harden the wire without making it unreasonably brittle, by means of a low-temperature heat treatment at about 400° C for not more than 10 minutes. This can be done in an oven, or by passing an electric current through the wire from an attachment to an orthodontic welder. The latter method is less controllable. The effect of this heat treatment is usually described as 'stress relieving' but also has the effect of causing a precipitation of cementite (iron carbide, Fe_3C), which further hardens the steel.

5. Austenitic steel is essentially non-magnetic, but if a magnet is applied to a piece of hard wire the latter will be found to remain to some extent magnetic, due to this precipitation of iron carbide.

6. Fortunately stainless steel, like all ferrous metals, is a poor conductor of heat and electricity. This means that the heating of a length of wire to weld or solder attachments can, with care, be localised; it also means that it is possible to weld the wire electrically.

7. If stainless steel is heated excessively, the chromium combines with the carbon to form a carbide of chromium which is deposited on the faces of the crystals of the metal, weakening their structure and reducing the stainless properties. In fact this feature, although widely quoted, is not a practical problem. It is the reason for the very low carbon content and also for the presence of small quantities of titanium or niobium which preferentially combine with the carbon, without having the undesirable properties of chromium carbide.

Precious metal

This is the term usually applied to alloys of gold and platinum which were widely used in the past. In their definitive form they had a comparatively high proportion of platinum or palladium, and were silver in colour. They had some advantages relative to stainless steel: they could be heat-treated to harden them, so that heavy lingual or labial arches could be bent in the soft state and then hardened in an oven. As will be explained later, a gold wire will produce a gentler pressure, other things being equal, than similar stainless steel but will be more prone to permanent distortion. In physical properties, stainless steel is superior for archwires, although gold might have advantages in the simpler techniques. In recent years relative cost has made its use prohibitive, although it has a certain scrap value.

'Elgiloy'

This was originally developed by the Elgin Watch Company of America as a material for the mainspring of watches, being advertised under the slogan 'The heart that never breaks'. The Rocky Mountain Company have the sole rights to its use for orthodontic purposes and it has recently taken a new lease of life due to its being recommended by Dr Ricketts for use with his technique.

It is essentially an alloy of chromium and cobalt, its composition being declared as Co 40 per cent, Cr 20 per cent Ni 15 per cent Fe about 10 per cent, with small quantities of Mo, Mn, Be and C. It responds to heat treatment, so that an arch may be bent up 'soft' and then hardened by heating to 510° C, although the effect of this heating is not great. It is supplied in four degrees of hardness, colour-coded (in increasing hardness) blue, yellow, green and red.

When first introduced, it was possible to obtain a harder wire in Elgiloy than in stainless steel, without undue brittleness, but this is no longer true with later advances in stainless steel. Like stainless steel, Elgiloy becomes soft if heated above the temperature of recrystallisation, and cannot easily be re-hardened. If a short length is softened, as in welding or soldering, the wire immediately adjacent to the softened portion becomes extremely brittle. It is not, therefore, practicable to weld or solder the two hardest grades. Its only present advantage is its ability to be worked in a comparatively soft condition and then hardened by heat-treatment.

Titanium Alloys

Recently a number of alloys of titanium have been introduced for orthodontic purposes which have certain advantages and, inevitably, certain disadvantages. The first of these was 'Nitinol', which is an intermetallic compound of approximately equal quantities of nickel and titanium (Ni 52 per cent, Ti 45 per cent and Co 3 per cent. It was evolved by the (American) Naval Ordnance Laboratory, hence the name; NIckel TItanium NOL. It has been adapted for orthodontic use by Dr George Andreasen of the University of Iowa.

Its physical properties are strange. If the wire is bent and then heated above a critical temperature it will return to its original shape, and it was initially advertised as 'the wire with a memory'. Although some attempt has been made to modify the material to have this effect at mouth temperature, it is not at present of clinical importance. As will be described in the next section, some of its properties are very attractive, but unfortunately it becomes brittle and breaks if it is bent to any extent. It is sold as preformed arch wires, and further bends should be very gentle; it is not possible to bend in closing loops, stops, etc., nor to weld or solder it. Moreover, if the wire is bent, and then activated in the opposite direction, as in a tip-back bend in the Begg technique, its elastic recovery is not superior to stainless steel. It may be used as an initial aligning arch, but even in this form it is sometimes disappointing, as shown in Figure 7.1.

Titanium–molybdenum alloy (TMA) has been developed at the University of Connecticut under the guidance of Dr Charles Burstone. Pure titanium is in the form of close-packed hexagonal crystals and is unsuitable for use in orthodontics, having properties inferior to stainless steel. As with stainless steel, it changes its form if heated above a critical temperature, in this case 890° C, when the titanium takes up the 'beta' form, and this can be maintained at room temperature by the addition of stabilisers such as molybdenum. Its constitution is probably Ti 79 per cent, Mo 11 per cent, Zr 6 per cent and Sn 4 per cent. Its properties, both advantageous and disadvantageous, lie between those of stainless steel and Nitinol. It can be formed into loops and stops, although care should be used, bending it round the round beaks of pliers. It may be welded but not soldered.

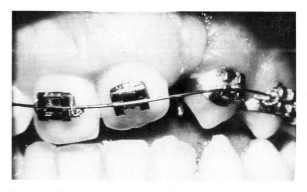

Fig. 7.1 Nitinol arch wire with permanent set 1 month after insertion to align /13. The tooth was later corrected with stainless steel wire.

Both the above alloys are the restrictive preserve of specific companies, and not surprisingly other companies have produced their own versions of titanium alloys. Basically these fall into one of the two types described. A recent development is Chinese NiTi wire, which was developed under the direction of Dr Tien Hua Cheng in Beijing, China. Its properties would seem to be somewhat superior to Nitinol in a number of respects. Doubtless there will be further developments of titanium- based wires in the near future.

PROPERTIES OF SPRING WIRE

The desirable properties of stainless steel or other wires used for construction of orthodontic springs are essentially the same whether the spring is a simple cantilever, such as is used to retract upper canines, or the most complicated archwire used in fully banded techniques.

Flexural rigidity (stiffness)

This property is dependent on two factors: Young's, modulus, which is an intrinsic property of the material used; and the (radius)^4 of the wire. Clearly a small increase in radius has a large effect in increasing flexural rigidity. It is a measure of the amount which a given length of wire would be deflected by a given load. Alternatively, it indicates the force which will be produced by a spring for a given deflection. It is usually considered desirable that the force should be as low as is reasonably possible, and also that the deflection to produce this force should be as great as possible, so that the spring remains active for a long period. It is therefore desirable that the flexural rigidity should be as low as possible.

A thin wire is desirable but clearly there is a limit. Gold has a low flexural rigidity; ordinary stainless steel has a lower value than high tensile stainless steel. Elgiloy is similar to high tensile steel. Nitinol has a very low value, so that a 0.018 inch (0.45 mm) Nitinol arch may be tied in much further than a similar SS arch, with the value for TMA lying about half-way between the two. Perhaps the lowest value is that for multistrand

wire, because of the narrow radius of the individual wires.

Elastic recovery (springback)

The basic principle on which all orthodontic springs work, whether they be cantilever springs on removable appliances or archwires, is essentially the same. The spring is deflected to the tooth and returns to its original position, carrying the tooth with it. In fact, it will never return completely to its original position but will bend to some extent. If soft wire were used, clearly it would adapt to the tooth and have no useful effect. For orthodontic springs, and especially for archwires, it is desirable that they should return as closely to their original position as possible. So far in this chapter this property has been referred to as 'hardness' of the wire, but a better term is 'elastic recovery' or 'springback'. An ideal wire, particularly for use with banded appliances, should have a high elastic recovery and low flexural rigidity. Unfortunately these are not mutually compatible.

Gold, although having a low flexural rigidity, has a low elastic recovery, even in the form of orthodontic alloys. Stainless steel has a moderate to good elastic recovery; the best heat-treated high tensile wires are very good. It is possible to draw stainless steel to a greater hardness without its becoming brittle if the wire is thin than if it is thick, and multistrand wire therefore has a high elastic recovery (and low flexural rigidity). Elgiloy, when heat-treated, is similar to the best stainless steel; certainly no better. Nitinol is excellent, with almost total recovery, although in this property, as in most, its behaviour is odd.

Length

The force which a spring applies to a tooth is a function, as has already been indicated, of the flexural rigidity; a light force is usually desirable. It is also a function of the length of the spring. In fact, it is proportional to the (length)^3, so that a small increase in length is almost as valuable as a small decrease in the thickness of the wire. In the case of cantilever springs, as used in removable appliances, this can be achieved by recurving the wire, as in a buccal canine retractor, and by the incorporation of coils in the spring. A coil in a cantilever spring has the obvious effect of lengthening the wire but it also has an intrinsic advantage apart from this, due to the increased work-hardening and stress set up in the wire, especially if it is deflected in the direction in which it is bent. A coil should therefore be opening in function, as is usually the case in a palatal canine retractor, as illustrated in Figures 7.2A and B, and the buccal retractor shown in Figure 7.2C is slightly less efficient.

In the case of archwires the length of the spring is represented by the distance between the brackets, and in this respect the narrow Begg bracket clearly has advantages over the wider edgewise bracket, especially the twin bracket. If a round wire of diameter 0.010 inch (0.25 mm) is deflected only 1 mm in order to tie it into the edgewise bracket, the force applied to the tooth will be over 1000 g. This force can be reduced by incorporating loops into the wire, as indicated in Figure 7.3A, producing the well-known 'swinging gate'. The vertical arms of the loops will increase the flexibility mesio-distally and labio-lingually. The (more or less) horizontal part of the loop, between

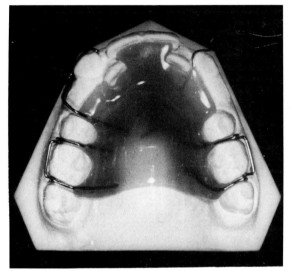

A

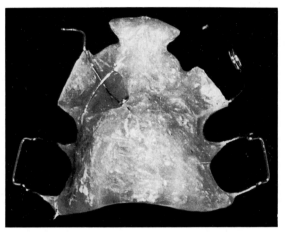

B

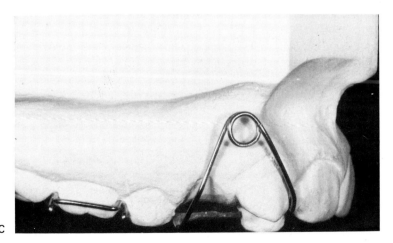

C

Fig. 7.2 Upper removable appliance to retract 3/3. A, Polished surface. B, Fitting surface. C, Buccal canine retractor on 3/.

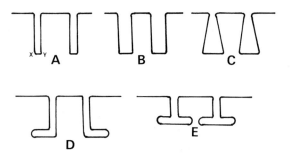

Fig. 7.3 Loops used on fixed appliance archwires. A, Standard vertical loops in 'swinging gate', B, Loops with wider horizontal section, C, Modification of B to maintain inter-bracket length. D, L-shaped or 'boot' loop. E, T-loops for depression of incisors.

X and Y in Figure 7.3A, undergoes torsion as the part between the loops is deflected into the bracket. Wire is resistant to torsion, so this horizontal part of the loop should be as long as possible, as illustrated in Figure 7.3B and C, even though this is not so neat as a narrower loop.

Vertical loops increase the flexibility of wire in the labio-lingual and mesio-distal directions, but have no effect in the vertical dimension. If, therefore, it is desired to depress or elevate a tooth or group of teeth, then the loop must have a horizontal component, as illustrated in Figure 7.3D and E.

Formability

It is obviously desirable that the wire may be formed into the required arch shape and that it may have loops, stops and other accessories bent into it. For removable appliances it must be possible to bend springs, clasps, etc., without fracture. This property is in some respects the converse of elastic recovery.

Gold is very formable, especially as it can be heat-treated after forming. It is easy to bend and does not easily fracture. The same is true of Elgiloy, at least in the softer grades, although the effect of heat treatment is relatively mild. Ordinary hard-drawn stainless steel (as used in removable appliances) is fairly difficult to bend and work-hardens readily, so that care is necessary in bending, for example, the arrow-head of an Adams clasp. High tensile stainless steel, being thinner, is reasonably easy to form but the hardest

grades are liable to fracture where bends are acute, as in tie-back stops and some loops. It is better to avoid sharp bends, by bending around the round beak of pliers, and to bend slowly. The same is even more true with TMA, which can be bent, with care. Nitinol cannot accept more than the mildest bends and is usually purchased as preformed archwires which require little modification. It is not possible to bend stops or loops into multistrand wire, which is used only for initial alignment.

The more formable the wire, and consequently the lower the elastic recovery, the more likely it is to be distorted, accidentally or otherwise, in the mouth.

Cost

This a property which should not be overlooked! Gold is very expensive, although it has a scrap value. Stainless steel is comparatively inexpensive if purchased in spools of 25 feet (7.6 m). TMA and Nitinol are costly, especially as they are usually provided as preformed archwires: stainless steel is costly in this form; about half the cost of titanium alloys.

WELDING

In the process of welding, two pieces of a similar metal are brought together under pressure and heat is applied. The simplest form is that used by the blacksmith, with his anvil. Under these conditions recrystallisation of the metal occurs across the join and the two pieces unite. The metal does not melt for this to occur.

In orthodontic practice the heat is produced electrically, taking advantage of the poor conductivity of all ferrous metals. The two pieces of stainless steel are brought together under pressure and an electric current passed through them. If the current is large enough, heat is produced. This has three effects:

1. The metals are welded together.

2. The work-hardening is destroyed and a short length of the wire becomes soft.

3. If the heat is applied for sufficient time 'weld decay', due to the production of chromium

carbide, will weaken the joint. As indicated above, this is largely of academic interest.

To reduce the softening of the wire, the time during which the current passes should be kept to a minimum; not more than one-hundredth of a second. If insufficient heat is produced to make the desired weld, the current and not the time should be increased.

An electric welder therefore consists of three parts:

1. A transformer. This produces a very large current at low voltage; usually about 6 volts. A high voltage has no advantage and obvious disadvantages. The current available should be 400 to 1 000 amperes.

2. A time switch. The earlier welders had a mechanical switch but these were not very consistent. Modern welders rely on the discharge from a capacitor or use electronic timing. The latter is used in all welders of British manufacture.

3. Electrodes, which should be clean and of suitable shape. Dirt between the electrode and the metal to be welded gives rise to resistance and therefore to additional heat. This serves no useful purpose but helps to produce the undesirable side-effects. The electrodes should contact the metal over the greatest possible area, in order to minimise resistance at this point — this involves using grooved electrodes when welding wire and flat electrodes for bands, brackets, etc. Finally, the electrode should be as bulky as possible, so that the heat will be conducted away from the join when the weld is complete. This may have to be sacrificed to some extent for convenience of electrode shape.

The electric current from the mains passes through a suitable time switch into a transformer. This reduces the voltage to 6 volts. If it is desired to have 400 amps available, this will take only 10 amps from a 240 volt socket, well within its capacity. Conductors from the transformer to the electrodes should be thick and of low resistance. The electrodes are brought together under pressure — at least 10 1b/sq. in. — either by a foot or hand control, and the current is then discharged, often by a further pressure on the control.

The softer and thicker grades of Elgiloy may be welded. Gold is too good a conductor to be welded satisfactorily and Nitinol cannot be welded. TMA may be welded.

SOLDERING

To construct a soldered joint, two pieces of metal are heated and the molten solder allowed to flow between them. To make a satisfactory joint the molten solder must 'wet' the metal, and for this to occur the metal must be absolutely clean of impurities, including oxides. The exact nature of a soldered joint is not clear; there is some physical union but there is also probably an atomic interchange between the solder and the metal to be soldered, and even possibly some recrystallsation across the boundary. There is not normally any appreciable alloying between solder and metal, and where this occurs (in soldering gold, for example) the joint is weakened. Contrary to earlier belief, stainless steel can be soldered quite normally, and such a joint is no different from any good soldered joint.

The first requirement in a soldered joint is cleanliness, and this presents a special problem with stainless steel because of the oxide layer which ensures its stainless properties. To penetrate this special fluxes are required containing a fluoride. A typical formula would consist of 50 per cent potassium fluoride, 30 per cent boric acid and small quantities of borax, silica and sodium carbonate. These fuse and form a bead of glass around the area to be soldered, isolating it from the air, while the fluoride content removes the oxide layer, allowing the molten solder to wet the surface.

The second problem again arises from the nature of stainless steel: its tendency to soften if heated above the recrystallization temperature. This can be minimised by using a low-fusing silver solder and by applying heat very locally to the area to be joined. A small, hot, reducing flame from a suitable blow-lamp should be used and the work quenched in cold water immediately after the solder 'flows'. Although the temperature should be kept to a minimum, more joints probably fail from too little than from too much heat. The work must glow cherry red but for as short a time and over as short a distance as possible.

Softening may be minimised by careful technique. If a spring is to be soldered to a 1 mm lingual arch, the arch is 'tinned' with a bead of solder, while the spring wire is only fluxed. The solder is melted, the spring brought into the molten solder and the joint withdrawn from the flame as soon as the molten solder flows on to the spring. Similarly, if a hook is to be soldered on to an archwire, the solder is first applied to the wire which is to form the hook, which is already soft, to keep heating of the spring archwire to a minimum. In both cases the spring wire receives less heat.

Frequently, as in the last case, it is desired to solder an attachment such as a hook to an archwire. For this electric soldering is to be preferred. This again takes advantage of the high resistance of steel. Electrodes are applied to each of the pieces of metal to be joined, close to the joint, so that a high current of low voltage flows, heating the metal sufficiently to melt the solder which has been added to the fluxed joint. Such a soldering machine is often an accessory to a welder, using many of the same components but eliminating the time switch. Since the procedure would require three hands, one of the pieces of metal is clamped in a vice which forms one electrode, while the second electrode is made of carbon, so that it does not itself become soldered to the joint. Hooks are usually made of brass wire, and electrodes of this metal, already tipped with solder, are commercially available, the electrode then being fashioned into a hook.

In addition to stainless steel, gold and Elgiloy (softer grades) may be soldered. Nitinol and TMA and other titanium alloys cannot be soldered.

FIXED APPLIANCES

The purpose of this section is to outline the basic principles underlying the use of fully banded (or bonded) appliances, in the hope that the reader will appreciate that these basic principles underlie the mode of action of even the most exotic appliance.

The history of banded appliances is usually traced back to the expansion arch of Dr E. H. Angle, shown in Figure 7.4, although he himself

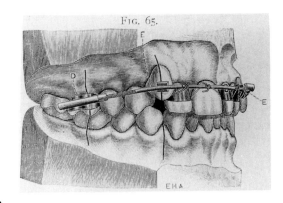

A

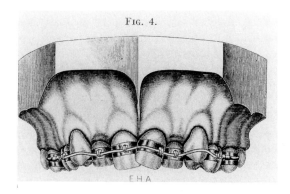

B

Fig. 7.4 Angle's appliances. A, The expansion arch. B, The ribbon arch.

traced its origins back at least as far as Pierre Fauchard in the early eighteenth century. The expansion arch consisted of a solid archwire passing through tubes on molar bands which were clamped to the first molars. Irregular teeth were then drawn on to this archwire by means of ligatures passing round the teeth and twisted tightly round the archwire. Various materials were used for ligatures, and Angle was probably the first to use metal, in the form of brass wire. This is basically the principle of all banded appliances, so far as tooth alignment is concerned. Dr Angle soon realised that the ligatures tied around the teeth were not satisfactory, and realised the need for a bracket in which to engage his fairly flexible German silver wire. His first design was the pin and tube appliance, but even Angle came to realise that few orthodontists had the necessary technical skill to use this demanding appliance. He therefore developed the ribbon arch appliance (Fig. 7.4B) which used a slotted bracket in which the wire could be held by means of a pin. Use of this bracket was taught by Dr Angle to Dr P. R. Begg who adapted it for use in his well-known technique, mainly by turning it upside-down. Angle's wire was no longer round but rectangular in cross-section and this fitted into the slot in his bracket with the longer dimension of the ribbon wire parallel to the long axis of the tooth. In American parlance it went into the bracket 'flat-wise'. This gave some control over bucco-lingual tilting, by means of torque forces transmitted in the wire. It did not completely satisfy Angle because of its lack of control over mesio-distal tilting, and in 1929 he introduced his definitive appliance with touching modesty as 'the latest and best in orthodontic mechanism'. This involved a new bracket into which the rectangular wire was inserted with its short dimension parallel to the long axis of the tooth; that is, it went in 'edgewise'. This edgewise appliance is the basis of the vast majority of fully banded appliances in use in the world today.

Its principal components are an archwire to bring about movement of the teeth and a series of brackets to bring it into close contact with the teeth. The latter may be welded to stainless steel bands around the teeth, or may be bonded directly on to the teeth themselves.

The original edgewise bracket was comparatively narrow mesio-distally, and had a slot 0.022 inch wide and 0.028 inch deep (0.55×0.7 mm). This controlled the tooth well for all required movements except for rotation, and for this purpose small eyelets were soldered mesially and distally to the bracket which could be ligated to the archwire. These were far from satisfactory and very liable to come off the band, apart from the initial difficulty in soldering them in place. Several attempts have been made to overcome this shortcoming, of which the most widely used nowadays is the Siamese twin bracket. Here two brackets are mounted side by side on the base, giving excellent control in all possible dimensions. Indeed, perhaps the edgewise bracket gives too much control. This was certainly the opinion of Dr Begg, who reverted to the ribbon arch bracket, which effectively attaches the tooth to the wire at

a single point. This allows the tooth to tilt freely, which makes for ease of tooth movement and for limited strain on the anchorage. On the other hand, problems arise when accurate control is required, and it becomes necessary to use additional auxiliary wires and springs, making for a very complicated and somewhat unhygienic arrangement in the later stages of treatment.

The second problem with the original bracket arises from the size of the slot. Angle originally used German silver wire, but by the time he designed the edgewise appliance he was using gold alloys which have a flexural rigidity considerably below that of stainless steel. To tie in a stainless steel wire 0.022×0.028 inch (0.55×0.7 mm) into a bracket of the same size would produce a quite unacceptable force, and a second type of bracket, with a slot measuring 0.018×0.025 inch (0.45×0.625 mm) has been introduced. Both brackets are widely used, with the older type in fact used by a slight majority of orthodontists, at least in North America. The larger bracket is used with wires which do not by any means fill it, and this allows for some degree of latitude in less skilled hands. It also offers less resistance to the mesio-distal movement of teeth along the archwire. On the other hand, with the smaller bracket it is possible to 'fill the bracket' at an earlier stage in treatment, thus giving better control throughout tooth movement. Both brackets are satisfactory, and the choice is a matter for the individual.

Bucco-lingual tooth movement

Bucco-lingual tooth movements are brought about in the bucco-lingual or labio-lingual direction in the alignment of displaced teeth. They were the only movements possible with the original expansion arch. It might seem that ideally one should select a wire with very low flexural rigidity and very high elastic recovery (which nevertheless was formable) and bend it into a simple arch shape. This could then be tied into all the brackets of the arch, displaced or otherwise, and would bring them back on to the ideal arch form. Even if such a wire existed it would not be quite this simple. The buccal surfaces of teeth, and therefore the bases of the brackets, do not lie on a simple curve. Lateral incisors are somewhat thinner labio-lingually than central incisors or canines, while premolars similarly do not project as far buccally as molars. For this reason bends or 'offsets' are necessary in even an ideal archwire if it is to fit into the brackets of an ideal dental arch without distortion. This is largely overcome in the straight wire edgewise technique, where the bases of the brackets are of varying thickness to compensate for the variation in the labial or buccal surface of the appropriate teeth.

An ideal wire does not exist. For tooth alignment maximum flexibility between the brackets is desirable, and the Siamese twin bracket, while excellent in other respects, has undesirable features in this context, since the distance between brackets is correspondingly reduced. The Begg bracket, on the other hand, maximises this distance. This problem can to some extent be overcome by a choice of wires. The original multistrand wire had three fine wires twisted together, but this has been developed further with a larger number of even finer wires, either twisted or braided together.

As already indicated, multistrand wire has low flexural rigidity and high elastic recovery. There are two reasons for this. It is possible to draw a fine wire to a greater degree of hardness without its becoming brittle, thus giving greater elastic recovery. Also, since flexural rigidity is proportional to the fourth power of its radius, each of, say, three fine wires will have a very low flexural rigidity. The total rigidity of the combined three strands will be only three times that of the fine components; much lower than a solid wire of comparable diameter. Some operators prefer to use a very fine single strand of 0.010 inch (0.25 mm), but this has a very inaccurate fit in the bracket, with limited control, and is liable to damage and distortion in the mouth. On the other hand, a multistrand wire of 0.018 inch (0.45 mm) will completely fill the bracket of the same size, giving good control. Because of its high elastic recovery it is not possible to form a multistrand wire into an arch. For tooth alignment a straight wire is therefore usually tied into the brackets, and while in theory this would cause expansion of the buccal segments of teeth, in practice I have never seen this happen, since such a wire is left in place for a comparatively short time.

This need for a wire of low flexural rigidity and high elastic recovery can be achieved to some extent by the use of titanium-based wire, discussed in the previous section, and again these have the advantage that the bracket can be filled at an early stage of treatment. Where teeth are markedly displaced and stainless steel wire is used, its flexibility may be increased by the incorporation of loops, as described in the previous section and illustrated in Figures 7.3 and 7.5. Multiple loops tend to become distorted in the mouth and to cause ulceration to the gingivae or the inner surface of the lip. Loops should therefore be used sparingly. A single loop, as indicated in Figure 7.6A. may be used for alignment of a rotated tooth or for mesial or distal movement of the tooth, but very often it is preferable to use two loops, this and the intervening length of wire being termed a 'swinging gate', acting much as a flapper spring on a removable appliance (Figs 7.3A–C and 7.5A). More elaborate loops, which control the tooth in several dimensions, are the box loop and cross-over loop, shown in Figure 7.5B and C.

Mesio-distal tooth movement

It is sometimes necessary to move teeth mesially or, more often, distally, as for example in retracting a canine following the extraction of a first premolar. This may be done in one of two ways. A vertical loop may be placed between the canine and first premolar, using a sectional arch. The simplest form is shown in Figure 7.5D, and diagrammatically in Figure 7.6A, and is often referred to as a Bull loop, after its inventor Harry Bull. It is somewhat inflexible and the extreme tip of the loop tends to work-harden, and therefore to break. To overcome this the tip of the loop may be widened in the 'teardrop' loop in Figure 7.6B. The reverse loop shown in Figure 7.6C lengthens the wire considerably, and also has the advantage that the loop acts in the more efficient opening direction. Other variants of the loop are shown in Figure 7.6D and E.

Any flexible wire will tend to bend during this type of activation, and retraction of the tooth will therefore be to a large extent by tilting. The more flexible the loop, the greater the tilting. This is not

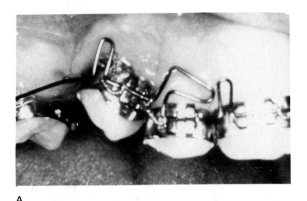

A

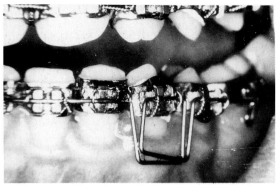

B

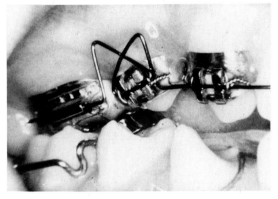

C

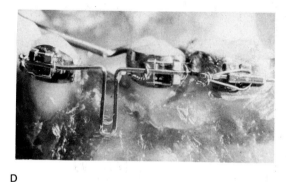

D

Fig. 7.5 Fixed appliance loops. A, Swinging gate with L-loop. B, Box loop. C, Cross-over loop. D, 'Bull' loop.

always desirable and can be controlled to some extent by 'tipping forward' the anterior end of the arch wire, so that, in theory, the tooth will be tipped mesially by the tilt in the anterior end of the wire, while being retracted distally, resulting in bodily distal movement.

Any of these loops may be used to retract the labial segment of teeth in order to reduce an overjet. In this case one would be placed on each side of the mouth, usually between the lateral

Fig. 7.6 A, 'Bull' loop. B, 'Tear-drop' loop. C, Reverse loop. D and E, Other modifications.

incisor and canine. Retraction loops should be placed as close as possible to the teeth to be moved, to allow the maximum amount of overall activation.

An alternative method of moving teeth distally is to slide the bracket along the archwire. This is sometimes referred to by the American term 'sliding mechanics'. The motive power is usually supplied by elastic chains between the brackets on either side of the space, that on the distal side being tied back to a number of more posterior teeth to increase the anchorage. Latex rubber bands may serve the same purpose from a hook on the archwire to the molar band. Alternatively, a coil spring anterior to the bracket may be used, and this compressed spring will provide a force on the tooth, but elastomeric chains have virtually made both this technique, and the coil-spring

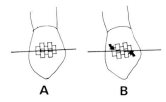

Fig. 7.7 A, Bracket before retraction to right side. B, As the tooth tilts, the archwire binds on the bracket as indicated.

pulling from the distal, obsolete. As the tooth slides along the archwire it will tend to tilt and become jammed across the bracket, as shown in Figure 7.7. To minimise this, an arch should be used which does not completely fill the bracket, and for this purpose the 0.022 inch (0.55 mm) bracket has some advantages, although with some inevitable loss of control.

Either of these methods of moving a tooth mesio-distally will tend to tilt the tooth considerably. Again, this may be minimised by appropriate bends in the main archwire. Bends of this type are sometimes called 'second- order bends'. (First-order bends are those in the bucco- lingual direction, although the latter term is seldom used.) To avoid the necessity for these bends, the brackets may be attached to the teeth at a slight angle, so that a straight wire has the effect of tipping the tooth in the appropriate direction. In the case of the straight wire appliance this tip is built into the bracket, since the slot is not quite at right angles to the long axis of the tooth.

Vertical tooth movement

Intrusion or extrusion of teeth may be achieved by placing the archwire so that it lies occlusal or gingival to the bracket on the tooth to be moved, and then displacing the wire into the bracket. This would, however, produce an unacceptably heavy force if the movement required was other than minimal. Here again, loops can be used to reduce the force, while allowing a reasonable range of activation. As explained previously, a loop does not increase flexibility if the activating force is along the long axis of the loop. For vertical movement, therefore, the loop should have a horizontal component. Examples of this are shown in the L-shaped loop between 2/ and 3/ in Figure 7.5A, and

also in the box loop and crossover loop in Figure 7.5B and C.

It is frequently desirable to depress, and occasionally to elevate, a group of teeth. The most common example is the 'depression' of lower incisors in order to reduce an overbite. The simplest form is illustrated in Figure 7.8A. The vertical loop does not increase the flexibility of the wire vertically, but serves another purpose. Both lower and upper incisors are usually proclined relative to the occlusal plane and therefore relative

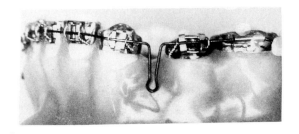

A

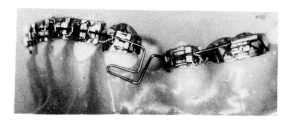

B

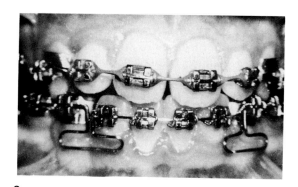

C

Fig. 7.8 Appliances to depress lower incisors. A, depends on a reverse Curve of Spee in the archwire; the loop prevents proclination of incisors. B, with a 'boot' loop, the additional wire assists depression. C, The T-loop, with rectangular wire, ensures a long-lasting gentle force while controlling the angulation of the incisors.

to the archwire. If a downwards force is placed on the brackets of the incisors, it will procline them, and the closing loop in Figure 7.8A, by exerting a gentle lingual force, prevents this proclination, albeit in a rather hit-and-miss fashion.

If greater flexibility is required in depression of these teeth, the L-shaped loop shown in Figure 7.8B may be used. This type of loop is sometimes called a 'boot' loop. A more satisfactory loop is the T-loop shown at the end of this stage of treatment in Figure 7.8C. This clearly has great flexibility, and is neat and atraumatic. It is constructed in rectangular wire, which controls the labio-lingual tilting of the teeth, and enables them to be depressed down the 'corridor' of cancellous bone.

Apical tooth movement

A force may be transmitted along a rod-shaped piece of metal by twisting one end of the rod. Such a force may be used in an orthodontic wire. The wire is adjusted relative to the bracket as shown in Figure 7.9A, so that it has to be twisted in order to insert it into the bracket, as shown in Figure 7.9B. This introduces a force into the wire which in this case would have the effect of tilting the incisor tooth, so as to move the apex palatally and the incisal edge labially. In practice the latter movement is prevented by the closing loops between lateral incisors and canines, and this type of adjustment is widely used in reducing overjets or in correcting the angulation of incisors in the Class II Division 2 type of incisal relation. A similar force may be used in a round wire if some feature is introduced to prevent the wire from rotating in the bracket, of which the best known is the spurs used with the Begg technique. The

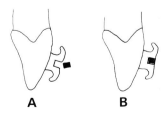

A   **B**

Fig. 7.9 Passive rectangular wire, when inserted in slot of edgewise bracket B, produces active torque force to move apices palatally.

nature of the force is the origin of such phrases as 'torquing the incisor teeth'.

The following features should be borne in mind when using torque forces to move upper incisors palatally.

1. Force on the tooth is produced by the third order of levers, and quite a strong force is necessary within the bracket in order to produce the minimal force at the apex of the tooth which will bring about its movement.

2. It is usual to employ a rectangular wire, somewhat smaller than the internal dimensions of the bracket. The wire will therefore rotate to some extent before having any effect on the bracket. This is more than would appear since the corners of rectangular wire are usually rounded.

3. The effect of a torque force on the incisor teeth, together with a palatal force from closing loops, tends to bring the incisal apices together, causing the incisors to tilt distally like the spokes of a cartwheel. This may be prevented by suitable bends in the wire, or more easily by offsetting the position of the brackets slightly.

4. The torque effect can be produced by altering the direction of the slot within the bracket, rather than by bending the wire. Similarly the cart-wheeling effect can be prevented by suitable mesio-distal tilting of the slot within the bracket. Both these features are built into modern brackets in the straight wire techniques.

Torque forces have many uses in fixed appliance techniques, by no means confined to the edgewise appliance. With the latter it is usually necessary to incorporate a torque force in the opposite direction, that is buccal root torque, on the posterior teeth, to maintain them in good position. A standard type of edgewise bracket lies parallel to the buccal surface of the tooth. The buccal surfaces of the premolars slope towards their occlusal surfaces, and the molars do so even more, so that a progressive twist is necessary in the wire to accommodate this. This necessity is again eliminated in straight wire appliances, where the brackets are constructed to take account of this fact.

In the case of the incisors the whole of the torque force lies in the short distance between the brackets on the anterior teeth, and this is one of the shortcomings of the appliance. This force may be reduced to some extent by the inclusion of loops between the lateral incisor and canine teeth. With the Begg appliance force is applied over a much greater length of wire in the so-called torquing auxiliary. Although orthodontists speak cheerfully of torquing upper apices palatally, this is more difficult than might appear, and in many cases the fact of merely maintaining the apex in its original position, while the crown is moved palatally, is sufficient to produce a good result. It should be borne in mind that for practical purposes the roots of the teeth may only be moved within the alveolar bone which is present at the beginning of treatment, as described in Chapter 10.

Anchorage

Newton's Third Law states that 'To every action there is an equal and opposite reaction'. Nowhere is this more true than in orthodontic treatment, and especially in the use of fixed appliances. Very occasionally it may be possible to move teeth adjacent to a space reciprocally, but usually it is desired to move those on one side of the space without moving those on the other side to the same extent. An obvious example is the retraction of anterior teeth, using the posterior teeth as anchorage, although the opposite does sometimes apply in the closure of extraction spaces. There is no such thing as stationary anchorage within an arch, although movement of anchor teeth can be substantially reduced by a number of methods.

One such method is to adjust the appliance so that the anchor teeth may only move bodily, which requires a much greater force, while the teeth to be moved are allowed to tip. In the Begg technique the ends of the archwire are tipped back, which would have the effect of tipping the molar teeth distally. At the same time an elastic force is tending to move them mesially, the combination of two forces resulting in bodily movement. On the other hand, the incisor teeth are moved palatally by pure tilting, and anchorage is thus considerably reinforced. The same effect may be produced with the edgewise appliance by means of second-order bends, and this was taken to extreme limits by Tweed, who had such a bend

on each of the posterior teeth. A similar effect can be produced where it is desired to bring forward the posterior teeth to close spaces, by putting lingual root torque into the wire where it affects the anterior teeth, so that these may only be moved bodily. In both of these cases the reciprocal effect, in the first case of depressing the anterior teeth and in the second of moving them lingually, is a usually desirable one.

A second method of reinforcing the anchorage takes advantage of the fact that mesial movement of the posterior teeth is not directly anterior but is anterior and medial. If, therefore, the intermolar width is maintained, as by a lingual or palatal arch, as these teeth come forwards they will come into contact with the outer plate of bone which will again reduce the anchorage loss. The same effect is produced by Ricketts in the bioprogressive technique, where his heavy utility arch is deliberately adjusted to bring the apices of the molars into contact with the buccal plate of bone.

Both these methods will reduce anchorage loss but will not eliminate it altogether. In many cases, therefore, it is necessary to reinforce it from outside the dental arch. Intermaxillary elastics from the lower arch will reinforce the anchorage to some extent in the upper arch but will, of course, have an effect on the former. It is therefore used comparatively little except in the Begg technique where it has the additional advantage of preventing undue distal tilting of the lower molars. The alternative is to use extra-oral anchorage, usually by means of a heavy Kloehn bow to a second tube on the upper molar bands, although anchorage may be added to the archwire itself, with so-called J-hooks attaching to a suitable loop or hook in the anterior region. This need for extra-oral anchorage in the edgewise technique is again one of its shortcomings, since it requires substantial cooperation from the patient. However, few types of orthodontic treatment will succeed without the patient's cooperation.

A variety of different types of cervical or occipital headgear is available from which force may be applied. It has been suggested by Merrifield and Cross that cervical traction has the effect of producing anterior open bites. This effect has undoubtedly been grossly exaggerated but a low-pull type of headgear should be avoided in patients who have a tendency to reduced overbite with an increased lower facial height. Alternatively the low-pull may be combined with a second elastic to a high headcap, so-called combination or 'combi' headgear, and this has the advantage of spreading the load on to two parts of the patient's head, which appears to be rather more comfortable.

REMOVABLE APPLIANCES

This section will deal only with active removable appliances, where teeth are moved by direct forces from springs or screws. The more passive types of appliance, usually called functional appliances in Europe but removable appliances in North America, are the subject of the next section.

Every orthodontic appliance inserted should be designed by the orthodontist who will use it, and some thought should be given to the design of even the most routine case. The appliance should usually be worn for all or most of the time. While cooperation of the wearer is essential, this will only be achieved if the design is such that the patient may reasonably be expected to tolerate it.

Fixation

This is the term which describes the parts of the appliance which hold it in the mouth; for the most part clasps. Alternative terms are 'retention' and 'anchorage', but both of these words have other meanings in an orthodontic context. The modified arrowhead clasp of Adams is so satisfactory that it has superseded other types, except for upper incisors. It is illustrated in Figure 7.10A, and is not always well made. The arrowheads should impinge on the tooth in the mildly undercut areas on the mesio-buccal and disto-buccal corners of the tooth. Seel has shown that an undercut of 1 mm is ideal. If the bridge is too short, as is often the case, the clasp will meet the tooth on its sloping buccal surface, where there is no undercut. Another common fault concerns the angulation of the arrowheads. The two arrowheads may be tilted slightly towards each other, but in the vertical dimensio they should be parallel to the occlusal plane, or inclined at not more than 30° thereto. One often sees clasps on which the arrowheads are almost vertical. This not only reduces

their grip on the tooth, but shortens the curved region where the wire passes over the contact point, and thus reduces the 'springiness' of the clasp. If the tooth is incompletely erupted in a young child, a little of the plaster gum may be removed on the model, so that the arrowhead lies close to the gingival crevice in the mouth, but the plaster tooth should not be trimmed. Where the crown of the tooth is long, as in an adult, the arrowhead may lie above the gingival margin, since the undercut may be too great at the gingival level for the plate to be inserted. While it is not normally necessary to survey the tooth to be clasped, this may be done by eye to some extent.

Almost any tooth may be clasped with an Adams clasp; an excellent clasp may be fitted on the canine, as in Figure 7.11A, if made in 0.6 mm wire, rather than the more usual 0.7 mm. An Adams clasp can be constructed for the incisor teeth, clasping the two central incisors as if they were a single tooth, but a neater and more efficient device is the 'Southend' clasp shown in

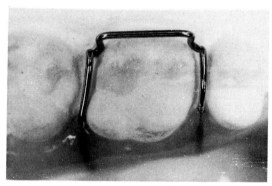

A

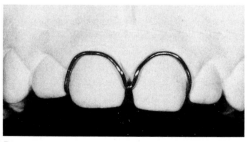

B

Fig. 7.10 A, The Adams modified arrowhead clasp. B, The Southend clasp.

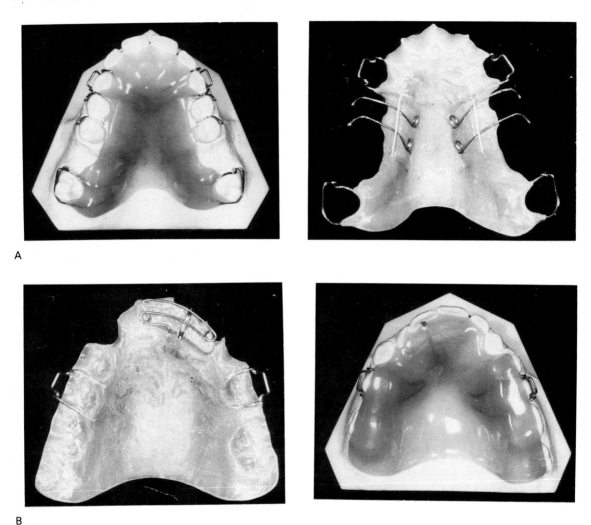

Fig. 7.11 A, Appliance to retract 54/45 following extraction of 6/6, with clasps on 73/37. B, Appliance to procline 21/1, with clasps on 4/4.

Figure 7.10B, designed by Di Biase and Leavis, and described by Stephens (1979). This should have a single arrowhead between the central incisors, and the wire then follows the gingival margins of the teeth. Its construction is not easy.

In many cases the first molar is the tooth of choice to clasp, as in Figure 7.2 for retraction of upper canines. This is not always the case. A spring to procline one or more incisor teeth will have an upward component, which will tend to displace the appliance downwards. The clasps should therefore be placed more anteriorly, on the first or second premolars, as in Figure 7.11B, or on the second deciduous molar in the mixed dentition. In the case illustrated in Figure 7.11A, where the first molars have been extracted, clasps on the second molars alone will be insufficient to hold up the appliance, and teeth further forward, premolars, incisors or, as here, canines should be clasped. Additional clasps are also necessary if the appliance is likely to be displaced by extra-oral forces, as in Figure 7.15, or orthodontic screws, as in Fig. 7.14.

The Base

This part of the appliance is normally made of acrylic resin. It is not uncommon to be asked to advise on a case in which treatment is not going well, partly due to insufficient wear of the appliance. On examination one finds an appliance so bulky that it is surprising it is worn at all. The purpose of the base is to hold together all the active components, and the acrylic should be as thin as possible for this purpose. The thickness of a sheet of pink wax is sufficient, and this may quite reasonably form ridges over the insertions of wire-work. It should not interfere with the occlusion unless it is intended to do so. If an anterior bite plane is required to reduce the over-bite, it should only be high enough to take the posterior teeth 2–3 mm out of occlusion. If necessary it may be increased later by the addition of cold-curing acrylic. The bite plane should extend lingually sufficiently to prevent the lower incisors from biting posterior to it, but no further.

If it is necessary to 'gag' the bite, by means of blocks over the posterior teeth (Fig. 7.11B), as is sometimes the case when one or a small number of teeth are locked inside the bite, then these bite-blocks should be trimmed until only just high enough to eliminate the overbite on the affected teeth. It is surprising how thin a layer of acrylic is required, and frequently trimming will produce holes in parts of the bite-blocks.

Finally, the acrylic base should be finished closely around the necks of the teeth, again being kept as thin as possible. This type of finish is sometimes called 'gum-stripping' in a partial denture, but this feature does not arise in a well-fitting appliance. It should be trimmed well clear of teeth which it is intended to move, unlike the situation illustrated in Figure 7.11A!

Springs

The springs on removable appliances are virtually all variants of the cantilever principle. In its simplest form, as in Figure 7.12A, this consists of a straight piece of wire embedded in the acrylic base-plate, the other end being deflected and placed in contact with the tooth. This is then moved as the spring returns to its passive position. The force applied to the tooth should be the smallest which will move the tooth; excessive force produces little but pain for the wearer. For a tipping action on a single rooted tooth, a force

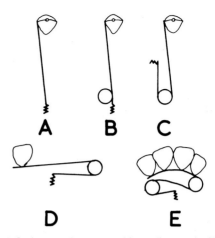

Fig. 7.12 Springs used on removable appliances. A, Simple cantilever, B, Cantilever with loop. C and D, Recurved cantilever. E, Doubly recurved cantilever.

equivalent to 30–50 g is ideal. It is also desirable that the force should be long-lasting, and nearly as great at the end of the period of wear as at the beginning.

Ideally this gentle force should, as indicated earlier in this chapter, be produced by a long thin spring. There is limited room for a spring in the mouth, but this may be overcome in a number of ways. A loop may be inserted within the wire, as illustrated in Figures 7.12B and 7.11A. This not only lengthens the spring but marginally increases its efficiency by virtue of the loop. The springs shown in Figures 7.2B and 7.11A, which uncoil in action, are again slightly more efficient than the type shown in Figure 7.2C, where the coil closes in action.

The spring may be further lengthened by recurving it, as in Figures 7.2C and 7.12C and D. If the spring is doubly recurved, as in Figures 7.11B and 7.12E, a number of teeth may be proclined in virtually parallel movement. This is also true in the trebly recurved Coffin spring in Figure 7.15A.

As already indicated, the majority of orthodontic springs are of the cantilever type. The Roberts retractor in Figure 7.13 is essentially two cantilever springs with loops, joined by a horizontal bar. A little thought will enable one to identify the cantilever principle in most springs used in both removable and fixed appliances.

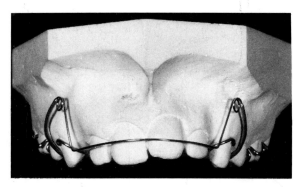

Fig. 7.13 The Roberts retractor.

Screw appliances

Screw appliances have a long history in the United Kingdom and underwent a new popularity in the period after the Second World War, when the ideas of Martin Schwarz were introduced by Dr W. Grossmann. A wide range of screws is available, many of which were reviewed some years ago by Haynes and Jackson (1963). They carry a central threaded rod, with a right-hand thread at one end and a left-hand thread at the other. This is housed in the two metal ends, which are embedded in the acrylic base, so that as the screw is turned the two ends move apart. In addition there are one or two guide rails, consisting of a plain rod sliding in a tube, which maintain rigidity and prevent the two housings from rotating relative to each other. The device is suitably positioned in the base-plate, and this is then cut at right angles to the direction of activation of the screw. The patient is given a key with which he can turn the screw, usually one quarter-turn per week. This is best done on a Saturday or Sunday, being days which are easily remembered.

Each quarter-turn moves the two parts of the plate apart by about 0.2 mm. When the appliance is inserted it compresses the periodontal membrane on each side of the screw to about half its width, and the teeth then move until the width of the membrane is restored.

Figure 7.14 shows some uses of the screw mechanism. In my hands it is most frequently used to reopen the space for a mildly impacted second premolar, as illustrated in Figure 7.14A and B, and for this purpose it is very satisfactory. Indeed it is one of the few removable appliances to be well

tolerated in the mandibular arch. It may similarly be used to move upper molars distally, especially if the condition is unilateral, although for this purpose it is rather slow, and usually requires extra-oral support. It may also be used in the midline, as illustrated in Figure 7.14C, for bilateral expansion. Figure 7.14D shows it used for the proclination of two incisors, and a similar arrangement may be used to move premolars buccally. The disadvantage of these latter cases is that the screw must be parallel to the occlusal plane, and the appliance therefore becomes rather bulky. The appliances illustrated in Figure 7.14 all employ the Glenross screw, but more modern screws, sadly of foreign manufacture, have the advantage of being less bulky and having a greater range of action.

Anchorage

Although removable appliances are less subject to anchorage loss than fully-banded fixed ones, if a spring or screw applies a force to a tooth or group of teeth, these apply an equal and opposite force to the spring or screw and therefore to the appliance as a whole. This is quite inescapable. It will be transmitted by the plate to the tissues to which the appliance is anchored. For example, in the case shown in Figure 7.2 for the retraction of upper canines, the reaction from the activation of the springs will be transmitted to the first molars, tending to bring them forward — usually the last thing one wants. If the acrylic fits accurately around the remaining teeth, the force will be transmitted to the second premolars, the incisors and the vault of the palate. Moreover, since the intermolar width is maintained, this will increase anchorage, in the same way as has already been described for a lingual arch, but even more efficiently. If a gentle force is used for tooth movement this force, distributed among all these factors, may well be dissipated without loss of anchorage.

Extra-oral traction

Anchorage may, where necessary, be augmented by intermaxillary or extra-oral traction, although the former is seldom used with removable

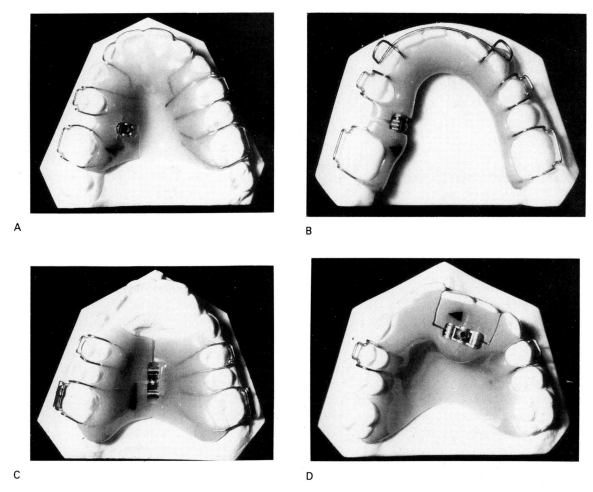

A

B

C

D

Fig. 7.14 Screw appliances. A, Upper appliance for distal movement of molars. B, Similar lower appliance. C, Appliance for mid-line expansion, with tubes for extra-oral traction. D, For proclination of /12.

appliances. Extra-oral traction may be used either as the motive force in moving blocks of teeth, usually distally, as shown in Figure 7.15A, or to reinforce anchorage as in Figure 7.15B. In the first case the extra-oral 'whisker' is permanently attached to the appliance, which is worn for about 12 hours a day, mostly in bed. To move teeth distally a purely posterior force is not sufficient; some lateral component is necessary, (the opposite of a situation discussed earlier: a fixed inter-molar width will not only reinforce anchorage, but will prevent distal movement of teeth). In the appliance shown in Figure 7.15A a Coffin spring is used to provide this, but an alternative would be the mid-line screw illustrated in Figure 7.14C.

In the appliance shown in Figure 7.15B an alternative method of attaching the 'whisker' to the appliance is illustrated. Tubes are soldered to the Adams clasps on the molars, into which a Kloehn type of bow is inserted. This enables the main part of the appliance to be worn full-time, and the extra-oral component to be attached as appropriate. In the case shown here, the buccal segments of the dentition were first moved distally by the appliance shown in Figure 7.15A. It would seem unwise now to use these teeth as anchorage for the retraction of the canines, so in this case, in Figure 7.15B, the extra-oral traction is used purely to reinforce anchorage, and not as a motive force.

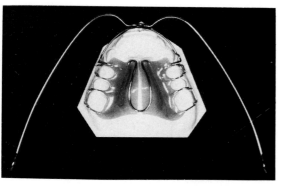

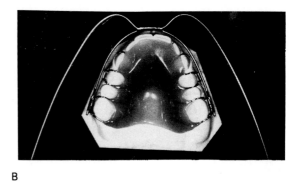

A

B

Fig. 7.15 A, 'En masse' appliance for distal movement of buccal segments using extra-oral traction. B, Subsequent appliance for retraction of 3/3, with extra-oral anchorage.

Elastic traction is applied to the whisker from either a neck strap or headcap, or a combination of the two. All these, and especially the first, have a tendency to displace the appliance, so fixation is important, and four clasps, as here, are usually required. As with fixed appliances. strong forces, up to 500 g on each side, are necessary, although it is wise to increase the force gradually over the first few visits, commencing with, perhaps, 200 g on each side. Somewhat lower forces may be used if the traction is only for anchorage reinforcement.

FUNCTIONAL APPLIANCES

These constitute a group of mostly removable appliances, in which the patient's own muscles are used to effect correction of a malocclusion. Their originators usually claim success in all types of case, but in practice they are mostly used in the treatment of Class 11 Division 1 malocclusion.

The Andresen appliance

This was the first functional appliance to be widely used. It was developed by Viggo Andresen in the period after the First World War. It is often claimed to owe its origin to the 'monobloc' of Pierre Robin, although this is disputed. The name 'monobloc' is sometimes incorrectly applied to the Andresen appliance, and other names are Norwegian plate and Activator.

It consists of a block of acrylic which is essen-

tially upper and lower base-plates joined together so as to hold the mandible in a protruded position, as shown in Figure 7.16A. The mandible being held in this protruded position tends to return to its centric relation. This force is transmitted by the acrylic to the upper teeth, tending to move them distally, or at least to minimise their forward movement due to normal growth. There is, of course, an 'equal and opposite reaction', which has the effect of moving the lower teeth forward, but this is usually less than one might fear. To minimise this it is customary to cap the incisal edges of the lower incisors.

Much controversy has raged over the correct method of trimming this appliance. It will probably work in the majority of cases if left untrimmed, but if so the posterior teeth are encased in what are virtually upper and lower cap splints. If the acrylic between the posterior teeth is widely trimmed away, as in Figire 7.16B, these teeth can erupt and thus reduce the overbite, and also can take the line of least resistance, along the cancellous trough of bone, to move to the required position.

The mode of action of the Andresen appliance is considered in Chapter 8, but the two conditions for success, in addition to correct treatment planning, are active growth of the patient and a high level of cooperation. The appliance must be tolerable; the acrylic should be as thin as possible, and also for this reason I personally construct the first appliance with the mandible displaced downwards and forwards only as far as is comfortable, almost

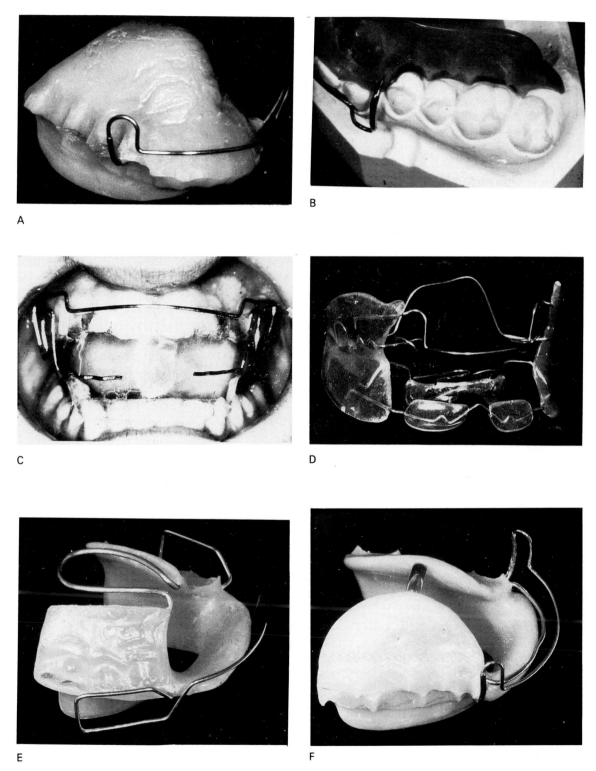

Fig. 7.16 A, The Andresen appliance. B, Trimming of upper buccal segments of Andresen appliance. C, The Harvold appliance in the mouth. D, The Fraenkel F.R.1 appliance. E, The Bionator. F, The Minator.

always proceeding to a second, more protruded appliance later.

The Harvold appliance

This was modified from the Andresen appliance by Egil Harvold. Again there are variations for most types of malocclusion, but Class 11 Division 1 is the most popular (Fig. 7.16C). The appliance is superficially similar to the Andresen activator, but is constructed with the mouth open beyond the rest position. Both upper and lower incisors are usually capped, and acrylic is widely removed above the lower cheek teeth, but is left in contact with the uppers. In addition to the other mechanisms it is intended to function by allowing the lower posterior teeth to erupt upwards and forwards, while those in the upper jaw are restrained, thus correcting the post-normal relation. For treatment of Class III malocclusion the situation is reversed, with acrylic removed above the occlusal surfaces of the upper posterior teeth only, while for treatment of open bite it is left in contact with both upper and lower cheek teeth, and removed incisally of the anterior teeth.

The Fraenkel appliance

Also known, in a translation from the German, as function regulators, these are the brain-child of Rolf Fraenkel and come from East Germany. They consist of a wire framework with acrylic shields in the buccal and labial sulci, and in some variants in the lower lingual sulcus. There are four main types, with individual variations. The F.R.1, shown in Figure 7.16D, is for use in Class II Division 1 malocclusion, and has several different versions. The F.R.2 is for Class II Division 2 malocclusion, the F.R.3 for Class III, and the F.R.4 for the treatment of open bite. They function somewhat differently from the appliances so far described since, in addition to holding the mandible in a protruded position (in the cases of the F.R.1 and F.R.2), the acrylic shields hold the cheeks and lips away from the teeth and alveoli, thus allowing expansion of the teeth and, according to its originator, the basal bone. There is little evidence to support or refute the latter claim. The appliance in function, and to some extent in design, bears some resemblance to the oral screen which was used by Caseley as a functional appliance immediately after the Second World War. Although some operators claim good results, my immediate colleagues have found it disappointing.

The Bionator

This was designed by Balters in Germany in the 1950s and has recently enjoyed considerable popularity. It is illustrated in Figure 7.16E. It might be described as a 'skeletal Andresen', and again is mainly used in the treatment of Class II Division 1 malocclusion, although other types have been described. It will be seen to have additional wire-work compared with the Andresen activator. The 'Coffin spring' in the palate is not intended to produce expansion; this would be impossible with a bar of acrylic behind the lower incisors. Its purpose is to encourage the tongue to lie in a more anterior position, a feature which the originator believed to be important. The labial bow is extended into the buccal sulci, to serve the same purpose as the acrylic shields in the Fraenkel appliance. A similar wire shield will be noticed in the Harvold appliance in Figure 7.16C.

The Bionator is a useful appliance. It is 'user-friendly' and apparently efficient. It has a tendency for the acrylic behind the lower incisors to break.

The Minator

This is my own contribution to the variants of the Andresen appliance (Figure 7.16F). The only difference from the conventional appliance is the elimination of the acrylic palate and its replacement by an oval wire, which should be placed about 2 mm from the palate, and not in contact therewith; in construction it is held away from the palate by a thickness of tinfoil. There is also a 1 mm lingual arch behind the upper incisor teeth which, in addition to strengthening this part of the appliance, minimises lingual tilting of these incisor teeth. The appliance is trimmed in the conventional manner.

The Herbst appliance

This is the only fixed functional appliance. It was first described by Herbst as long ago as 1905, but was forgotten until redescribed by Pancherz. In its classical form it consists of bands on upper and lower first premolars and molars — indeed, originally only on the upper first premolars and lower first molars. The bands were held together with upper and lower lingual arches. These were then joined to each other by means of a telescopic device, with the mandible in a protruded position. The mandible could be opened and closed but not retruded, and there was no lateral movement apart from that permitted by slackness in the joints.

The appliance has proved unacceptably liable to damage and various modifications have been produced, including the use of open cap splints made from cobalt–chromium alloy. The effect on the skeletal pattern would appear to be dramatic, but there are reports of damage to the articular head of the condyle, which are rather worrying.

In addition to the above types of functional appliances there is a large number, mostly from Germany but an increasing number from America, whose use appears to be localised to the immediate environment of their creator. Among these are the Bimmler appliance, Kinetor, Propulsor and L.S.U. activator.

SUGGESTED READING

Adams C P 1984 The design, construction and use of removable orthodontic appliances. John Wright, Bristol

Andrews L F 1972 Six keys to normal occlusion. American Journal of Orthodontics 62: 296–309

Berman M 1976 Directional forces. British Journal of Orthodontics 3: 131–7

Brown M 1984 Controlled space closure with the edgewise appliance. British Journal of Orthodontics 11: 92–9

Burstone C J, Goldberg A 1980 Beta titanium: a new orthodontic alloy. American Journal of Orthodontics 77: 121–32

Cadman C R 1975 A vade-mecum of the Begg technique. American Journal of Orthodontics 67: 447–512 and 601–24

Fletcher G G T 1981 The Begg appliance and technique. John Wright Bristol

Isaacson K G, Williams J K, 1984 An introduction to fixed appliances. John Wright, Bristol

Levason J A 1978 Simple controlled tooth movement with the edgewise appliance. British Journal of Orthodontics 5: 5–12

Muir J D, Reed R T 1979 Tooth movement with removable appliances. Pitman Medical, Tunbridge Wells

Orton H S 1977 An introduction to the Kingston approach to edgewise treatment. British Journal of Orthodontics 4: 109–19

Ricketts R M 1976 Bioprogressive therapy as an answer to orthodontic needs. American Journal of Orthodontics 70: 241–68 and 359–97

Waters N E, Stephens C D, Houston W J B 1975 Physical characteristics of orthodontic wires and archwires. British Journal of Orthodontics 2: 15–24 and 73–84

8

Treatment planning in orthodontics

Before proceeding to a consideration of individual types of malocclusion and their treatment, there are certain basic principles involved in this treatment which apply to a greater or lesser extent to all types of malocclusion. In considering the following dogma, it should be borne in mind, certainly in orthodontics, that there are exceptions to all rules (even this one!).

THE SKELETAL PATTERN

The jaws are related to each other in three dimensions of space, as previously discussed, and claims have been made in the past for bringing about changes in all of these.

The antero-posterior relationship

This is the subject of some confusion. The base of the jaws may be represented in the maxilla by structures such as the anterior nasal spine and pterygo-maxillary fissure and in the lower jaw by the lower part of the symphysis and the angle of the mandible. The dento-alveolar structures include the teeth and their surrounding bone and it is widely accepted that the alveolar bone tends to follow the teeth, at least to some extent, during tooth movement. Downs' points A and B, mentioned in the last chapter, are closely associated with the apices of the teeth and are therefore alveolar points, although they may be referred to as 'the dental base' or 'apical base'.

There is some controversy about the possibility or otherwise of changing the skeletal pattern by means of orthodontic appliances. Such a form of treatment is often described as 'orthopaedic' to differentiate it from 'orthodontic' treatment, the latter being confined to the movement of teeth through bone.

The maxilla is attached to the rest of the skull by means of sutures which are, like the periodontal ligament, a modified form of periosteum. Logically, if pressure is exerted on a suture, resorption of bone will take place and the maxilla will move, just as does a tooth following pressure on a periodontal ligament. In practice, even if the normal forward growth of the maxilla could be eliminated or reduced, a useful effect would be produced. In animal experiments posterior movement of the maxilla has been demonstrated, in addition to movement of teeth through the bone and tilting of the maxilla. In human subjects the force can only be applied through the teeth, which move through the bone. When the desired occlusion has been achieved, this stage of treatment is complete (unlike the situation in animal experiments) and in practice little bony movement takes place.

Wieslander, in a series of cephalometric investigations, found an average posterior displacement of the pterygo-maxillary fissure of rather less than 2 mm, which seemed to be permanent. Bernstein et al. (1978), using metal implants in the maxilla in six individuals, with 1000 g of force applied to a closely adapted splint, found no appreciable bony movement. Melsen (1978), also using metal implants, found reduced forward growth during treatment, which was cancelled by a 'catching-up' process later.

The effect of functional appliances in causing either additional growth of the mandible or anterior displacement of the glenoid fossa, is also equivocal. Histological investigations using animals tend to be purely descriptive, although McNamara and also Petrovic have undoubtedly shown changes in the pattern of growth. Recent work by Meikle's team (Tonge et al., 1982; Tewson et al., 1983) using radioactive labelling, has failed to show any greater amount of condylar growth in experimental than in control animals.

There have been numerous investigations based on cephalometric radiographs, some of which I reviewed in 1983. The cases analysed are usually successful results in which growth may have been particularly favourable. They are usually compared with an untreated group which is seldom comparable in age, type or severity of malocclusion. Nevertheless there is a surprising uniformity in their findings, with the experimental group showing 0.5 to 1.0 mm greater growth per annum in length of the mandible than does the control group. A surprising finding is that most if not all of this increase appears to be in the vertical rather than the horizontal ramus, while Hunt in unpublished work on the Bionator has suggested that the effect, here again, may be transient.

Recently it has been suggested that the effect may involve a recontouring of the glenoid fossa, an idea originally advanced by Breitner over 40 years ago. There is also a suggestion of damage to the condylar head, especially in those appliances which are worn more or less continuously.

It would seem that the controversy lies between those who have apparently shown no change in the skeletal pattern (probably an extreme view with modern knowledge) and those who claim an average favourable change of a millimetre or two. Because of the variation in natural growth in both amount and direction, it is only possible to compare averages: it is not difficult to find an individual case which will 'prove' any point. It is important to remember that half any sample of cases will react less favourably than the average. This is well illustrated by Creekmore and Radney (1983) who showed, for example, that the angle ANB decreased more, on average, in cases treated with the Fraenkel appliance than in an untreated group. Nevertheless, in both groups the largest number — nearly half the whole — showed no change in this angle. While more showed a reduction of the angle in the treated group, by chance

the greatest favourable change was in an untreated individual!

On the other hand the dento-alveolar structures can be changed and with modern, sophisticated appliances, the teeth may be moved bodily, producing a very substantial change in the dental base relationships. As we shall see, when we come to consider Class II malocclusions, there is a limit to the amount of change of this type which can be obtained.

The vertical relationship

During the period when orthodontic treatment is normally carried out, the amount of vertical growth of the face is greater than the horizontal growth, although there is of course considerable individual variation. Here again, orthodontists have claimed that it is possible to change this vertical dimension of the face permanently as discussed in the preceding paragraph. Again a policy of cheerful pessimism would seem indicated. For example, if the overbite is reduced by causing the posterior buccal segments to develop excessively, rather than by intruding the incisors (and this is almost always the case) then a situation arises similar to that produced by fitting 'over-opened' dentures. The mandible will rotate downwards and backwards unless the face grows sufficiently to accommodate the increased vertical dimension which has been produced. Such an 'over-opening' without a compensatory growth is liable to relapse and this is doubtless one of the causes of such a relapse in some cases of deep overbite. It seems doubtful whether a permanent change in vertical jaw relationships can be achieved, as a result of orthodontic treatment, at least predictably. This is an aspect of treatment presently giving rise to much interest, and in which future developments are probable.

The lateral relationship

Here again claims have been made for the increase in width of the maxillary base, especially when brought about by rapid expansion opening the mid-line suture. This will be dealt with in detail later but there is no doubt that such a result can be obtained. Again, firm evidence is lacking about its permanence. What little there is would seem to indicate that, surprisingly, the expansion of the skeletal base is more permanent than the expansion of the dental arches.

In general, therefore, it would be wise to assume that the skeletal pattern cannot be changed to any worthwhile clinical extent, except of course by surgical procedures. Certainly the extravagant claims made for certain esoteric techniques, depend largely on the observation of normal favourable growth changes through rose coloured spectacles.

THE QUESTION OF EXTRACTIONS

The size of the teeth and to a slightly lesser extent the size of the jaws, are determined at a very early stage and largely by genetic factors. We cannot substantially change the size of the teeth and it should also be regarded as axiomatic that we cannot appreciably change the size of the jaws. Crowding of the teeth will therefore occur if the teeth are too large for the jaws, and spacing in the opposite condition. Fortunately, the former can be permanently corrected by the extraction of teeth and one wonders why there are still some orthodontists who seem opposed to this very satisfactory form of treatment. Ideally, teeth should only be extracted for this reason — the relief of crowding. In a few special cases, which will be mentioned later, they may be extracted for other reasons.

THE PLANNING OF ORTHODONTIC TREATMENT

In planning treatment of malocclusion, it is helpful to have a datum — some structure which we believe we cannot change permanently — around which we can arrange the rest of the dentition. I showed some years ago (Mills, 1968) that the lower incisors appear to be in a rather stable position labio-lingually, and that attempts to move them more than a very small amount in either of these directions are likely to be followed by relapse. There are a few minor exceptions to this rule which will be mentioned in their appro-

priate places. Treatment planning may be illustrated by considering the case shown by the models in Figure 8.1. This patient exhibits some incease in overjet and quite severe crowding. Planning of the treatment, therefore, commenced by considering the lower labial segment of teeth. It should be emphasised that the procedure which follows is purely a planning exercise and that actual tooth movement may, at a later stage, be carried out in quite a different order.

Accepting the principle that the labio-lingual position of the lower incisors cannot be changed to any extent, crowding will be reduced by moving the canines distally along the arch. If crowding is present this is the only way to reduce it. In order to move the canines distally, it is necessary to have space behind them and this would virtually always be produced by the extraction of suitable teeth. The choice of extractions will be considered in the next section. In the present case, the first premolars were the teeth of choice. The premolar having been extracted, the canine is moved distally sufficiently to allow the alignment of the lower incisors, as shown on the right side of the model in Figure 8.2. This procedure would normally be carried out in the mind's eye although it has been illustrated here by setting the teeth in wax. Such a wax set-up can indeed be useful in difficult cases. It will be observed in this segment, that there is a small amount of residual space between the lower right canine and second premolar and assessment of this residual space gives some idea of the care necessary in retracting the canine. In treatment of this case, there are two possible tooth movements. The teeth of the labial segment may move distally, which is desired, or the teeth of the buccal segments may move mesially. The latter is all too easily achieved and is usually undesirable. If some space closure is desired, it should be left until the anterior teeth are in their final position. In this case some forward movement of the lower posterior teeth is desirable to prevent residual spacing, and this may be balanced against the retraction of the anteriors. This problem of anchorage balance is one of the most important in considering orthodontic treatment.

Having mentally corrected the lower arch, we then consider the tooth movement required in the

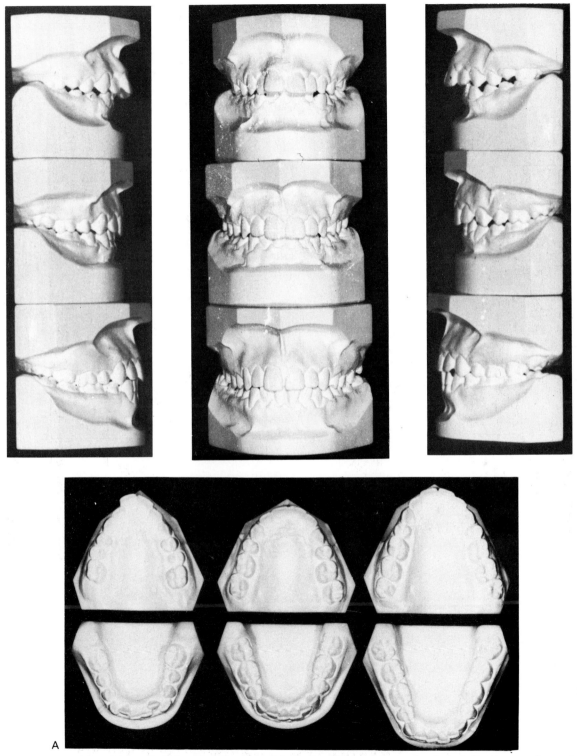

Fig. 8.1 A, Models and B (overleaf), lateral skull radiographs of patient Howard before and at the end of treatment and some 3 years out of retention.

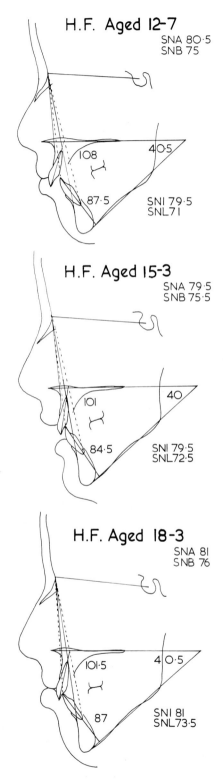

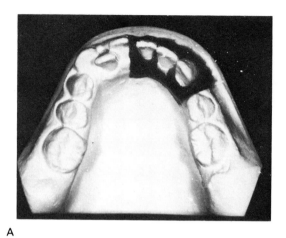

A

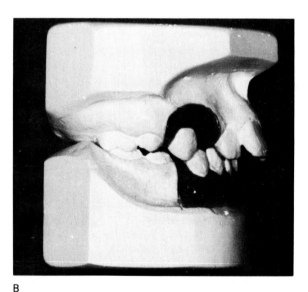

B

Fig. 8.2 Initial models of patient Howard. On the right side the first premolars have been 'extracted', and the lower canine and incisors 'aligned'. The upper canine has then been 'retracted' to its correct position. A, Occlusal view of lower model. B, Right lateral view to show planned position of 3/.

Fig. 8.1 (cont'd)

upper jaw. The key here is the upper permanent canine. There are some exceptions, but for most cases the final position of the upper canine should be in normal relationship to the lower canine, that is occluding between this tooth and the tooth immediately distal to it. Such a position is seen in Figure 8.2B and again space is necessary behind the canine tooth and this has been achieved by extracting the first premolar. In this case, however, we have no residual space. The width of the extracted first premolar will be completely taken up by retraction of the upper canine and the upper buccal segments cannot be allowed to move mesially at all. It is important to know that at the commencement of treatment so that adequate precautions, probably involving the use of extra-oral anchorage, may be instituted.

All that remains is the planning of the treatment of the upper labial segment which may involve the relief of crowding, the reduction of the overjet and/or overbite. This will be dealt with in the appropriate sections of this work. Finally, consideration should be given to the need for closing any residual spaces.

It is again emphasised that this exercise is intended to plan the necessary tooth movements. The actual order or method of carrying out treatment may vary in individual cases. The technique applies with modifications to virtually all types of malocclusion, although superficially, it may appear to have less application in Class III malocclusion than elsewhere.

THE CHOICE OF EXTRACTIONS

As already indicated, extractions are invariably required for the relief of crowding brought about by an adverse tooth/tissue ratio and in an ideal world, this would be the only reason for such extractions. In assessing this crowding, a note should be made whether this is anterior or posterior to the first molar (or both) and generally extractions would be in the same segment. With this initial proviso, the individual teeth will be considered. It is almost always desirable to balance the extractions, that is to extract the same tooth in each quadrant of the arch.

First premolars

These are usually the teeth of choice and we have already seen an example where they were in fact extracted. Figure 8.1 shows the records of the treatment of that patient, illustrated by means of study models before treatment, at the end of treatment and some 3 years out of retention, together with tracings of the appropriate lateral skull radiographs. First premolars provide the space near to the front of the mouth but at the same time do not involve the loss of an obvious 'front tooth', which might be aesthetically unacceptable. The second premolar bears a strong resemblance to the first premolar, both aesthetically and functionally and usually provides a good contact point with the canine. The main exceptions to the general rule 'first premolars, why not?' arise when crowding is very slight, when it is confined to the area behind the first molars, or where other teeth are to be preferred because of caries or other pathological conditions.

Second premolars

The second premolar is traditionally chosen in those mouths where crowding is comparatively slight. In the past this was probably to ensure that residual spacing would be out of sight. Where the spaces were allowed to close by natural drifting, this could give rise to a somewhat unsatisfactory contact point between the first premolar and the first molar. This often took the form of a 'slack contact' with food impaction and pocket formation. However, with modern appliances it should be possible to bring the teeth together and to provide an adequate contact point without undue tilting. The loss of a second premolar rather than a first premolar, alters the 'anchorage balance'. Before retracting the canine, it is necessary to retract the first premolar, while a premolar has been removed from the posterior segment which forms the anchorage for these movements. There is therefore a greater tendency to mesial movement of the molars and space is more readily closed in cases of comparatively mild crowding.

There is, therefore, a case for the extraction of second premolars in a minority of cases where crowding is slight, and a typical case is shown in Figure 8.10. It is also of course very often the tooth of choice where the health of the second premolar is unsatisfactory due to caries or hypoplasia, while lower second premolars are not infrequently congenitally absent and the space thus provided may obviate the need for any extractions in the lower arch. In this case, the missing lower second premolar would be balanced by the extrac-

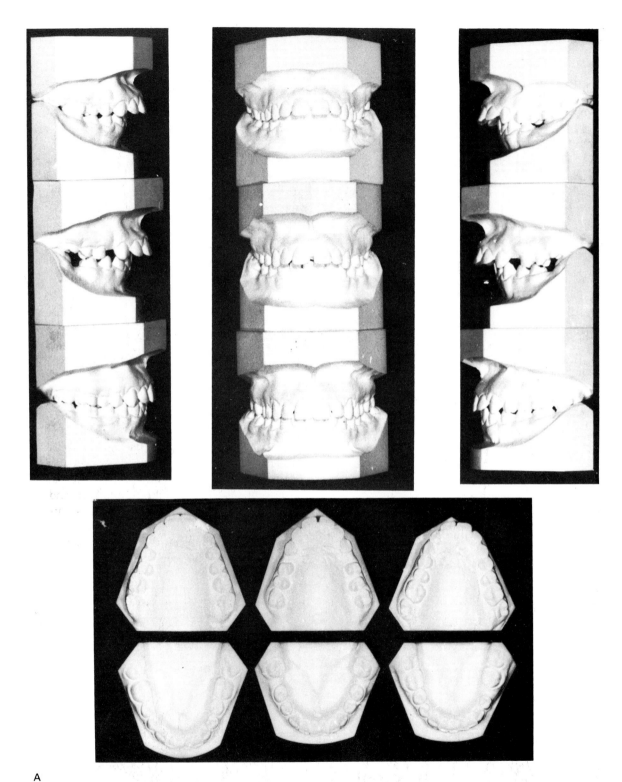

A

Fig. 8.3 Records of the patient Valerie, in whom first molars were extracted as part of orthodontic treatment. A, Models before treatment. The second models after retraction of $\overline{54/45}$. At this stage no treatment apart from extractions had been carried out in the lower arch. The final models are 4 years out of retention. B, Tracings of lateral skull radiograph at age 18 years, superimposed on initial radiograph.

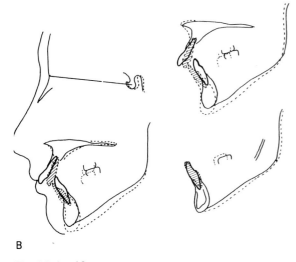

B

Fig. 8.3 (*cont'd*)

tion of a corresponding upper tooth, or occasionally, by the loss of the upper first premolar.

First permanent molars

Some years ago, I coined the phrase that the extraction of first permanent molars in orthodontic treatment 'doubles the treatment time and halves the prognosis'. This tooth is the first of the permanent teeth to erupt, at the age of 6 years, and is often not recognised as a permanent tooth by the child or its parents. It is very prone to caries and by the time orthodontic treatment commences, may have been filled or have a carious cavity. The general dentist would like this tooth to be included in the plan for extractions, but this does make the treatment very much more difficult and prolonged. There is nothing more annoying to the orthodontist than to see a new patient arrive with all first molars recently extracted and the sockets barely healed — unless it be to see one of his own patients some years after the completion of treatment with four first premolars very properly missing but at least one first molar also extracted.

The problems differ in the two jaws and can be clearly seen in the case illustrated in Figure 8.3. This girl had only fairly minor crowding but both lower first molars were very heavily filled and one of them had further caries which had resulted in

an exposure of the pulp. It was therefore decided to relieve the lower crowding and reduce the overjet with the extraction of all four of these teeth.

The main problem in the upper arch concerns control of the second permanent molar. If this tooth is unerupted at the time of the extraction of the first molar, it need change its direction of eruption only slightly to erupt in a very mesial position — indeed, not infrequently, in contact with the second premolar. This may be overcome by delaying treatment until the second permanent molar has erupted and this should be regarded as the normal procedure. The problem here is that in a crowded mouth the patient is often well past the thirteenth birthday before the second molar erupts and when it does so, it is far back in the mouth and difficult to clasp. Banding or direct bonding is even more difficult. Such a clasp will not provide adequate fixation of the appliance and further clasping will be necessary in a more anterior part of the mouth. In the case shown in Figure 8.4A a clasp has been placed on the upper permanent canine, the alternatives being the first premolar or teeth in the labial segment. The next problem concerns the retraction of the premolars, and, especially if removable appliances are used, there is a strong tendency for these teeth to tilt. While natural correction of this tilting frequently occurs (as in the case here), it is quite difficult to retract a second premolar through it own width. Extraction of first molars does not give more, but rather less space in the anterior part of the arch, although it almost invariably allows the third molar to erupt normally.

In the lower dental arch on the other hand the lower second molar does not move mesially as rapidly as one would hope. We have dealt with this in some detail in Chapter 4. Occasionally in a very crowded mouth, especially if the second premolar is impacted, the space will close to a reasonably acceptable position. But where the crowding is less severe, as in the case illustrated here, the second molar will tilt mesially and will lock itself firmly behind the upper second molar, where it will remain. In practice this means that if the first molar has been extracted in the lower arch a rather prolonged period of fixed appliance treatment is almost inevitable. Premolars and

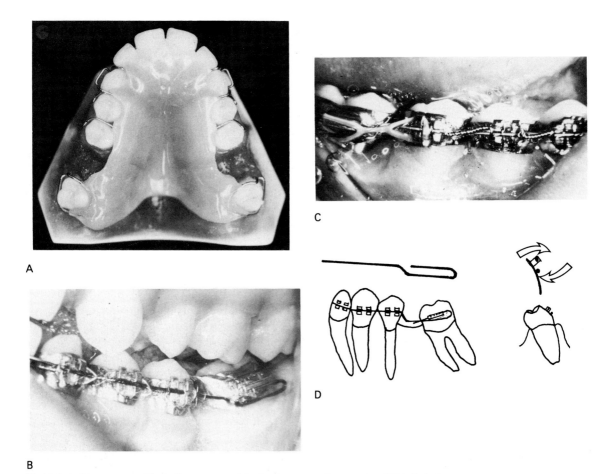

Fig. 8.4 A, Upper removable appliance, as used in the first stage of treatment of Valerie in Fig. 8.3. B, Lower recurved arch to bring forward /7̄. C, The same arch on 7̄/ showing the addition of elastic chain to provide motive power. D, Diagrammatic representation of recurved arch.

canines may be retracted as necessary, but ultimately it is usually necessary to bring the second molar forward into contact with the second premolar, and this is one of the most difficult tooth movements in fixed appliance therapy. Without adequate control, the tooth tends to tilt mesially, to rotate mesiolingually and especially to roll lingually, that is the occlusal surface tilts in a lingual direction. This lingual rolling is almost always the result of unskilled treatment with banded appliances and is extremely difficult to correct. It is, therefore, important to keep control in this dimension throughout treatment, either by using a rectangular wire in a rectangular tube or if round wire is used, the end may be recurved as shown in Figure 8.4B and C, so that the tooth moves along the recurved wire, while the lower of

the two parallel wires presses firmly on the band gingivally to the tube as shown diagrammatically (Fig. 8.4D). Retraction of the premolars and canines is less of a problem in the lower than in the upper arch, and once again it is unusual for the third molars to present any problem where the first molar has been extracted.

So the extraction of first molars has the advantage of removing very caries-prone teeth and of relieving impaction of the third molars. Inevitably, it involves the retraction of two premolars in each quadrant in addition to the canines and therefore lengthens treatment considerably. It cannot be emphasised too strongly that anchorage may readily be lost in the upper arch, with the second molar coming forward to an unsatisfactory extent. While this anchorage may be reinforced by extra-oral apparatus, this does not wholly solve the problem. The extraction of first molars is therefore usually restricted to those cases where they may not be permanently saved.

Second permanent molars

Extraction of second permanent molars is usually indicated in those cases where crowding is confined to the area distal to the first permanent molars or where crowding anterior to these teeth is very mild. It will be seen in Chapters 10 and 11 that extraction of upper second molars often facilitates the distal movement of upper buccal segments in cases where posterior crowding would otherwise prevent it.

Before considering the extraction of any teeth, it is of course necessary to ensure that all other permanent teeth are present and developing normally. Extraction of second molars is not usually indicated unless the third molar teeth are developing in a good position and are of a reasonable size. If this is the case, then following the early extraction of the second molar, the upper third molar will usually erupt to replace it, often well before its usual time. The situation is much less satisfactory in the lower arch where the third molar may well erupt impacted against the first permanent molar to a greater or lesser extent. While such an impaction can be corrected orthodontically, it is usually difficult to persuade a patient, who has already had 2 or 3 years orthodontic treatment, to submit to a further period of treatment for the sake of something at the back of the mouth, the importance of which seems to the patient slight. In considering the extraction of lower second molars, certain factors are of assistance and the following suggestions are based partly on the work of Cryer (1967).

1. The best time for extraction of the second molar is at the stage when the whole of the crown of the third molar is calcified but the root has not yet begun calcification. This is seen in Figure 8.5. This feature is one of the most important indicators.

2. The third molar should be well forward in contact with the second molar or, better still, overlapping it to a reasonable extent. It is by no means uncommon to find the developing crown of

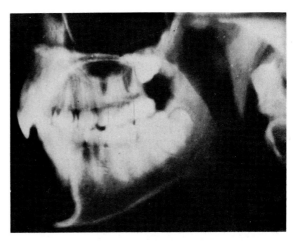

A

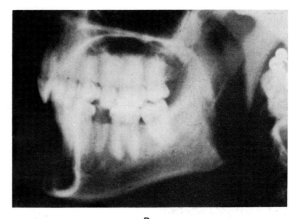

B

Fig. 8.5 Radiographs of the same patient A, before and B, some years after the extraction for orthodontic reasons of $\overline{7}|\overline{7}$.

the third molar overlapping the second molar when seen in a radiograph, and this is not radiographic distortion: the tooth often develops on the buccal side of the second molar.

3. The normal developmental position of the third molar is mesially inclined but it seems undesirable that the long axis of the third molar should have an angle greater than about 30 degrees to the long axis of the first molar.

4. It is advantageous if the third molar is developing at a lower level than those teeth which have erupted. This is however unusual. The third molar usually develops in the vertical ramus of the mandible immediately behind the remaining molar teeth.

If these criteria are observed the third molar will usually take the place of the second molar, if the latter tooth is extracted. The main advantage of doing so is to allow the eruption of the third molar or possibly to relieve impaction of a second premolar. Distal movement of complete lower buccal segments is a prolonged and difficult procedure which is usually better avoided.

Third permanent molars

Both the third molar and the space for its accommodation develop too late to be of any great help in orthodontic treatment. It has been suggested that this tooth can readily be enucleated when the crown is in the early stages of calcification. This may be a simple surgical procedure but it involves the admission of a child to hospital which would seem to be a procedure to be avoided unless absolutely necessary. From the orthodontic point of view the operation is worthless. It does not give space for alignment of crowded teeth and the third molar would seem to play little part in the development of late crowding.

Anterior teeth

Anterior teeth would seldom be the teeth of choice for extractions but their loss is sometimes dictated by factors outside our control. Upper central incisors may be lost as a result of trauma and in this case the space may be closed (see Fig. 4.4). The lateral incisor on the appropriate side may be crowned or built-up with composite filling material to stimulate a central, although this is a skilled and difficult technical procedure and the long-term prognosis for such teeth is not known. Moreover care and skill are necessary to move the lateral incisor to the desired position without displacing the centre-line (Fig. 8.7). Upper lateral incisors may be extracted if they are grossly misplaced or malformed and are not infrequently congenitally absent. If this is the case in a crowded mouth, the space may be used to align the teeth, with the upper canines taking the place of the upper lateral incisors (Fig. 8.6A). Upper canines would only be extracted if grossly displaced and where it is not possible to position them in the arch. If the upper lateral incisor and first premolar

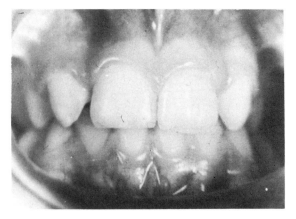

A

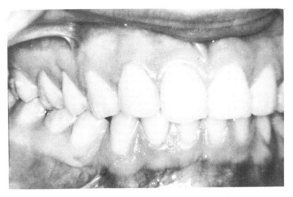

B

Fig. 8.6 A, The grossly misplaced 2/2 have been extracted and 3/3 moved forward to replace them. B, 3/ was grossly misplaced in the palate. 4/ brought forward to replace 3/.

are already in contact then a reasonable result can often be shown (Fig. 8.6B) but if the space has to be closed mechanically, although this can be achieved, there is a strong tendency for a small space to re-open. Lower canines, again, would seldom be extracted unless grossly misplaced and it is difficult to achieve a good contact point between the lower lateral incisor and first premolar.

The extraction of one or more lower incisors presents special problems and is worthy of some note. Superficially, if the arches are well aligned apart from crowding in the lower labial segment, a condition by no means uncommon in the older patient, it is very tempting to extract a single lower incisor. This has two unfortunate sequels.

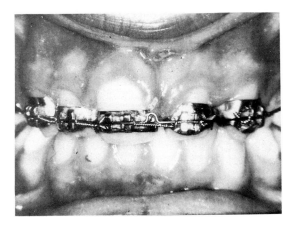

A

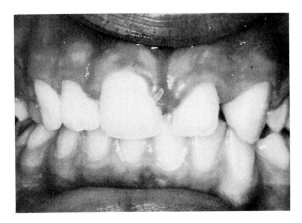

B

Firstly, it is frequently found that although the space may be closed comparatively easily we are left with three crowded lower incisors instead of four crowded lower incisors! This is because they drop lingually a matter of a millimetre or so and therefore have to take up a smaller part of the arch. This lingual movement of the lower incisors may sometimes be followed by a similar movement of the upper incisors so that the upper labial segment also becomes crowded. For these reasons the extraction of lower incisors has a bad reputation but nevertheless can be the treatment of choice if care is taken. It is important to measure the space available and to make sure that three incisors will fit comfortably into this area, preferably with a little residual spacing. Having extracted the lower incisor, the remaining teeth must be aligned with a fixed appliance and care taken to bring the apices together and to ensure good contact points. 'Stripping' of the contact points serves to render tham flat, and to increase the contact area, and would to some extent help to ensure that they remain well aligned. The extraction of the lower incisor may be indicated where the posterior occlusion is excellent and the upper incisors well aligned but with a deep overbite. It may also be indicated where the angulation of one or both lower canines is particularly unfavourable (Fig. 8.8). If it is proposed to extract one lower incisor, thought should be given as to whether it would not in fact be better to extract two lower incisors.

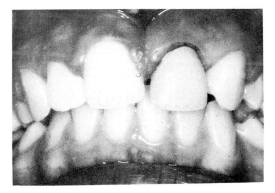

C

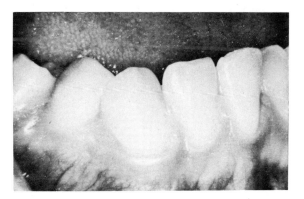

Fig. 8.7 /1 was lost as a result of trauma. A, /2 has been moved to the position of /1 maintaining position of the centre-line. B, Immediately before, and C, immediately after, building up with composite resin.

Fig. 8.8 Lower labial crowded, with distally inclined lower canine. The extraction of a lower incisor might well be indicated.

The 'stripping' of lower incisors

As an alternative to the extraction of lower incisors, various authorities, notably Peck & Peck (1975) have advocated the reduction of their width by removal of tooth substance from the contact areas mesially and distally. As already indicated, a flattening of the contact areas may reduce the tendency for contacts to slip. The practice is known in North America as 'reproximation', but a long name does not make a doubtful procedure respectable.

If the width of the teeth is unduly reduced, and the spaces closed, the roots of the teeth will be brought closely together and the interdental septum of bone may be completely resorbed, giving rise to pocket formation later. Interdental stripping should probably be limited to the amount which might be lost by natural wear over adult life, and while such an amount may occasionally be helpful, it will not relieve any serious crowding.

Multiple extractions

Both the dental bases and the teeth have finite sizes. Cases occasionally arise where the extraction of four teeth, especially four first premolars, does not give sufficient space to align the remainder. In these cases extraction of more than four teeth may be indicated. Such cases are rare and the fact that multiple extractions are sometimes justified should not be used as an excuse for additional extractions where careless anchorage control has allowed the buccal segments of teeth to come forward to an undue extent. The teeth of choice are probably first premolars and second molars, although followers of the Begg technique prefer to extract first premolars and first permanent molars. With careful anchorage control, it should almost always be possible to avoid such multiple extractions, although it is by no means uncommon to find that following loss of four premolars, the third molars remain impacted.

EXTRACTIONS AND THE FACIAL PROFILE

In recent years there has been increasing interest in the facial profile and the effect thereon of orthodontic treatment, especially that involving the extraction of teeth. While one should always strive for the best possible result, it is important to remember that facial form varies between individuals, and it is not possible to make everyone conform to a common ideal.

Looi, a graduate student at the Eastman Dental Hospital, London, compared a group of patients with Class II Division 1 malocclusions treated by the Andresen appliance, without extractions, with a second group treated with the Begg appliance and the loss of four premolars. These were chosen to represent the extreme effects of treatment on the soft tissues, and were contrasted with an untreated group of similar malocclusions. Both treated groups showed a falling back of the upper lip, which had been held forward by the prominent incisors, but the difference between the two treated groups was of the order of a millimetre, although the lower lip followed the retraction of lower incisor in the Begg group rather more closely. Papert, also at the Eastman, could find no appreciable difference in the effect on the lip of the extraction of first premolars, compared with that of second premolars or first molars.

It would seem that the upper lip has a natural resting position, from which it may be held forward by prominent incisors, but to which it will return when the incisors are retracted, irrespective of the amount of retraction. The 'dishing in' of facial profiles probably owes more to pubertal growth of nose and chin than to orthodontic treatment.

ROTATION OF TEETH

The rotation of teeth is a common condition which is comparatively easily corrected with fixed appliances. In the case of posterior teeth, the correction is often permanent because the occlusion holds the teeth in this new position. In the case of incisor teeth, the tendency to relapse is very high. The reason for this strong tendency to relapse may not be fully understood but it would seem that an important factor lies in the fibres of the periodontal ligament. It should be remembered that the periodontal ligament is a part of the periosteum of the jaw and is in every way continuous with the mucoperiosteum which covers the alveolar processes. Reitan (1959) has shown that when a tooth is rotated, the fibres become arranged tangentially. This initially applies to all the fibres of the periodontal ligament but, after a period of approximately 4 months, those fibres which run from the tooth to the alveolar bone become re-arranged into their normal position. However, those fibres which run into the mucoperiosteum and transeptally to the adjacent teeth recover very much more slowly. In an experiment on dogs by Reitan after 250 days there was little change in these free gingival fibres. Edwards (1970) has shown in human subjects that if tattoo marks are placed on the gingivae above a rotated premolar, as the tooth is rotated, these tattoo marks follow the rotating tooth to a decreasing extent as they move away from the gingival margin. The logical step following the discovery was to cut through these free gingival fibres and this operation is known in the United Kingdom as pericision and in the American continent as circumferential supercrestal fiberotomy (sic). With a local anaesthetic a fine scalpel blade is inserted down the periodontal membrane until the tip of the blade touches the alveolar crest. In a child this is considerably further than one would expect since the gingival margin does not coincide with the anatomical margin of the crown and considerable crypt is still present. The blade is then moved around the tooth, keeping in contact with the alveolar crest, and including a section of the transeptal fibres. The operation takes about 5 minutes and gives rise to little or no after pain. No dressing is necessary, and there is no permanent loss of attachment, but long-term results do not entirely support early optimism (Bellardie, 1985).

This does not of course deal with those fibres which run into the alveolar bone and it is therefore necessary to retain the teeth in position until these fibres have had an opportunity to reform in a more desirable position. Both from the work of Reitan and the clinical experience of Pinson & Strahan (1974) and Walsh (1975) it would seem that about 4 months allows this to happen. It would therefore seem to be wise to be on the safe side and to retain the teeth in position for some 6 months. These teeth have a strong tendency to relapse and a

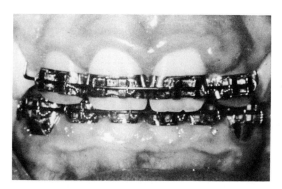

Fig. 8.9 Upper and lower fixed sectional retainers to prevent rotational relapse of teeth.

removable retainer is not usually satisfactory. It is advisable to leave bands or bonds on the appropriate teeth and to retain by means of a short sectional fixed retainer (Fig. 8.9).

Even with these precautions, the rotated incisors will relapse to a small extent. To overcome this it may be desirable to over-correct the teeth by about 10°: a procedure which is easier said than done.

Figure 8.10 shows the records of Androulla, a Greek Cypriot girl who presented at the age of 15 years with some crowding and marked rotation of the upper incisors, especially 1/. She was treated by the extraction of second premolars, since crowding was not severe, and upper and lower fixed appliances. 1/ was slightly over-corrected and the final condition was retained with upper and lower fixed retainers (Fig. 8.9), for 6 months, 1/ being pericised during the early part of retention. The small amount of relapse which took place is typical.

It will be seen from Figure 8.10B that the condition is otherwise unchanged, growth having apparently ceased in this girl.

SUGGESTED READING

Bellardie H 1985 The effect of pericision on the relapse of rotational upper incisors. British Journal of Orthodontics 12: 49

Creekmore T D, Radney L J 1983 Fraenkel appliance therapy: orthopedic or orthodontic? American Journal of Orthodontics 83: 89–108

Cryer B S 1967 Third molar eruption and the effect of extraction of adjacent teeth. Dental Practitioner 17: 405–18

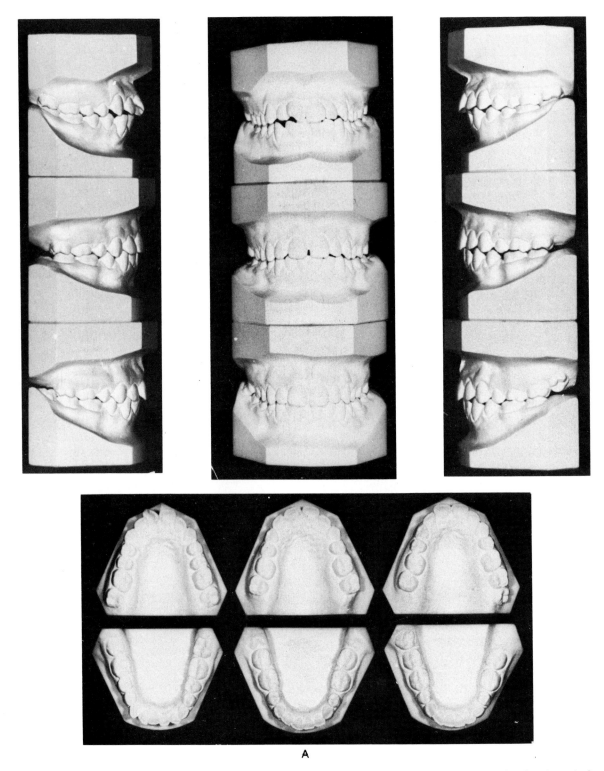

A

Fig. 8.10 A, Models of dentition of Androulla taken before treatment, at the end of retention and 18 months after the end of retention. B (opposite) Lateral skull tracings at the same stages.

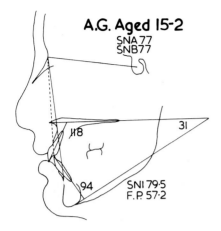

A.G. Aged 15·2

SNA 77
SNB 77

31

118

94

SNI 79·5
F.P. 57·2

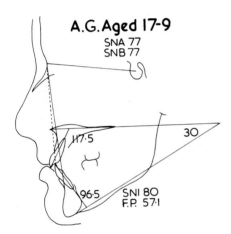

A.G. Aged 17·9

SNA 77
SNB 77

30

117·5

96·5

SNI 80
F.P. 57·1

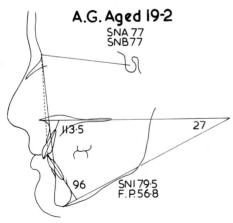

A.G. Aged 19·2

SNA 77
SNB 77

27

113·5

96

SNI 79·5
F.P. 56·8

B

Fig. 8.10 (cont'd)

Melson B 1978 Effects of cervical anchorage during and after treatment: an implant study. American Journal of Orthodontics 73: 526–40

Mills J R E 1968 The stability of the lower labial segment. Dental Practitioner 18: 293–305

Mills J R E 1978 The effect of orthodontic treatment on the skeletal pattern. British Journal of Orthodontics 5: 133–43

Mills J R E 1983 Clinical control of craniofacial growth: a skeptic's viewpoint. In: McNamara J. (ed.) Clinical alteration of the growing face. Center for Growth and Development, Michigan, Ann Arbor

Peck H, Peck S 1975 Reproximation (enamel stripping) as an essential orthodontic treatment ingredient. In: Cook J T (ed.) Transactions of the Third International Orthodontic Congress. Crosby Lockwood Staples, London

Pinson R R, Strahan J D 1974 The effect on the relapse of orthodontically rotated teeth of surgical division of the gingival fibres — pericision. British Journal of Orthodontics 1: 87–92

Reitan K 1959 Tissue rearrangement during retention of orthodontically rotated teeth. Angle Orthodontist 29: 105–33

Tulloch J F C 1978 Treatment following loss of second premolars. British Journal of Orthodontics 5: 29–34

9

The treatment of Class I malocclusion

Angle defined his classification of malocclusion on the basis of the relationship of the first permanent molars. Class I comprised those cases in which the mesio-distal occlusion of the first permanent molars was normal, that is with the mesio-buccal cusp of the lower first molar occluding between the mesio-buccal cusp of the upper first molar and the buccal cusp of the second premolar. The British Standard incisor classification (BS4492) defines Class I as 'the lower incisor edges occlude with or lie immediately below the cingulum plateau (middle part of the palatal surface) of the upper central incisors'. It comprises therefore all those patients in whom the antero-posterior relationship of the dental arches is normal and the abnormality is within, rather than between, the arches.

CROWDING

Aetiology

As already indicated in Chapter 4, crowding of the teeth is the result of the inheritance of comparatively large teeth in small jaws. The size of the teeth is finally determined when the calcification of the occlusal surface is complete and it would seem that this is regulated almost entirely by genetic factors. The size of the jaws is also largely genetically determined but it may be that environment has some effect in this context. There is, however, no evidence that the size of the jaw can be in any way increased by normal orthodontic procedures.

Treatment

The basic principles of the treatment of crowding

have been covered in some detail in the previous chapter and it is not proposed to repeat them here. The practical application of these principles can be shown by consideration of the treatment of Ruby shown in Figure 9.1.

Ruby first presented shortly before her thirteenth birthday, that is at a slightly older age than the majority of patients. It will be seen from Figure 9.1B that she had a Class I skeletal pattern with a normal relationship of the arches both antero-posteriorly and vertically. The posterior occlusion was Class I but there was crowding in both upper and lower labial segments. In the upper incisor region this had caused 2/2 to be displaced palatally and to occlude inside the bite. Fortunately, the crowding did not involve the rotation of any of the teeth.

Looking at the occlusal view of the lower arch in Figure 9.1A it will be seen that there is some crowding of the incisor region and this could be relieved by moving the lower canine teeth distally. This would necessitate the extraction of teeth posteriorly to the canine and the obvious choice would be the first premolar on each side. In the absence of any reason to the contrary these teeth were chosen. It will also be noted that this would leave substantial residual space and anchorage would not appear to be a problem.

Turning now to the upper arch, the plan would be to move the upper canines into a Class I relationship with the uncrowded position of the lower canines. Here again, there would appear to be some residual spacing and anchorage would not prove too great a problem except possibly in the upper right segment where care should be taken. Following these extractions and preliminary tooth movements, the anterior teeth could be aligned

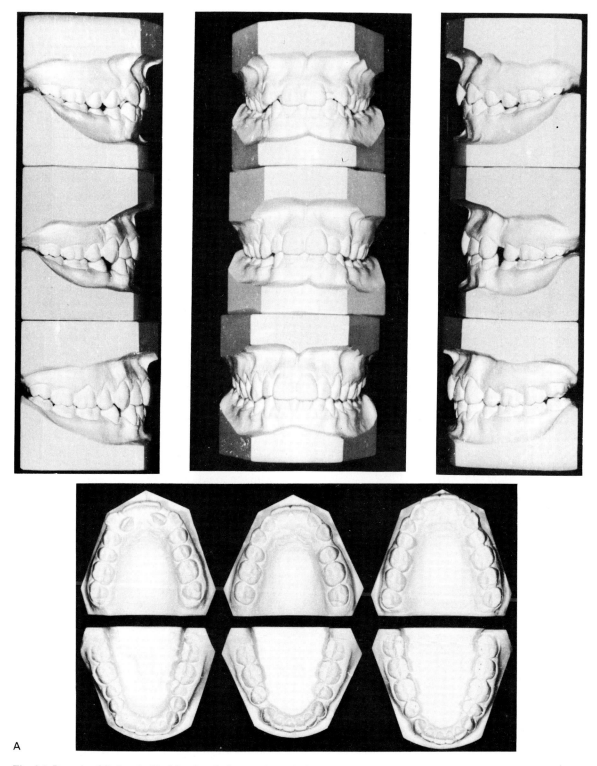

Fig. 9.1 Records of Ruby. A, Models taken before, at the end of treatment and over 5 years after all appliances removed. B, Tracings of lateral skull radiographs at the same stages (overleaf).

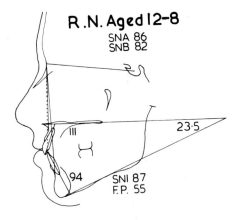

R.N. Aged 12-8
SNA 86
SNB 82

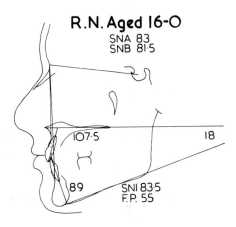

R.N. Aged 16-0
SNA 83
SNB 81·5

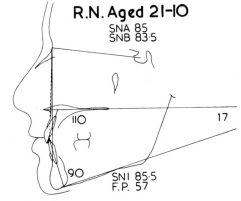

R.N. Aged 21-10
SNA 85
SNB 83·5

B

Fig. 9.1 (*cont'd*)

and this would involve proclining 2/2 over the bite. Looking at the upper model in Figure 9.1A (before treatment) it will be noted that approximately the same amount of the palatal surface of both the central and lateral incisors is visible, if anything rather more of the lateral incisors. This would indicate that these latter teeth are displaced bodily in a palatal direction and may complicate treatment to some extent. If they had been merely tilted lingually, so that less of the lingual surface was visible in this view, treatment would have been easier.

Active treatment took 11 months and involved the use of three upper removable appliances only. An impression for the first of these was taken before the practitioner was asked to carry out the extractions, so that the appliance illustrated in Figure 9.2A could be fitted very shortly after this had been completed. It is advisable to fit an appliance within 2 or 3 weeks of the extraction of teeth since otherwise, occasionally, the upper posterior teeth may move forward and the appliance will not then fit. In considering the retraction of upper canine teeth — and indeed of any other teeth — it is important to observe the angulation of the teeth relative to the occlusal plane. Turning for a moment from Ruby, in Figure 9.3 are shown two upper canines in separate patients. Figure 9.3A shows a canine which is very mesially inclined and in this case, as in Ruby's it could be retracted by means of a removable appliance using a tilting action only. The canine shown in Figure 9.3B on the other hand, is already distally inclined and if an attempt were made to retract it by a pure tilting movement it will be grossly tilted distally by the time it is in its correct position. In this latter case therefore it will be necessary to move the tooth bodily and this will involve the use of a fixed appliance. Perhaps more important, it should be borne in mind that the bodily movement of a tooth requires much greater anchorage than does a mere tilting action and it is probable that any appliance would have to be reinforced with extra-oral anchorage.

Ruby had two upper incisors occluding inside the bite. Where this is the case it is by no means uncommon to find that a premature contact takes place on these instanding teeth with a forward displacement of the mandible on closing. This was so here. If 2/2 had been extracted the mandible would have immediately returned to true centric jaw relationship with the development of a small overjet on the upper central incisors. This will also occur when the positions of 2/2 have been

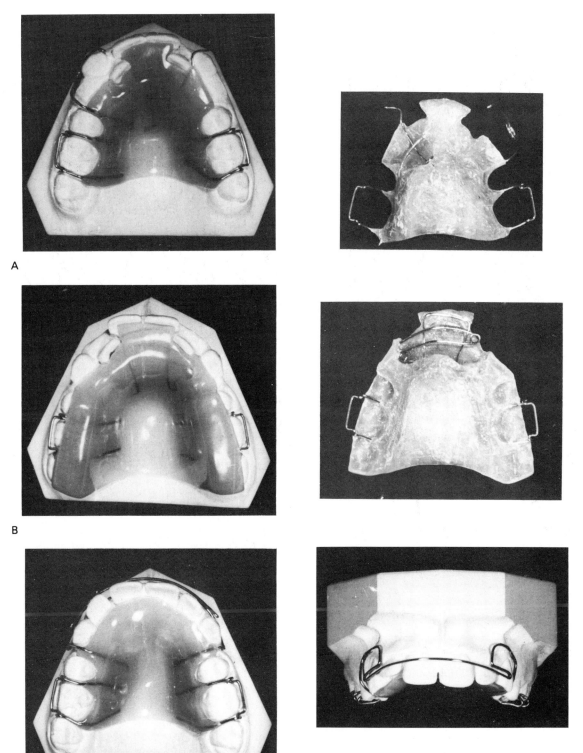

Fig. 9.2 A, Replica of upper removable appliance to retract
3/3. B, Second appliance to procline 2/2. C, Third appliance
with labial bow for final alignment of upper incisors.

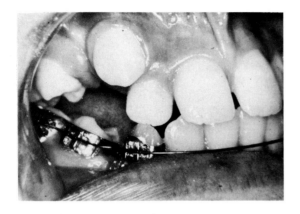

A

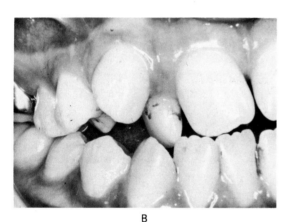

B

Fig. 9.3 A, Upper labially placed canine which is mesially inclined and may be easily retracted. B, Distally inclined canine which poses a more difficult problem.

corrected and it is necessary to have sufficient space available for the elimination of this small overjet. It may therefore be desirable to retract 3/3 very slightly further than would at first sight seem necessary.

The next stage is to move 2/2 over the bite and here a second removable appliance was used. It will be seen from Figure 9.2B that the posterior teeth have been covered with an occlusal bite plane in order to eliminate the overbite. In most cases, with the exception of those where there is an extremely deep overbite on the instanding teeth, it is not essential to 'gag' the bite in this way. Nevertheless, I feel that the elimination of the overbite, and of the occlusion which would otherwise oppose the action of the spring, must hasten treatment and make it somewhat less trau-

matic. If the posterior teeth are capped then this posterior bite plane should only be sufficiently thick to eliminate the overbite on the instanding teeth. In practice, this means that it has to be trimmed using articulating paper and a large acrylic burr and in most cases the posterior part of the bite block is perforated in some places during this procedure. It is advisable to draw the patient's attention to these holes, since otherwise he returns a few days later convinced that he has broken the appliance!

Following correction of 2/2 some mild irregularity of the upper incisors remained, with, as already explained, a small overjet of 1/1 and the canines slightly buccally placed. A third appliance, illustrated in Figure 9.2C, was therefore placed to complete alignment of the upper incisors, although this final alignment might well have occurred spontaneously over the ensuing months.

In the lower arch following the extraction of lower first premolars, no appliance therapy was instituted. The lower canines have a stronger tendency to drift distally than do the corresponding upper teeth and it is almost always good practice to leave the lower arch for a period following the extraction of premolars. During this time some natural reduction of crowding will take place and this may in a proportion of cases be sufficient to carry out the treatment required. Rotated incisors will seldom correct themselves spontaneously. If this practice is followed, however, a close watch should be kept on the lower arch with several points in mind.

1. At each visit the operator should check that there is still sufficient room for the lower incisors to align and indeed slightly more space than this. If the lower posterior teeth are moving mesially so as to endanger alignment of the lower incisors, a lower lingual arch may be fitted as a space maintainer. Indeed this may be done initially if anchorage is at all critical.

2. Again at each appointment, the lower labial segment should be checked to see that crowding is in fact reducing spontaneously. It is unlikely that this will continue for more than about 12 months after the extraction of the premolars. If natural alignment does not occur, or has ceased, then it will be necessary to fit a fixed appliance in the lower arch to retract the lower canines and

possibly to subsequently align the lower incisors.

3. A close watch should also be kept on the angulation of the lower second premolars. In some cases they tend to tilt mesially and to impact under the distal aspect of the lower canines. If this is occurring, then at the appropriate stage, a lower banded appliance should be inserted to upright the teeth and ensure a good contact point between the lower canines and second premolars.

The condition at the end of treatment and the final condition, when the patient was approaching 22 years of age, are seen in Figure 9.1. It will be noted that at the end of treatment some residual space remained between the canines and second premolars. In this case it was probably rather more than is desirable but spacing will usually close spontaneously and in the lower arch certainly it is good practice to leave a space of about 2–3 mm between the canine and second premolar as a 'safety valve' against late crowding of the lower labial segment. If the posterior occlusion is in Class I relation inevitably some spacing must be left in the upper arch also.

In this case no retention was considered necessary. As already indicated, prolonged retention is essential where rotation of teeth has been carried out, but labial and lingual movement of teeth does not usually require any great amount of retention. An exception to this is where a lower incisor has been substantially displaced in a lingual direction. If this corrects itself spontaneously following distal movement of the lower canines, then clearly no retention is needed. If, however, it is necessary to align the tooth by means of a fixed appliance, then it will have a strong tendency to relapse to some extent. To prevent this a lower lingual arch retainer should be fitted as shown in Figure 9.4. This consists of bands on the lower canines, or sometimes $\overline{2/2}$ or $\overline{4/4}$, and a 1 mm close-fitting lingual arch lying on the cingula of the incisors and soldered to these two bands. Alternatively, the arch may be bonded to the lingual surface of the appropriate teeth, and suitable equipment, with pads for direct bonding, is commercially available, in a selection of sizes. It may be necessary to wear such a retainer for about 12 months but the prolonged wearing of these appliances, as practised in some quarters, would seem to be undesirable.

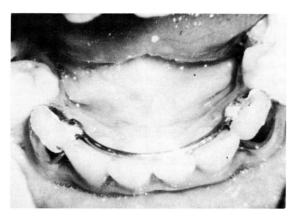

Fig. 9.4 Lower lingual arch on $\overline{3/3}$ to retain lingually placed lower incisors.

Serial extraction

In the previous section, it has been implied that the treatment of crowding is normally carried out in the complete permanent dentition. This practice has much to recommend it in the majority of cases. In 1948, Kjellgren suggested the technique which has come to be known as serial extraction as a method of intercepting crowding of the dentition at an early stage. Briefly, the technique consists of the extraction of four deciduous canines to allow some natural alignment of the crowded incisors. This is followed by the extraction of four deciduous molars to encourage the eruption of the first premolars which are then in their turn extracted.

It would seem that this technique has a limited application although it has been occasionally applied with some success. One should bear in mind that permanent incisors are usually somewhat crowded as they erupt and although this crowding disappears during their eruption, it may persist for a time after the incisors are fully erupted but still eventually correct itself. This is a rare occurrence and does not constitute a major snag. The principal objection would seem to be:

1. The extraction of deciduous canines, although relieving crowding in the labial segment, does in fact cause a slight mesial drift of the buccal segments and therefore a slight overall crowding in the arch.

2. It is somewhat unpredictable and requires monitoring at reasonably frequent intervals — say

every 3 months — and this is liable to use up the patient's cooperation.

3. Although it may produce a substantial amount of improvement, it is comparatively uncommon for this procedure to produce a perfect alignment and a shortened period of appliance therapy is likely to be necessary when all the teeth have erupted. This is less likely to be successful if the patient's co-operation has already been exhausted as indicated above.

4. The extraction of 12 teeth on three separate occasions is an ordeal for any child.

If it is proposed to follow this line of treatment, it is suggested that it should be confined to those cases with a Class I skeletal and dental pattern. Crowding should only be mild or moderate and preferably should not involve the rotation of any incisor teeth. The four deciduous canines are extracted first and this should not be carried out until at least two thirds of the roots of the permanent canines have calcified. Also before extracting any teeth, it should be checked radiographically, that all permanent teeth are present and are in their normal developmental position. The latter applies particularly to upper canines.

This extraction of deciduous canines will allow some natural alignment of the incisor teeth, especially in the lower arch. I have never been responsible for the extraction of first deciduous molars in this context and would recommend that this stage be eliminated. When the first premolars have erupted they may be extracted and as soon as this has been carried out, the posterior teeth will start to drift mesially, especially in the upper jaw. It is therefore essential to fit an upper space maintainer, usually in the form of a removable appliance with clasps on the first molars and an acrylic palate. It may conveniently carry a bite plane to commence overbite reduction. The condition is less urgent in the lower jaw and unless space is critical, it is usually sufficient to keep the dentition under observation. If space is, or becomes critical then the fitting of a lower lingual arch may act as a not wholly efficient space maintainer.

A patient in whom this technique was carried out is illustrated in Figure 9.5. In this case there was only mild crowding and space maintainers were not therefore fitted even in the upper jaw.

Nevertheless, the case was closely observed especially after the extraction of the first premolars. It will be seen from the superimposed tracings in Figure 9.5B that the distal drifting of the permanent canine is noticeably more marked in the lower than in the upper jaw.

Modifications of this technique have been used. In particular the last stage, that is the early extraction of four first premolars shortly after their eruption, can play a useful part to allow some spontaneous alignment in many cases of comparatively mild crowding. Here again, however, the need for space maintenance, especially in the upper jaw, should be borne in mind.

It has been suggested, not normally by orthodontists, that crowding may be eliminated by the early extraction of first deciduous molars and the surgical removal of the developing first premolars at the same time. This involves the admission of the child to hospital, which is a procedure always to be avoided where possible. Moreover, the removal of alveolar bone which is inevitable if unerupted premolars are to be extracted, is liable to lead to a poor contact point between the canine and second premolar at a later stage. It is unlikely to provide a complete alignment of teeth but would involve the wearing of a space maintainer for a prolonged period, or more probably the loss of space due to the patient's failure to wear this. I can see nothing to recommend this barbarous practice.

SPACING OF TEETH

A generalised spacing of teeth, at least in Western Europe is an uncommon occurrence and one which cannot satisfactorily be treated orthodontically. A case such as that shown in Figure 9.6A is probably best treated by our conservative colleagues. In this case the upper central and lateral incisors were built up with composite resins to produce the result shown in Figure 9.6B. Occasionally, orthodontic assistance is required to close the anterior spaces and to localise remaining space, usually between the canine and first premolar, where a bridge may be fitted to effectively insert an additional tooth on each side. This would normally be confined to the upper arch.

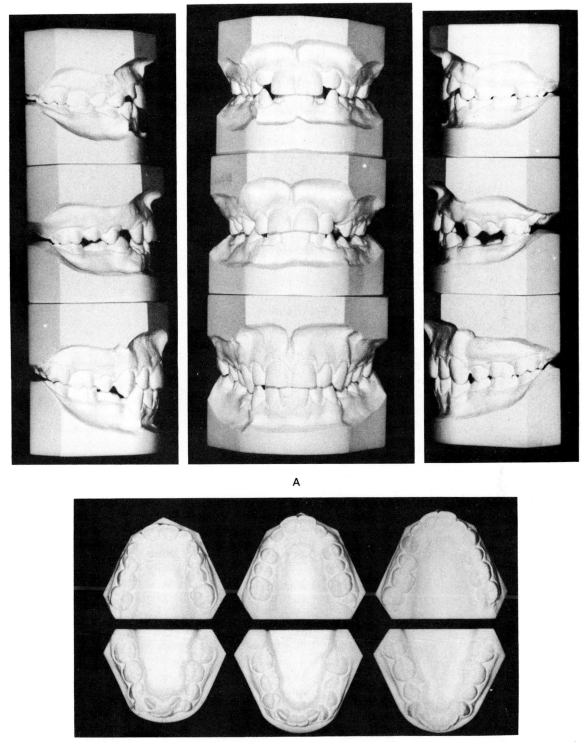

A

Fig. 9.5 Gary, treated by serial extraction of deciduous canines and the first premolars. A, Note the macrodent lower second premolars. B, Lateral skull tracings of final condition superimposed on the initial tracing. Note the distal drifting of canines, shown by heavy outline in initial tracing and cross-hatched in later one (overleaf).

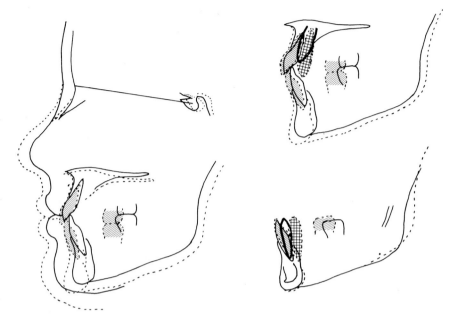

Fig. 9.5 (*Cont'd*)

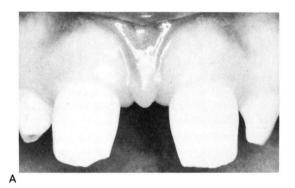

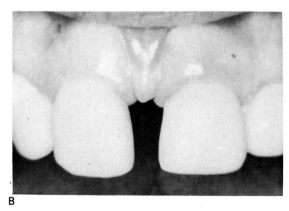

Fig. 9.6 A, Generalised spacing of the teeth with microdont 2/2. B, The same after building up of incisors with composite material.

Of more frequent occurrence is the median diastema in the upper arch. This is one of the more trying occurrences to befall the orthodontist. Closure of the space is easy but it is very much more difficult to prevent it from re-opening.

The teeth throughout the dental arch generally are held in contact by the transeptal fibres of the periodontal membrane. If a tooth is extracted the transeptal fibres reform between the remaining teeth and tend to pull these together. Although no histological evidene is available, clinically it would appear that this factor does not usually operate between the two upper central incisors. If therefore there is a lack of mesial pressure on the distal contact points of the upper central incisors, a space will normally exist between them. This lack of pressure may be due to generally small teeth, small lateral incisors, absent lateral incisors or the existence of an overjet in an uncrowded mouth. Even in the absence of this pressure, the central incisors may remain in contact and it is tempting to believe that in such cases the suture has closed prematurely.

The existence of a median diastema is frequently blamed on persistence of a labial fraenum and this blame is often unjust. As described in detail in Chapter 4, at birth the labial fraenum is attached to the incisive papilla, dividing the labial sulcus into two. When the deciduous incisors erupt they are usually spaced and the fraenum remains. When they are replaced by the permanent incisors these are normally in contact and the fraenum recedes. If however the space remains between the central incisors then the fraenum will remain attached to the incisive papilla and in the vast majority of cases is not the cause of the diastema but rather an effect. The large space between the two central incisors in Figure 9.6 is not the result of the low fraenum but clearly derives from the small size of the teeth. The space is far too wide to be caused by the fraenum.

It does seem however that occasionally a fraenum is seen which actually causes the diastema. Such a case was shown in Figure 4.15. Here the fraenum runs directly horizontally from the crest of the alveolus to be attached to the vermilion margin of the lip dividing the labial sulcus into two. It is the same width as the space between the teeth or very slightly narrower, while the anterior teeth generally are crowded rather than spaced. The radiograph shown in Figure 4.15B is diagnostic. There is no alveolar crest between the two central incisors but rather a 'V' shaped defect which is of course occupied by the fibrous tissue of the fraenum. In these very rare cases it would seem advisable to remove the fraenum, dissecting out the material thoroughly between the two central incisors and improving hygiene locally by establishing a labial sulcus in the mid-line. In such a case the incisors will tend to close of their own accord or may be brought together by means of an appliance. Even in such a case, the prognosis for complete permanent closure should be guarded, although the width of the diastema will certainly be reduced.

There can be little doubt that a very large number of fraenectomies have been performed unnecesarily. Bergstrom and co-workers (1973) have followed up the result of fraenectomy and shown that after a short time span the diastema had closed more effectively in those cases where the fraenectomy had been carried out than in a comparable group where it had not. However, by the end of the teens there was no difference between the two groups and in fact in many cases mid-line diastemata do close without treatment. In those where they do not, premanent closure is difficult to achieve.

Recently various methods have been recommended for permanently retaining such a contact between the two central incisors using composite resins. Merely to stick the two teeth together with a composite resin is not adequate and the material, being rather brittle breaks down in weeks or months.

It has been suggested that the teeth should actually be held together with something more flexible, such as closely fitting stainless steel gauze or multistrand wire (Fig. 9.7A). This would then be attached to the two teeth with composite filling material. This appears more satisfactory, but unless oral hygiene is scrupulous, there is some danger of plaque collecting around the composite material with decalcification such as can occur, all too easily, around directly bonded attachments on the more accessible labial surfaces of the teeth.

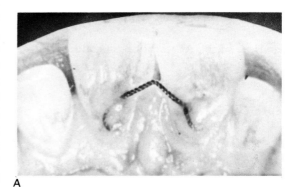

A

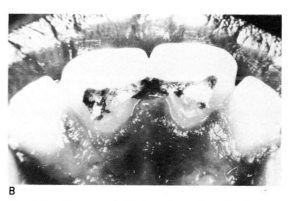

B

Fig. 9.7 A, Upper central incisors fastened together by multistrand wire bonded to the lingual surfaces of the teeth. B, Incisors held together by gold pinlays in their lingual surfaces.

Alternatively, gold inlays which are fused together may be inserted (Fig. 9.7B). The danger with all these procedures is that, with the slight mobility of the teeth, one attachement may become loose while the other remains fixed, with resultant caries in the one which has failed. The inlays in Figure 9.7B are retained by means of pins, and a simple 'key' would be quite inadequate for this purpose.

DISPLACED CANINES

The upper permanent canine tooth commences its calcification within the first year of life, before that of the lateral incisor. Like all permanent teeth the formation of the tooth germ commences on the lingual side of the deciduous tooth and from this position the developing canine has a long and tortuous journey to eruption. It must first move labially over the roots of the deciduous teeth to take up a position in the labial sulcus usually somewhat mesial of its final position. By the time that the permanent lateral incisor has erupted the canine is often lying over the distal aspect of the root of the lateral. It erupts after its neighbours and if there is a shortage of space it will tend to be crowded out of the arch.

It is emphasised that when any patient first presents, the presence and position of all unerupted teeth should be identified. This is particularly true in the case of permanent canines. If there is any doubt about the position of the unerupted tooth the following procedure should be carried out:

1. The initial examination should be clinical. In many cases it is possible to identify the position of the unerupted canine in the labial sulcus by means of palpation. It is often possible to locate the tooth from an evident bulge in the labial sulcus, but care is necessary. Where a canine is displaced the root of the deciduous tooth may not have resorbed normally and the resultant canine eminence may be mistaken for an unerupted permanent tooth. If the canine is displaced palatally, palpation may serve to confirm a diagnosis made by other means, but it is never reliable as the sole means of positioning the tooth. A more reliable indication comes from the angulation of

adjacent teeth and especially of the upper lateral incisor. The crown of the permanent canine will have the effect of displacing the root of the lateral incisor and its crown will therefore usually be displaced in the opposite direction. This can be seen in Figure 9.8, where the distal 'fanning' of the lateral incisor would indicate that the crown of the canine is lying on the distal aspect of its root. Subsequent surgical exposure has confirmed this.

2. The main part of the diagnosis must inevitably be radiographic. A single intra-oral X-ray, as shown for the two sides of the same mouth in Figure 9.9A will give limited information. It will indicate that the two permanent canines are present (and occasionally permanent canines are congenitally absent even where all the teeth otherwise are present in the mouth). It shows that they are to some extent related to the root apices of the lateral incisors but gives no indication whether they are on the labial or palatal side or directly distal. It will be noticed in this figure, that on the right hand side the deciduous canine has resorbed almost completely and that between it and the crown of the permanent canine is a black area with no bone present. This can be taken as some evidence that the permanent canine is erupting in the desired direction, whereas on the other side of the mouth although the decidous canine has resorbed to some extent, there is bone and even a lamina dura around the whole of the

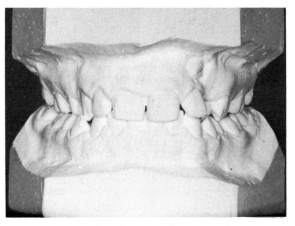

Fig. 9.8 Note the distal fanning of /2 and lingual displacement of its root apex indicating the position of the crown of /3. This tooth has been surgically exposed.

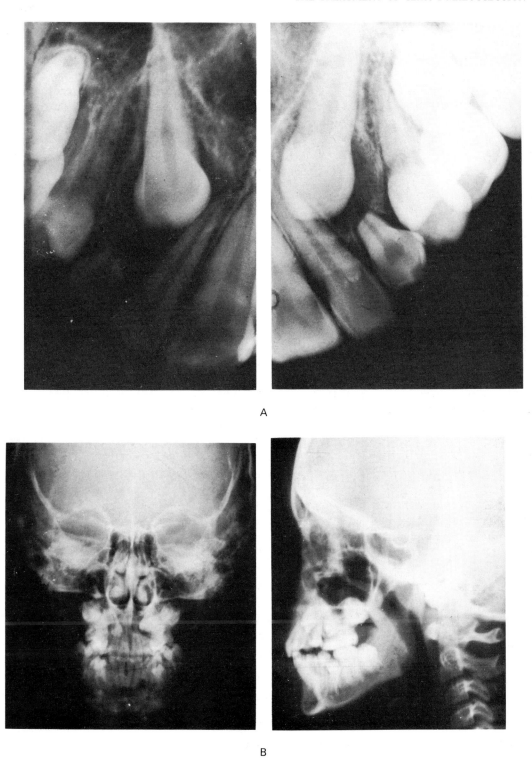

A

B

Fig. 9.9 A, Intra-oral radiographs of two buried canines, apparently in similar positions. B, Postero-anterior and lateral skull radiographs indicating that 3/ is palatally but /3 labially placed. C, Study models taken after the teeth had been surgically exposed (overleaf).

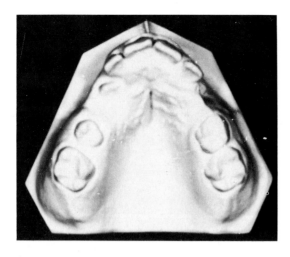

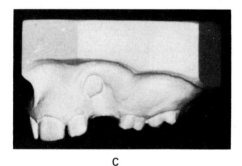

C

Fig. 9.9 (*contd*)

root, and it would seem that the permanent canine is no longer moving towards its correct position. If the unerupted canine appears somewhat fore-shortened (which is not the case here) this is an indication that it is displaced in a labio-palatal direction.

Probably the best method of positioning the unerupted tooth is by means of a lateral skull radiograph and a corresponding postero-anterior radiograph. These are shown for the same patient in Figure 9.9B. In the postero-anterior radiograph on the left, both permanent canines appear well above the occlusal plane with that on the patient's left being higher than the one on his right. They therefore indicate the position of these two teeth in two dimensions: they are too close to the mid-line and too high. Turning now to the lateral skull radiograph the two teeth may be identified since the higher one is on the patient's left. Quite

clearly the lower one, on the patient's right, is placed somewhat lingually to the root of the lateral incisor but the higher one would appear to be lying over the apex of the lateral and therefore in the labial sulcus, although at a very high level. Both these teeth were surgically exposed and the study model in Figure 9.9C shows their actual location. It is appreciated that not all orthodontists have the necessary cephalostat for the taking of true skull radiographs, but the same effect can be achieved with care by the use of a half-plate cassette. The patient steadies this on top of the headrest of the chair, placing the side of this face against the cassette, and the tube is centred over the first permanent molar. The second film is taken with the cassette touching the patient's nose, again steadied on top of the headrest, and the tube at the back of the patient's head.

These two pictures will give a clear indication of the position of the permanent canine and, with a single intra-oral radiograph, are often all that are required. If, however, there is any doubt about the relationship of the permanent canine crown to the roots of the adjacent teeth, then a second intra-oral film should be taken. The usual problem concerns the relative position of the canine and the root of the lateral incisor. Two intra-oral radio-graphs are taken as shown in Figure 9.10A using the 'tube shift' method of localisation. Ideally, the films should be placed in the identical position for both exposure, although some liberties may be taken. In this case the films have also been used to give a detailed outline of the teeth, but suffi-cient overlap is present to use the principle of parallax Considering the patient's right canine (on the left of the picture), and looking first at the left-hand radiograph, the tip of its crown exactly superimposes on the pulp-chamber of the central incisor. The central ray has been pointed at the bone between the central and lateral incisors on that side. Turning to the right-hand radiograph, the central ray is now pointing at the opposite lateral incisor, the right canine now overlies the mid-line suture of the maxilla, that is, it has moved in the same direction as the tube. A little thought, or a few moments experimenting with two pencils held vertically in front of one eye, will indicate that the canine is closer to the film than its neighbours, that is, it is palatally placed.

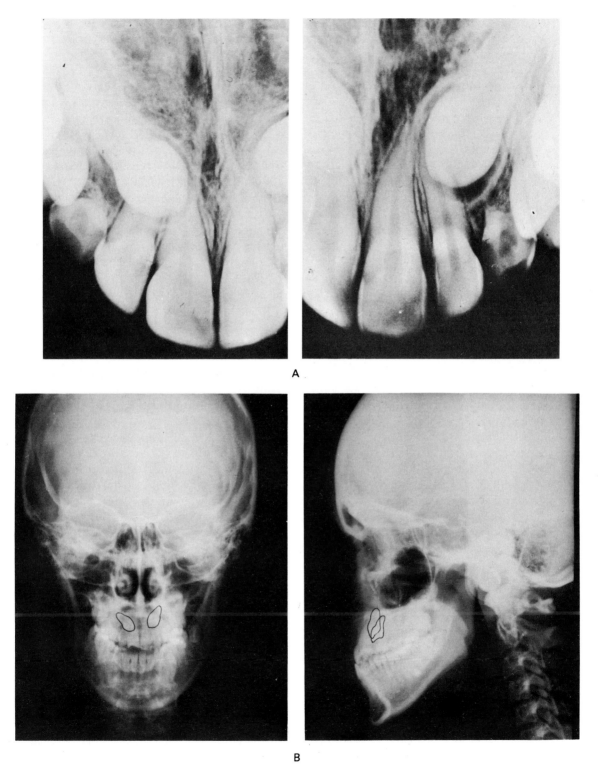

Fig. 9.10 A, 'Tube-shift' radiographs of Miriam to isolate position of 3/3. B, Postero-anterior and lateral skull radiographs of the same patient. The canines have been outlined.

Applying the same principle to the opposite canine, the same result is achieved, although the canine apparently moves somewhat more than its fellow. This would indicate that its displacement from the arch is greater. If the buried tooth does not appear to move relative to its neighbours, and the tube has been moved adequately between the two exposures, then the canine is in the line of the arch. If it moves in the opposite direction it is, of course, labial to its neighbours.

Turning to the individual radiographs, it can be seen that there is no obvious resorption of adjacent teeth, that the crypts of the developing canines are of normal size, that their roots are normal in shape and size. The deciduous canines have largely resorbed, but this process has ceased and bone is present against the resorbed surfaces of roots: the buried canines are not moving in the right direction.

Turning to the skull radiographs in Figure 9.10B, in the postero-anterior view on the left it will be seen that the crowns of the canines are lying above the contact points between the central and lateral incisors, with that on the patient's left being substantially higher than its opposite number. From the lateral view the palatal position of both is confirmed.

A method formerly much favoured for positioning these teeth is the vertex occlusal radiograph. This method is in fact very far from satisfactory. An occlusal radiograph involves a heavy X-ray dosage and moreover the centre ray is pointing directly downwards towards the gonads. On these grounds alone it is undesirable. To be of any value at all the X-rays must pass directly down the full length of the pulp chambers of the adjacent teeth. This is not easy to achieve and even then merely tells one whether the canine is labially or buccally placed and gives no idea of its accurate position. Unfortunately, in many cases although the rays appear to go down the pulp chambers of most of the incisor teeth, the lateral incisor is slightly elongated, since it is not parallel to the remaining incisors and the picture is then obscure. The condition shown in Figure 9.8 is a case in point. An occlusal radiograph in this case would very probably show the canine tooth to be palatal to the general line of the arch and one has known of cases where this has given rise to misinterpretation

and an approach being made from the palatal side only to reveal the root of a lateral incisor.

Labially placed canines

Generally speaking those canines which are placed labially to the line of the arch are either very easy to correct or very difficult. The vast majority erupt in the labial sulcus from which they can be moved into their correct position (examples are seen in Fig. 9.3). A few however, lie very high in the labial sulcus as in Figure 9.9 and 9.11. In this case they have comparatively little tendency to erupt and it is necessary to use orthodontic means to bring them down into the line of the arch. A suitable appliance, either fixed or removable, is constructed with a stout wire lying in the labial sulcus and attached to a crib or band on the first molar on the appropriate side. If a fixed appliance is used a lingual arch should connect this molar to that on the opposite side. The canine is then exposed conservatively (Fig. 9.11A) so as to leave an area of the surface of the tooth visible in the mouth and a pack is inserted while healing takes place — for a couple of weeks. It is then necessary to attach some form of hook to the very partially erupted tooth. In the present case, /3 of the case illustrated in Figure 9.9, and treated some years ago, a silver cap was made (Fig. 9.11B and C). A good alginate impression was taken of the whole mouth extending up into this area and a small cap, with the appropriate hook, fashioned in inlay wax and cast in silver. This can then be cemented with oxyphosphate cement to the tooth and traction applied to it by means of an elastic band. Alternatively, an orthodontic attachment, such as a Begg bracket, or lingual button, may be directly bonded to the exposed tooth and is a simpler method of doing the same operation, provided an adequately dry field can be obtained. In either case, a tooth may be brought down as shown in Figure 9.11D, and finally positioned in the arch.

In considering the exposure of any tooth in the labial sulcus, two structures should be safeguarded to the maximum. The outer plate of alveolar bone does not regenerate if lost, nor does the keratinised attached gingiva. Any exposure should therefore be minimal. A possible technique is the make the incision for the unerupted tooth as low down,

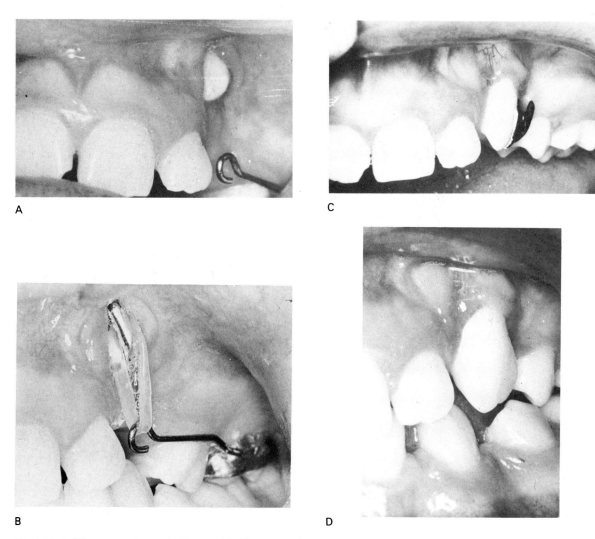

Fig. 9.11 A, The same patient as is illustrated in Fig. 9.9. A, /3 has been exposed. B, Silver cap cemented to the tooth and gentle traction applied. C, The tooth almost in position. Note silver cap and also unkeratinised gingival tissue. D, Finally positioned tooth.

towards the final position of the tooth, as possible. The gingival is then displaced and bunched upward and sutured towards the gingival margin of the crown. Minimal bone should be removed. The technique is not easy but good results have been obtained. An alternative is to reflect a flap and bond an attachment to the crown of the tooth (a Begg bracket is ideal). Two pieces of ligature wire are then attached through the hole in the bracket and the flap replaced. Gentle traction will then cause the tooth to erupt — provided that the bracket remains attached to the tooth!

In the present case although the result is an excellent one, the gingiva is not fully keratinised, as may be seen in Figure 9.11C, and the clinical crown is somewhat elongated.

Palatally placed canines

These present rather more of a problem in decision-making, since they vary in position from very mild displacement to virtually horizontal. The radiographs of Miriam have already been considered in Figure 9.10 where it was seen that the two canines were palatally placed to a considerable extent, and were quite high relative to the adjacent teeth. The left canine, in particular, is close to the limit which I would recommend for orthodontic correction. Other factors will enter into the decision. A keen and co-operative patient is essential for this procedure. If the lateral incisor and first premolar are already in, or close to, contact in a crowded mouth, then such an appearance may be acceptable (but not in conjunction with a deep overbite of the incisors). It is usual to state that the root apex should lie in its correct position, but in fact it is seldom otherwise.

The first stage in repositioning the tooth is its surgical exposure. This should be much wider than in the labial sulcus; the whole surface (usually the lingual one) of the crown should be uncovered, with a little bone removed down the sides of the tooth. The wound should then be packed with a zinc-oxide based dressing, which should be left in place for 2 weeks and then removed.

Orthodontists are acutely conscious of the fact that bone is a most labile tissue, but oral surgeons have less experience of this aspect of it. Left to their own devices they are apt to 'help things along' by digging channels through the alveolus for the passage of the tooth, and by 'giving it a shake'. These procedures are both counter-productive and should be discouraged.

When the packs are removed, the canines will be in view (Fig. 9.12B). They should then be allowed to erupt naturally, usually for about 3 months, until they reach the stage seen in Figure 9.12. Various techniques involving pins, screws, and chains have been evolved to pull these teeth down. All are successful, since the tooth will erupt adequately without them.

It is then necessary to move the teeth to their final positions. If they are grossly displaced, as in Miriam's case, this should be commenced from the lingual aspect. Removable appliances are not always satisfactory and I prefer to use a lingual arch with auxiliary springs (Fig. 9.12C). Such a spring will tend to slip over the tooth, and also to depress it. These may be prevented by bonding a suitable attachment to the tooth, under which the spring lies. Not only does this prevent

depression of the tooth, but its eruption can be mildly encouraged.

When the tooth is close to the line of the arch it may be finally positioned from the labial side, often using a banded appliance which has already been employed to provide adequate space for the tooth. It is not unusual for a palatally displaced canine to be severely rotated, and this may be corrected at this stage. Also, the root apex may be palatally displaced, and this should also be corrected. If the clinical crown appears short, a little trimming of the gingival margin is indicated.

The final condition for Miriam is seen in Figure 9.12E.

Resorption of adjacent teeth

Occasionally it will be found that the unerupted canine has caused the resorption of the root of the lateral and even the central incisors. This is very uncommon and would seem only to occur when the canine is unable to escape from a head-on collision with the root of the affected tooth. It would seem to occur at a very early stage and if no resorption is present by the tenth birthday, it can safely be assumed that it will not develop. Where the canine is well to the lingual or labial of adjacent teeth all is safe. If the displaced canine is identified at an early age when it is high in the alveolus, it is not usually advisable to interfere but the tooth should be kept under observation by 6-monthly radiographs. Occasionally, a quite badly displaced tooth will erupt normally and in most cases its position will improve substantially so that exposure can take place when it is closer to the surface.

Transplantation of canines

The transplantation of teeth is by no means new and over the centuries has acquired an unfortunate reputation. Recently, it has again been attempted apparently with rather greater success. It would seem to be a possible solution in cases where the canine is so displaced that it cannot be corrected by orthodontic means or where the patient is unwilling to persevere to the requisite extent. The important feature in achieving success would seem to be that the tooth should be handled as little as

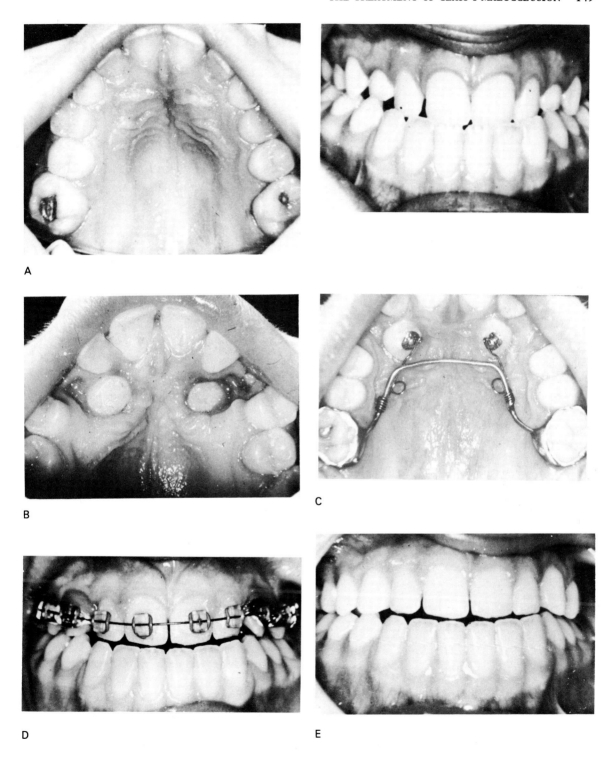

Fig. 9.12 Intra-oral photographs showing treatment of buried canines for Miriam. A, Before treatment: note mild Class III malocclusion. B, Shortly after exposure of 3/3. C, Palatal arch in place to commence tooth movement. D, Teeth have been finally positioned by banded appliance. E, Final condition after treatment.

possible (and the root not at all) and that it should not be allowed to dry. The tooth is first removed carefully from the bone, with the minimum of trauma. Some authorities believe that the best chance of success is obtained if a quantity of the patient's blood is converted into serum and the tooth placed immediately into this at body temperature. A socket is then produced in the appropriate part of the alveolus and the tooth firmly pushed into the sockot where it may be splinted, either by means of a silver cap splint or from bands on adjacent teeth. No attempt should be made to root-fill the tooth at this stage and indeed such a procedure should only be carried out if the tooth becomes obviously infected. While the success rate has improved from this approach, the patient should be warned that the prognosis is by no means perfect and resorption with anky-losis does occur in many cases, often some years after the operation.

SUPERNUMERARY TEETH

The importance of supernumerary teeth in the aetiology of malocclusion has already been discussed at some length in Chapter 4. In this section it is proposed to confine discussion to those supernumeraries occurring near the mid-line in the upper arch. As previously indicated, these fall into two broad types. The first which is usually peg-shaped, is associated with a displace-ment of the central incisor of the same side. This displacement may involve the crown, the root or both. The supernumerary tooth itself may have erupted but is frequently lying unerupted and usually on the palatal side of the remaining incisor teeth. If one or both central incisors is displaced, and there is no obvious reason for this displace-ment, then an intra-oral radiograph should always be taken to eliminate the possibility of one of these small supernumeraries. This applies particularly if the roots are displaced as seen in Figure 4.11. If a supernumerary is revealed then its position should be ascertained in much the same way as we have already described for unerupted permanent canines. It may then be removed, usually from the palatal aspect, and the appropriate teeth aligned. Unfortunately, where the teeth are displaced in

association with a supernumerary tooth, they show tittle tendency to stay in the correct position when this has been achieved, and prolonged retention is required.

Rather more may be said about the second type of supernumerary which is usually of more defi-nite shape, resembling a small incisor or even a molar, and is a associated with a failure of a corresponding central incisor to erupt. The typical picture is of a patient presenting at an age when one would expect the central to be present and when the remaining incisors have erupted. There is no history of the missing tooth having been extracted and the space for it may well have closed to a greater or lesser extent. Occasionally (as in Fig. 9.13) the condition is bilateral.

As in all orthodontic conditions, the first exam-ination should be clinical. Palpation of the area where one would expect to find the central incisor occasionally reveals its outline lying just under the mucosa. In these conditions it does not usually erupt within the next few weeks as one might expect. The palpation should be carried up into the labial sulcus and in some cases the outline of the tooth may be felt in this situation. Neverthe-less, the main part of the examination will inevi-tably be radiographic. There is much to be said for an initial intra-oral radiograph to give some idea of what is happening and to allow a differ-ential diagnosis of the various possible reasons for the absence of the tooth from the mouth. The principal such reasons are:

1. The central incisor may have failed to develop normally and may be revealed in the form of a grossly dilacerated tooth. Where this is found it is usually associated with a history of an acci-dent in infancy to this part of the mouth but such a history cannot always be elicited. In theory the tooth may be represented as an odontome although I have personally never seen such a case.

2. Occasionally a perfectly normal central incisor simply fails to erupt for no very good reason. When space is made it comes down and it may be in these cases that the lateral incisor has erupted before the central, moved mesially and impacted it.

3. There is a possibility of the tooth becoming involved in a dentigerous cyst or with a neoplasm

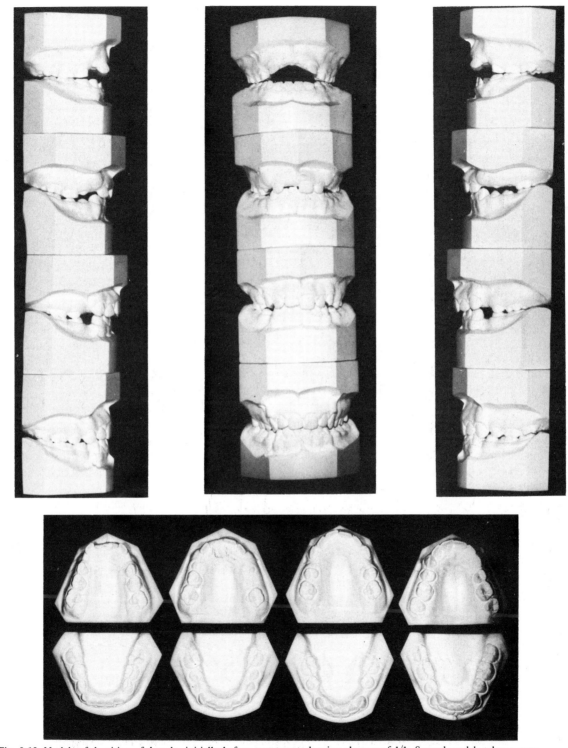

Fig. 9.13 Models of dentition of Angela, initially before treatment, showing absence of 1/1. Second models taken a year after removal of supernumeraries. /1 has erupted but not 1/, which was then conservatively exposed. Third models taken three months later. Final models 12 months after all appliances removed.

of a more sinister nature, although again, such a condition is excessively rare.

4. In practice, where such a history is elicited of the failure of the central incisor to erupt, it is almost invariably due to the associated presence of a supernumerary tooth.

If such a tooth is found it is then again necessary to locate its exact position. It is usually either lying on the palatal side of the permanent incisor or between the two central incisors. A lateral skull radiograph will show its position fairly accurately and this may be supplemented by a postero-anterior radiograph, although these are not always very clear in this situation and probably a second intra-oral radiograph using the tube shift technique (Fig. 9.14A) is equally satisfactory.

Treatment

The first stage of treatment in this type of case is to remove the supernumerary tooth, preferably from the palatal aspect. Having done this, the wound is then sutured closed. It cannot be emphasised too strongly that the unerupted tooth should not be exposed at this stage. This applies particularly if the tooth is lying high in the labial sulcus and it should always be remembered that the outer plate of bone is the tooth's most valuable possession, but its second most valuable is the labial mucosa. If the tooth is allowed or encouraged to erupt through the labial plate of bone, difficulty may be encountered in persuading the tooth to come down to its normal level. In some cases, in fact, it may fail to do so. A typical case is shown in Figure 9.15A. The left central incisor following removal of an associated supernumerary, erupted spontaneously in the labial sulcus from which position it gradually came down into approximately the situation shown. It would be noted that its clinical crown is somewhat longer than that of the contralateral central incisor although this condition is often more extreme than is seen here. Since the tooth failed to move further, an appliance was fitted, which without difficulty, brought the tooth down into line with the remaining incisors and indeed it was taken a little further so as to overcorrect the condition. The bands were left on the incisor teeth so that

the left central could be retained for a total of 6 months. The bands were then removed and within a very short time the tooth had returned to the position seen here.

So the supernumerary teeth are removed and orthodontic treatment instituted as necessary in order to make sufficient space in the arch for the central incisor or incisors to erupt. This may involve the extraction of premolars or in a younger child, of the upper deciduous canines. It is then necessary to wait. In the case shown in Figures 9.13 and 9.14, the left central incisor erupted after 3 months into a good position but 13 months later still, the upper right central incisor had not erupted. By this stage the tooth had moved down to lie only just under the mucosa and in a proportion of cases, this will happen but the tooth will then stop, apparently lacking the eruptive power to penetrate the mucous membrane. At this stage it is advisable to expose the crown but this should be done very conservatively. It is only necessary to make a half-moon-shaped opening around the incisal edge and in many cases the incision can be made more or less along the incisal edge with a piece of gingiva removed on the lingual rather than on the labial side of the tooth. With this assistance, the tooth will usually erupt and in fact in the case shown in Figure 9.13, it had come down to the position seen in the third set of study models only three months after the exposure.

It has already been stated that where the peg-shaped type of tooth has caused displacement of the permanent incisor, then these teeth show little tendency to remain aligned after their correction. With this second type of supernumerary, however, the permanent incisor will often erupt normally and into a good position requiring only a minimal amount of orthodontic treatment, if any, to align it completely.

Occasionally, the affected central will erupt through the labial plate of bone and move down a short distance and will then stop. In such a case a suitable attachment should be placed on the tooth, either as in Figure 9.15B, by means of a band or more probably nowadays, by direct bonding. Very gentle elastic traction will then usually bring the tooth down, although as already indicated, some problem may arise in keeping it at its correct final position. It is emphasised that

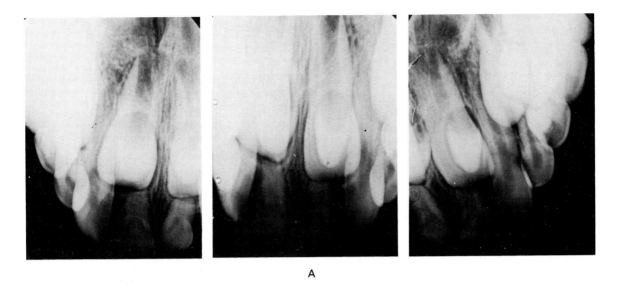

A

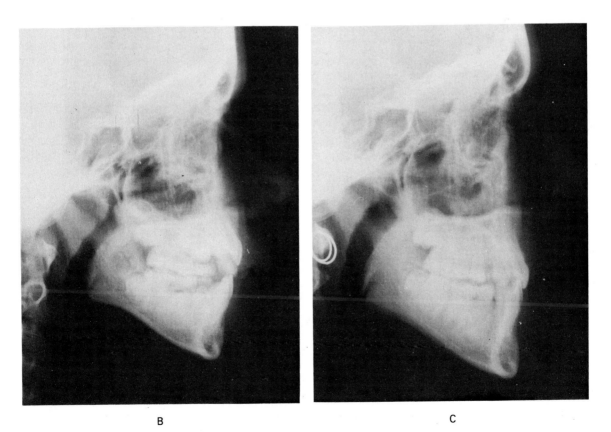

B   C

Fig. 9.14 A, Intra-oral radiographs of $\underline{1}/1$ of Angela, to show tube-shift method of positioning supernumeraries. B, Section of lateral skull radiograph; the central incisors are in a good position for eruption. C, Second lateral skull radiograph to show final position of $\underline{1}/1$.

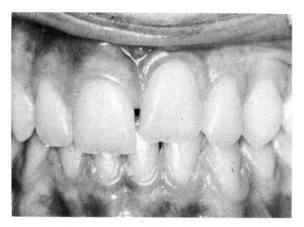

A

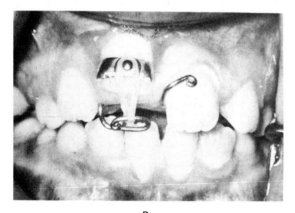

B

Fig. 9.15 A, Following removal of a supernumerary tooth /1 erupted and came down to about this height. Following correction by appliance, it relapsed as shown. Note long clinical crown. B, 1/ erupted as shown but failed to move further when space had been provided. Band fitted to tooth and traction to removable appliance. Note very gentle elastic force.

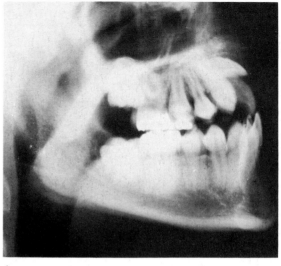

A

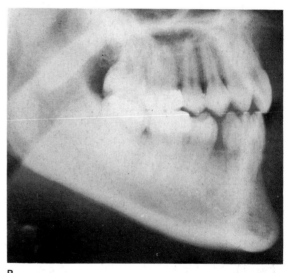

B

Fig. 9.16 A, Upper central incisor lying horizontally placed in the floor of the nose, associated with supernumerary. B, Position to which the tooth erupted when adequate space was made. No form of traction was employed.

the elastic force should be minimal to encourage the mucosa to follow the tooth.

The case shown in Figure 9.13 was a straight-forward one. The permanent central incisors were both in a good position for eruption (Fig. 9.14B). Cases will sometimes be seen where the central incisor is lying horizontal or even beyond the horizontal position in the floor of the nose. Provided the tooth is of normal shape and size, and the patient is still a child, it is well worth while carrying out the normal procedure of removing the supernumerary tooth and creating

sufficient space (and preferably rather more than sufficient space) for it to erupt. Apparently hope-lessly positioned teeth will often come down into the arch with little or no assistance, although in such a case the prognosis should obviously be somewhat guarded. Such a case is shown in Figure 9.16.

SUGGESTED READING

Bergstrom K, Jensen R, Martensen B 1973 The effect of superior labial frenectomy in cases of midline diastema. American Journal of Orthodontics 63: 633–8

Broadway R T, Gould D G 1960 Surgical requirements of the orthodontist. British Dental Journal 108: 187–93

Chan K C, Andreasen G F 1975 Conservative retention for spaced maxillary central incisors. American Journal of Orthodontics 67: 324–9

Dewel B F 1969 Pre-requisites in serial extraction. American Journal of Orthodontics 55: 633–9

Edwards J G 1970 A surgical procedure to eliminate rotational relapse. American Journal of Orthodontics 57: 35–46

Kjellgren B 1948 Serial extraction as a corrective procedure in dental orthopedic therapy. Transactions of the European Orthodontic Society 134–60

Moorrees C F A, Fanning E A, Grøn A M 1963 The consideration of dental development in serial extraction. Angle Orthodontist 33: 44–59

Perston C M 1973 Periodic observation of the relapse of upper incisors which had been rotated with an appliance. Journal of Dentistry 1: 125–33

Pinson R R Strahan J D 1974 The effect on the relapse of orthodontically rotated teeth of surgical division of the gingival fibres — pericision. British Journal of Orthodontics 1: 87–92

Reinhardt J W, Denehy G E, Chan K C 1979 Acid etch bonded case orthodontic retainers. American Journal of Orthodontics 75: 138–42

Ringenberg Q M 1967 Influence of serial extraction on growth and development of the maxilla and mandible. American Journal of Orthodontics 53: 19–26

Thonner K E 1970 Autogenous transplantation of unerupted maxillary canines: a clinical and histological investigation over five years. Transactions of the British Society for the Study of Orthodontics 56: 159–65

Wraith K W L 1969 Methods of repositioning the misplaced canine. Dental Practitioner 19: 387–93

10

The treatment of Class II Division 1 malocclusion

Angle's original definition of malocclusion was based on the relationship of the first permanent molars so that in Class II malocclusion the mesio-buccal cusps of the lower first permanent molar occluded between the two buccal cusps of the upper first permanent molar, that is the occlusion was postnormal by the width of one cusp. Division 1 involves those cases where there is an increased overjet. The more recent British Standard classification is based solely on incisor relationship. It defines Class II as 'the lower incisor edges lie posterior to the cingulum plateau of the upper incisors'. Division 1 is defined as 'there is an increase in overjet and the upper central incisors are usually proclined'.

AETIOLOGY

The cause of Class II Division 1 malocclusion results from the interaction, to a greater or lesser extent, of the three main factors:

Skeletal pattern

The skeletal pattern can fall into any of the three classes shown in Figure 10.1, but we usually find that the patient has a Class II skeletal pattern. In its simplest form, an individual may inherit a large maxilla and small mandible resulting in an antero-posterior discrepancy between the dental bases. However, it has been shown by several authors, including Bjork (1974) and James (1963) that the discrepancy more often lies remote from the jaws themselves. An abnormality in the base of the skull can ensure that the horizontal distance from the glenoid fossa to the maxilla is too great for the particular individual. Thus, a mandible of size comparable to the maxilla is placed too far posteriorly for normal occlusion to develop, the lower teeth erupting in a position posterior to that which will produce a normal occlusion. As soon as they erupt they come under the influence of the soft tissues as will be described in the next section.

The vertical relationship of dental bases is also of importance, especially in assessing the prognosis. As soon as they erupt as we shall see later, those cases with a large lower facial height and also those with an exceptionally small lower facial heights, give rise to difficulties in treatment and stability.

The soft tissues

As soon as the teeth erupt into the mouth, they come under the influence of the soft tissues. If the lips are competent and the skeletal pattern within normal limits, the effect of the lips, and secondarily of the tongue, will be to bring the incisor teeth together into a normal relationship. If the lips are incompetent, as already described in Chapter 3, the patient may find some difficulty in providing a seal by bringing them together. This applies especially if there is a Class II skeletal pattern. In such a case the seal may well be formed by contact between the lower lip and the tongue. If the lower facial height is reduced then the seal will largely be provided by the lower lip resting against the lower incisors and under the erupting upper incisors as shown in Figure 3.7. The overjet which has been produced by the skeletal pattern is worsened by the action of the lower lip which may procline the upper incisors and to some extent retrocline the lowers. On the other

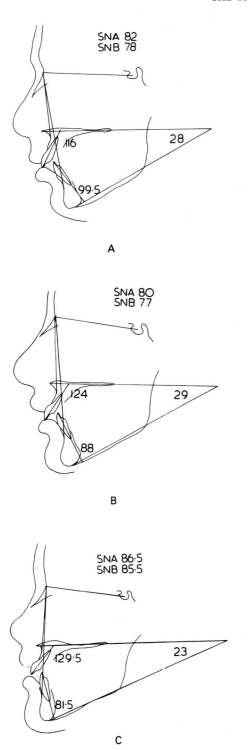

SNA 82
SNB 78

16   28

99·5

A

SNA 80
SNB 77

24   29

88

B

SNA 86·5
SNB 85·5

29·5   23

81·5

C

Fig. 10.1 Lateral skull tracings to show Class II Division 1 malocclusion on: A, Class II skeletal pattern, B, Class I skeletal pattern and C, Class III skeletal pattern.

hand, if the lip line is not unduly high, it can be used to advantage as a permanent retainer to maintain the position of the upper incisors following their retraction. If, however, the lower facial height is increased, then the lower lip will probably lie in a low position relative to the upper incisors. In this case the anterior seal will largely be provided by the tongue which may exacerbate any tendency to an incomplete overbite but will not affect the upper incisors which will be essentially at their normal angle to their base. The overjet will exactly reflect the skeletal pattern and when it has been reduced the lower lip will do nothing to maintain the new position of the teeth. It will be seen that the soft tissues may therefore serve to worsen a malocclusion produced by the skeletal pattern but it should not be forgotten that they may have the reverse affect and to some extent compensate for the skeletal discrepancy. It is by no means uncommon to find that the lower incisors are proclined where the skeletal pattern is Class II and, as discussed in the next chapter, the upper incisors may also be retroclined producing an acceptable incisor relationship.

In Chapter 3 a description was given of the type of hyperactive lower lip behaviour which may also produce an increase in overjet. Such an overjet is quite largely due to a posterior position, either by tilting or bodily displacement, of the lower incisors. It is a type of case which is very difficult to treat. Proclination of the lower incisors is followed by relapse while if the upper incisors are moved posteriorly into contact with the lowers, this tends to give an unsightly appearance with the patient appearing edentulous. Considerable thought should be given to this type of case before undertaking treatment and in many cases it is probably better to leave it untreated.

The dentition

It is by no means uncommon in Class II Division 1 malocclusion, as in all cases, to find that the individual is inherently crowded. It would seem that if crowding is present there will be insufficient room for the upper incisor teeth to be aligned normally. In other circumstances this might simply give rise to incisor crowding and imbrication but where there is some degree of skeletal discrepancy and/or incompetence of the lips there is a tendency for the central incisors at least to be pushed forward. This type of case, where crowding is an aetiological factor in producing the overjet, usually responds well to treatment and seldom relapses. It is a general finding that those cases of Class II Division 1 malocclusion with crowded dentitions are more likely to be stable following treatment than those with well aligned or spaced dentitions.

Digit-sucking

There is no doubt that the sucking of the thumb or finger can cause proclination of the upper incisors but the importance of this aetiological factor has been greatly exaggerated in the past. This matter has been dealt with in Chapter 4. Those cases in which digit-sucking is a major aetiological factor are exceptionally easy patients to treat, with the condition having a strong tendency to correct itself once the habit ceases. Efforts to 'break' the habit are usually unsuccessful and the best approach is to ignore the condition and carry on with orthodontic treatment as though it did not exist. With an orthodontic appliance in the mouth the habit usually disappears and treatment proceeds well.

TREATMENT

The planning of treatment

Once again the key to the planning of treatment lies in the lower arch and particularly with the lower incisors. Mills (1968) has shown that with a very few exceptions the lower incisors may not be successfully proclined or retroclined to any worthwhile extent. It is therefore wise to accept their labio-lingual position. If they are crowded, then two alternatives are open to us: to accept this crowding if it is slight (with the knowledge that it is likely to get worse during adolescence) or to relieve the lower crowding by moving the lower canines distally.

As with Class I malocclusion the solution to this normally lies in the extraction of teeth posterior to the canines. These canines may then be retracted, but here again it sometimes pays to wait for some time to see the extent to which a natural alignment of the lower arch will take place. Very occasionally, if the lower canines are very distally inclined or otherwise misplaced, it may be desirable to extract in the labial segment.

It was mentioned in Chapter 8 that a small proportion of patients will tolerate some proclination of the lower incisors. Many of the these in fact fall into the category of Class II Division 1 malocclusion where they form a small minority. The sucking of a digit may retrocline the lower incisors and if so they can clearly be proclined to their correct position: indeed they may do so spontaneously. The other category is the type of patient shown in Figure 10.2. Here the lower incisors appear to have been trapped within the vault of the palate and it would seem that as growth has taken place, the incisal edges have been restrained by this feature. If the overbite is reduced they may readily be proclined, the only problem being to know how far this should be done. It is emphasised that in the vast majority of cases the lower labial segment should be left strictly alone in the labio-lingual dimension.

Having, *in our mind's eye*, planned the lower arch, we then turn to the upper. As with Class I malocclusion the upper canine should usually be placed in a Class I relationship to the lower canine, although where the skeletal pattern is markedly Class II, the canines will probably end up in a slight postnormal relationship. Again space will be required distal to the upper canine in order to move it into the Class I position and this may be achieved either by the extraction of teeth or by distal movement of the upper buccal segments. Basically, the choice between these two approaches lies in the length of the dental bases relative to the size of the teeth, that is, to the presence or otherwise of crowding (Fig. 10.3). If the dental bases are short extractions will be necessary, whereas if they are long, distal movement of the upper buccal segments may be attempted. Sometimes if good, well positioned third molars are present and there is a lack of space posterior to the first molars, the upper second molars are extracted to facilitate this movement and to relieve the impaction of the wisdom teeth.

If the buccal segments are in Class II relation, it is possible to correct the canine relationship by

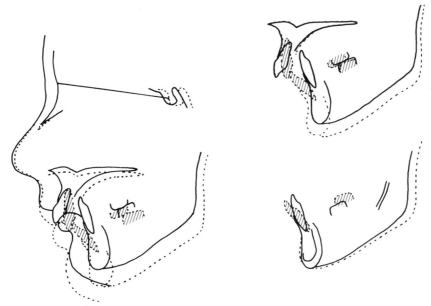

Fig. 10.2 Superimposed tracings of Class II Division 1 malocclusion in whom the lower incisors were 'trapped' in the vault of the palate (solid outline) and 4 years after their successful proclination (broken outline).

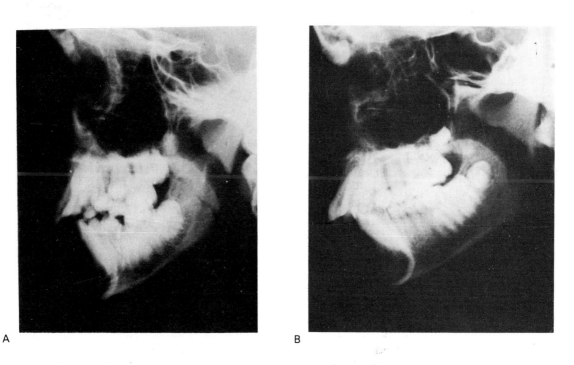

A   B

Fig. 10.3 Lateral skull radiographs of two boys, both aged $11\frac{1}{2}$ years with identical overjets. A, With short dental base; note 'stacking' or molars. B, With long dental bases.

extracting only the upper first premolars, with no lower extractions. This involves accepting a Class II posterior occlusion, which is a perfectly functional one. Experience shows that this is very frequently followed by late crowding of the lower labial segment. It should be carried out only in patients with very long dental bases, in whom there is a full unit of postnormal occlusion of the buccal segments and in whom the rather lengthy treatment involved in distal movement of buccal segments is not indicated. This applies particularly in adult patients who are no longer growing. In such cases there is some risk of residual spacing either in the upper incisor region or between the upper canine and second premolar. A case where this treatment was followed successfully is shown in Figure 10.4. This patient had a Class II Division 1 malocclusion with long dental bases on a Class II skeletal pattern. One would have expected the case to respond well to distal movement of the upper buccal segments and a functional appliance was initially used. This was completely unsuccessful, largely owing to a lack of co-operation by the patient. After 6 months, 4/4 were extracted and the upper canines retracted with reduction of overbite and overjet. This produced the acceptable result which is shown 4 years out of retention in the lowest models (Fig. 10.4). This was stable and the postnormal occlusion of the buccal teeth was acceptable. In this case crowding did not occur in the lower arch since the dental bases were long and indeed the teeth initially spaced. Equally, the patient was not left with spacing in the upper arch because of some unintentional mesial movement of the upper buccal segments so that in the final models the teeth are more than one unit postnormal in occlusion.

Occasionally, a patient presents with the buccal segments, including the first molars and canines in full Class II relation, and with crowding of the lower arch in the region anterior to the first molars. Such a case is shown in Figure 10.5. The standard approach would be to extract the lower first premolars and move back the lower canines sufficiently to align the lower labial segment. It can be visualised that the relationship of the canines would now be more than one unit postnormal and if the upper first premolars were extracted, there would be insufficient space to move the canines into a Class I relationship with their antagonists. Such cases are always difficult to treat, but generally it is necessary to move the upper molars distally (Fig. 10.5), in addition to extraction of the four premolars. Such a distal movement is usually achieved before extraction of the premolars and in this type of case it may well be necessary to extract four upper teeth, the second molars in addition to the first premolars.

The final stage in treatment planning involves the reduction of the overjet. If the overbite is complete, and the lower incisors are impinging on the cingulum of the upper incisors, or even on the palate, they will prevent lingual movement of these upper incisors. Such a situation is shown in Figure 10.6A. If a force is applied to move the incisor edges palatally, the the upper incisors will pivot about the lower incisor edges (Fig. 10.6B), producing an unsightly and often traumatic condition. To prevent this from occurring, the overbite should first be reduced by 'depressing' the lower incisors relative to the lower buccal segments. In such a case the curve of von Spee is usually excessive and the incisors should be depressed until they lie on the level plane with the buccal segments. The upper labial segment may then be moved palatally as indicated in Figures 10.6C and D.

In moving these teeth palatally, if the overjet is not too great and the teeth are proclined, a tipping action is all that is requires. Some degree of retroclination of the upper incisors is not unacceptable functionally or aesthetically but if they are tilted below an angle of, say, 95° to the maxillary plane, they will be either unstable, unsightly or traumatic. It is necessary therefore to judge whether a purely tilting action will be sufficient. With gentle forces the tooth would tilt about a point roughly one third of the way up the root from the apex, although stronger forces will increase the tilting and move the fulcrum closer to the incisal edge. If the condition is too severe for a pure tilting action, then bodily movement of the upper incisor must be attempted. This is more difficult to achieve and will require the use of a fixed appliance. Even for this there is a limit. Edwards (1976) has demonstrated that it is not possible to move the apex of the upper incisor indefinitely. Although the alveolar crest will reform as the

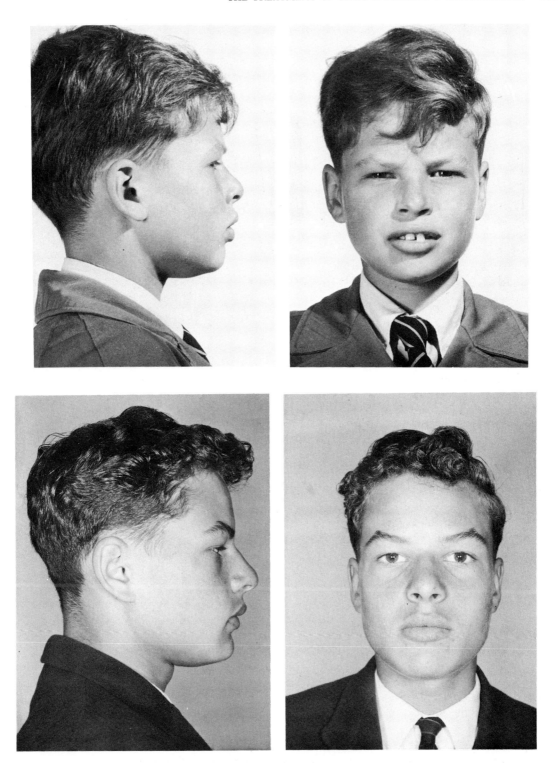

A

Fig. 10.4 Paul. A, Photographs before and after treatment; note different lip postures. B, Models taken before and after treatment and 4 years out of retention. C, Superimposed tracings before treatment (solid outline) and at the end of retention. D, Superimposed tracings at end of retention and 4 years later (B, C and D overleaf).

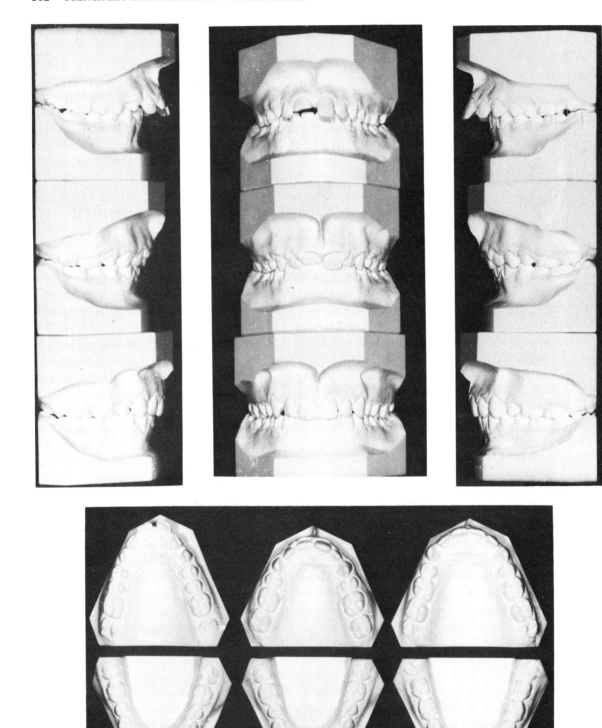

B

Fig. 10.4 (*cont'd*)

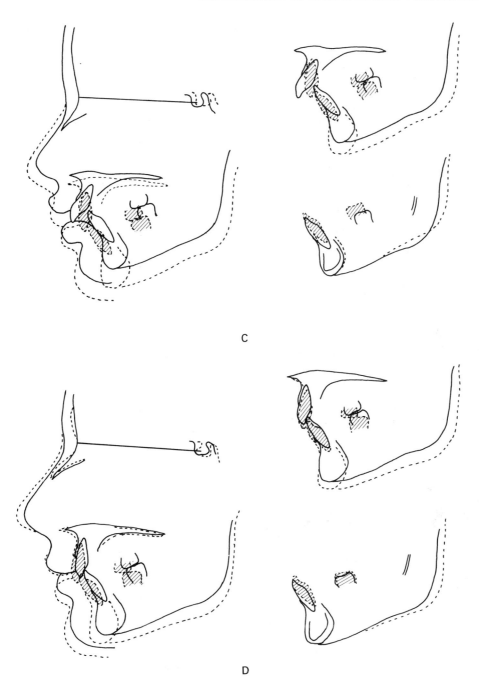

C

D

Fig. 10.4 (*cont'd*)

tooth is moved palatally, as has been shown by Ten Hoeve & Mulie (1976) the bone of the palatal vault does not follow the movement of the incisor to any appreciable extent and acts as a restriction to its movement: indeed, it is very likely to be

associated with resorption of the incisor apices. Figure 10.7 therefore illustrates the problem. In this case the alveolar ridge is comparatively narrow. The upper incisors are not proclined at the beginning of treatment and if the teeth were tilted palatally about the most favourable point, the ultimate result would be as shown in Figure 10.7B, clearly not acceptable. If on the other hand, the teeth were moved bodily the result shown in Figure 10.7C would result. The tooth would have moved completely out of the supporting bone and of course in practice this would be impossible. This is an extreme case

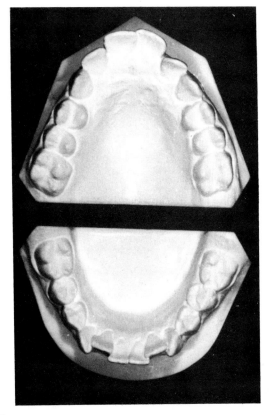

A

where the solution involved a compromise of some degree of tilting with the maximum possible amount of apical movement. Before attempting bodily movement of the upper incisors, it is desirable to examine a lateral skull radiograph to estimate the amount of bone available for their reception.

Having reduced the overjet and overbite, all that remains is to consider the necessity for space closure. Generally, provided the teeth are parallel there is much to be said for leaving some residual space especially in the lower arch. This will close naturally and will provide something of a safety valve against late crowding of the lower incisors. However, if the molar occlusion is initially Class II, then the lower molars must be brought forward into a Class I relationship since they are unlikely to do this satisfactorily by natural drifting processes.

'Orthopaedic movement'

Many orthodontists claim that by applying a strong force, of between 500 and 2000 grammes, to the upper first molars, it is possible to move the whole maxillary complex in a posterior direction. This is often referred to as orthopaedic movement to differentiate it from a purely dental or orthodontic tooth movement. The treatment is usually undertaken in the fairly early mixed dentition and produces a prolonged treatment period lasting perhaps from the age of 8 years to 13 or 14 years, and somewhat similar claims are made by the protagonists of functional appliances such as the Andresen appliance. This has already been

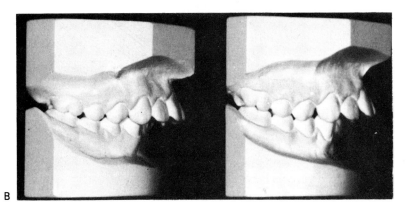

B

Fig. 10.5 Diane. A, The lower arch is crowded anterior to $\overline{6|6}$, but B, the posterior occlusion is one unit postnormal. It was therefore necessary to move the upper buccal segments distally as shown on the right, before extracting first premolars.

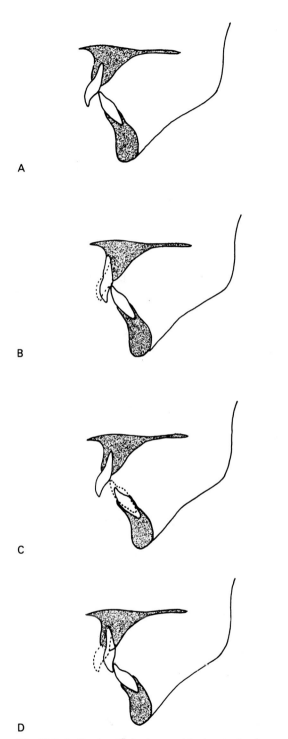

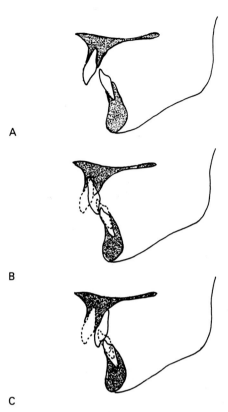

Fig. 10.7 A, Class II Division 1 malocclusion on severe Class II skeletal pattern. B, The overbite has been reduced and the upper incisors tilted lingually to produce an unacceptable result. C, The upper incisors have been moved bodily — out of the bone.

Fig. 10.6 A, Tracing of the jaws and incisor teeth of a typical Class II Division 1 malocclusion. B, The result of tipping the teeth palatally without reducing the overbite. C, The overbite is reduced and D, the overjet then reduced satisfactorily.

discussed in some detail in Chapter 8, but the orthodontist is well advised to assume that his treatment will be confined to movement of teeth through bone. If growth helps, this should be regarded as a bonus although it is certainly possible with modern appliances to affect, to a limited extent, the dental base, as represented by the cephalometric points B and, especially, A.

It is emphasised that so far we have been talking about the planning of treatment, and the actual treatment may be carried out in a different order from that so far described.

Practical treatment

It is customary, especially in North America, to divide the treatment of Class II Division 1 malocclusions into 'extraction cases' and 'non-extraction cases'. This is perhaps an over-simplification since in the latter case, if crowding is present distal to the first molars, and the third molars are in a good position, the second molars may be extracted. It is proposed here, therefore, to divide the treatment into those cases where the dental bases are short (Fig. 10.3A) and where crowding is present in the more anterior part of the arch, and secondly into those with long dental bases where the dental arches are uncrowded or crowding is confined to the tuberosity region and the corresponding part of the lower arch (Fig. 10.3B). The question of which teeth to extract has been extensively covered in Chapter 7 and it is not proposed to repeat the exercise here.

The difficulty of treatment and therefore the prognosis for a successful result is decided largely by the skeletal pattern and to a lesser extent by the sost tissues.

Thus Julie, illustrated in Figure 10.8, was a fairly straightforward case. Her skeletal pattern, antero-posteriorly, was only mildly Class II, with the lower facial height slightly increased. Both upper and lower arches were crowded and this, together with the skeletal discrepancy, caused the upper incisors, and especially the central incisors, to be proclined. Proclination was then further increased by an adverse effect of the lower lip. Nevertheless the overjet, of 8 mm was not severe. The upper incisors were at an angle of 118° to the maxillary plane, and could therefore be corrected by tilting rather than bodily movement.

All four first premolars were extracted and an upper removable appliance fitted to retract 3/3, which were mesially inclined. Although the overbite was not quite complete on the central incisors, it was complete on the more lingually placed lateral incisors. The lower incisors impinged on this bite plane, which held the posterior teeth out of occlusion. These teeth and their alveolus therefore developed vertically, reducing the overbite. This has the effect of causing the mandible to rotate downwards and backwards, a situation analogous to the fitting of an 'over-opened' denture. In the latter case the mandible will tend to return to its original height as a result of resorption of the alveolar crest, but fortunately most of our patients are growing children, and the lower face will usually increase in height sufficiently to accommodate the increased vertical dimension. It will be seen in Figure 10.8C that here this occurred to only a slight extent, since little overbite reduction was necessary, and vertical growth had compensated for the rotational effect of bite-opening by the end of treatment.

Mention has already been made of the need for gentle forces in moving teeth by removable appliances, and this is well illustrated in Julie's case. With a force of 30 to 50 g the canines were retracted without the need to reinforce anchorage, since such a force — dissipated between upper molars, second premolars, incisors and the vault of the palate — was probably below the threshold for their movement. The opposite of this is seen in Figure 10.9, where too strong a force was used to retract the canines. Although in Figure 10.9A the canines have apparently moved distally almost into contact with the second premolar, in fact the reverse has taken place. The canine in Figure 10.9B has tilted badly, but has not moved distally to any extent, and the space has been closed almost entirely by forward movement of the buccal segments.

Returning to Julie, the canines having been fully retracted, the overjet was reduced and the incisors aligned with a second removable appliance carrying a flexible labial bow. To prevent re-establishment of the overbite, a bite-plane was necessary on this second appliance, which was trimmed away carefully from the anterior edge to allow retraction of the incisors. In doing so the operator must be careful that a sharp corner is not left between the part which has been cut by the bur and the fitting surface of the appliance. The acrylic should be trimmed back approximately twice the distance which it is expected that the teeth will move, and the cut area should be smoothed and rounded into the fitting surface.

Here again, gentle forces have minimised tilting of the teeth so that at the end of treatment they were at an acceptable 98° to the maxillary plane, and were retained in this position by an adequately high lower lip-line, following a short period of wearing a removable Hawley retainer.

Apart from the extraction of first premolars, there was no active treatment in the lower arch, which aligned spontaneously. It is emphasised that, if this practice is followed, the lower arch should be examined *before* the upper at each visit. Firstly, is there sufficient space remaining for the teeth to align, and a little more? If not, a lower space maintainer should be fitted. Secondly, are the anterior teeth continuing to align? Thirdly, are the lower second premolars tending to tilt mesially to an unacceptable extent? If either of the last two questions cannot be answered satisfactorily, a lower fixed appliance should be fitted.

Two further features of this case will be noted.

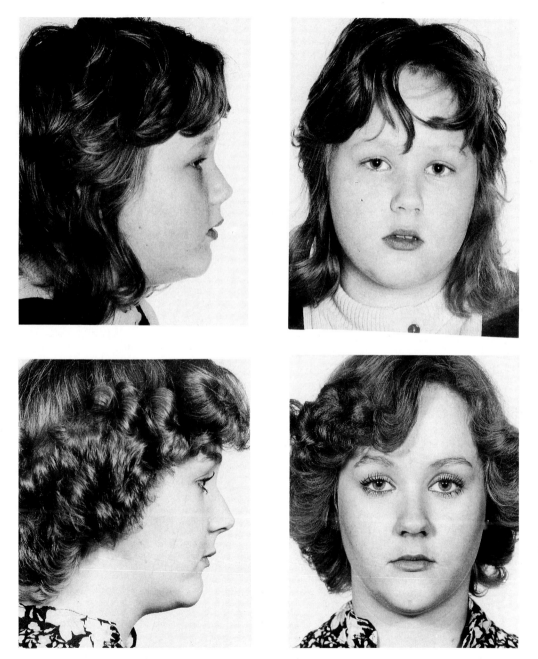

A

Fig. 10.8 Julie. A, Photographs before and after treatment. B, Study models taken before treatment, at end of retention and 7½ years later. C, Tracings before treatment superimposed on end of retention. D, Tracing at end of retention on 7½ years later (B, C and D overleaf).

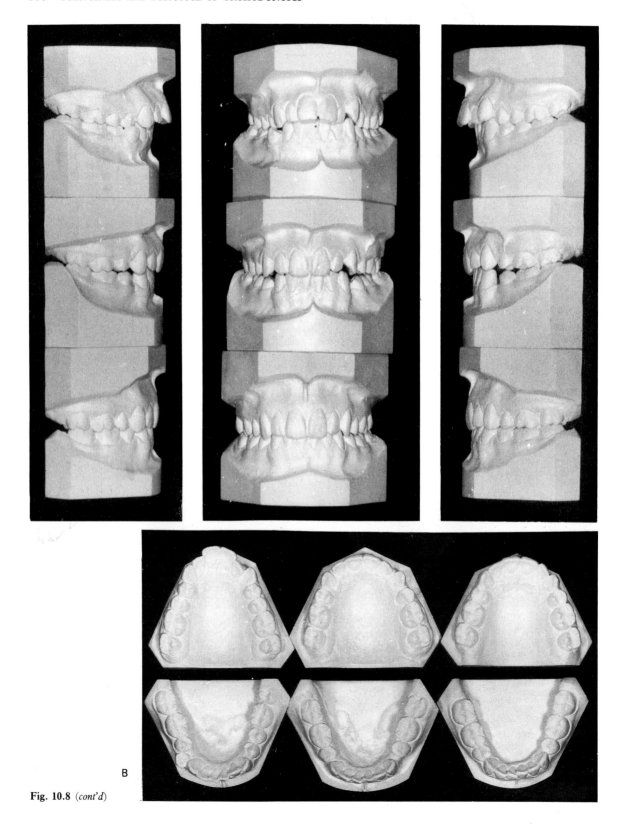

B

Fig. 10.8 *(cont'd)*

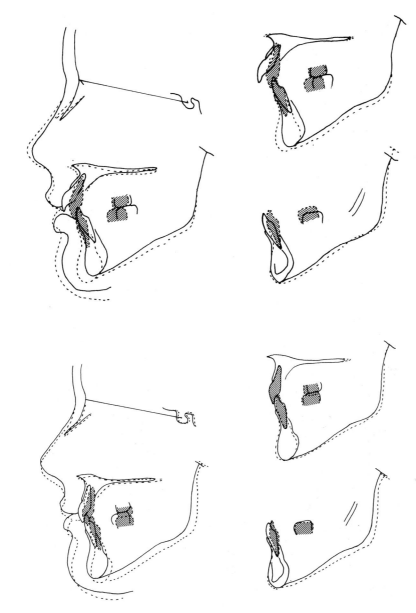

C

D

Fig. 10.8 (*cont'd*)

As in many (but not all) Class II malocclusions, there was improvement in the skeletal pattern, with forward growth of the mandible during the time in which treatment took place. Secondly, although the result at the end of treatment was far from ideal, there was considerable improvement in the 7 years before final records were taken.

The result achieved in Figure 10.8 was good for one achieved using only removable appliances. Nevertheless it was not perfect. The posterior occlusion was still slightly postnormal on the left side, and the incisors were somewhat retroclined, while the lower incisors were less than perfectly aligned. The result might have been somewhat better if upper and lower fixed appliances had been used. On the other hand the occlusion is

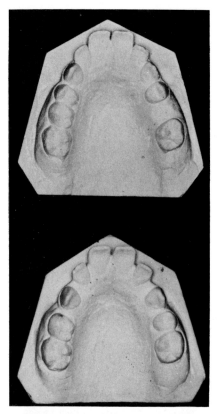

A

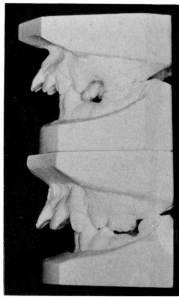

B

Fig. 10.9 A, Upper dental arch of patient with Class II Division 1 malocclusion, before and after retraction of 3/3. B, The same stages seen in occlusion: Note that retraction of 3/3 has been minimal, although the teeth have tilted excessively and the buccal segments have come forward, due to use of excessive force.

healthy and aesthetically satisfactory. The orthodontist should always remember that these are his goals, and not merely to produce final study models for his own satisfaction.

The case shown in Figure 10.10 presents rather different problems. Mandy has a severe Class II skeletal pattern with a reduced lower facial height. Both of these are reflected in the incisor relationship. The overjet was increased to 13 mm: anything over 10 mm can be regarded as severe and unlikely to respond to removable appliances. The overbite was excessively deep. The canines were not mesially tilted, indeed slightly distally inclined. The posterior occlusion was in fact slightly more than one unit postnormal so that no loss of anchorage was permissible — indeed mild distal movement of the upper molars would be desirable. Mandy was therefore treated throughout with fixed appliances. Bands were fitted to the first molars and a Kloehn bow with neck strap was used primarily to reinforce the anchorage but initially to gain slight distal movement of the first molars. Bands were selected for the lower arch and after preliminary alignment, a rectangular arch was fitted in order to 'depress' the lower incisors, of the type illustrated in Figure 7.8C. Although some depression was achieved, it will be seen from Figure 10.10C that the main affect here, as in the previous case, was elevation of the posterior teeth, with, in the absence of appreciable growth, a downwards and backwards rotation of the mandible. This 'over-opening' relapsed in Figure 10.10D. In using a banded appliance to depress lower incisors, a natural tendency is usually to procline these teeth so that the apex of the incisors comes into contact with the lingual plate of bone and the cervical part of the root with the alveolar crest. By using a rectangular arch this proclination can be prevented and the tooth depressed into the 'corridor' of cancellous bone. Even so it should be appreciated that genuine depression of teeth is very difficult to achieve. What we usually do is to bring about elevation of the posterior teeth while preventing the normal vertical development of the anteriors associated with growth. Having flattened the occlusal curve in the lower arch, the banded appliance was used to close the lower spaces.

Turning to the upper arch, the canine teeth

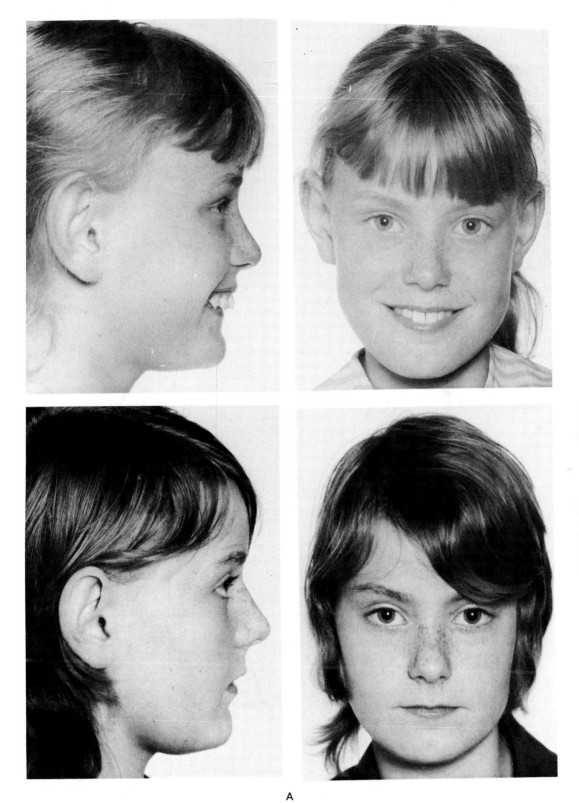

A

Fig. 10.10 Mandy. A, Photographs before and after treatment. B Study models before treatment, at end of retention and $5\frac{1}{2}$ years later. C, Tracings before treatment superimposed on those at end of retention. Note minimal growth of upper face but rotation of mandible. D, End of retention superimposed on tracing $5\frac{1}{2}$ years later. Note relapse of mandibular rotation (B, C and D overleaf).

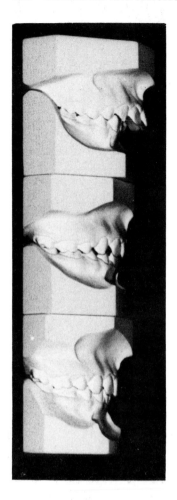
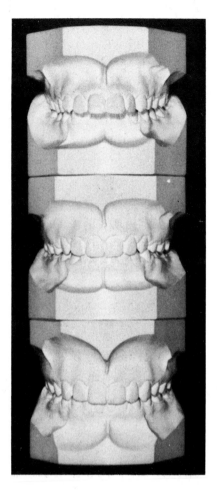
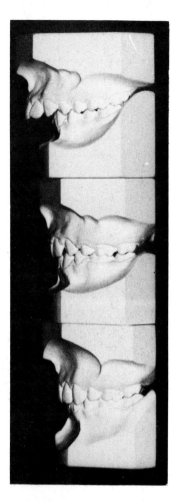

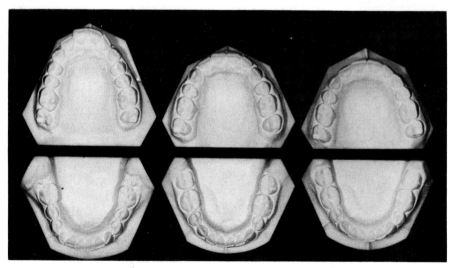

B

Fig. 10.10 (*cont'd*)

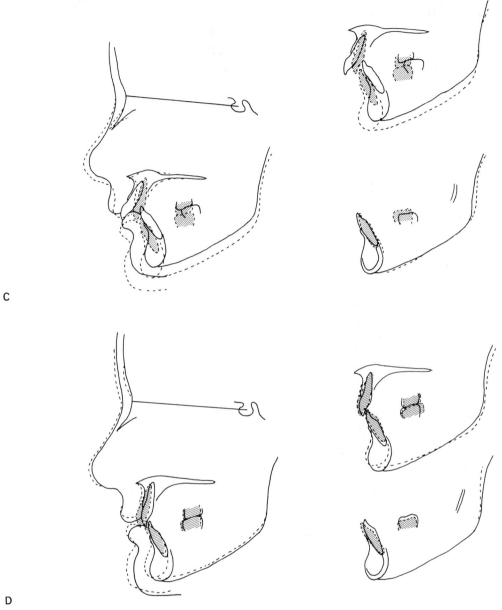

C

D

Fig. 10.10 (*cont'd*)

were retracted by means of sectional arches which enabled these teeth to be moved bodily. The canine has an exceptionally long root and to move any tooth bodily involves a very great 'equal and opposite reaction'. For this purpose, anchorage must be supported by substantial extra-oral traction as was done here. When the canines had been retracted into Class I relation with the lower arch,

the obvious next stage was to retract the upper labial segment. After preliminary alignment, it was appreciated that although the lower occlusal curve was now level, the overbite had not been reduced sufficiently to enable the upper incisors to be moved bodily in a lingual direction. It has already been remarked that where the lower lip is resting behind the upper incisors, as in this case, this can form a valuable permanent retainer following completion of treatment. In Mandy's case however, the lower lip had a very high relation to the upper incisors and had they merely been retracted inside this lower lip, they would have taken up a Class II Division 2 relationship as in the next chapter. It was therefore felt that in this case the overbite could be reduced further by an attempt to intrude these upper incisors, and this was carried out again by means of a headgear, in this case of the 'high pull' type which is acting at about 45° to the occlusal plane similar to that shown in Figure 13.6. As in the lower arch it was necessary to control the angulation of the teeth so that a rectangular archwire was used, not only to attempt to intrude the incisor teeth, but also to move them bodily lingually and the result shown in Figure 10.10 was achieved. Bodily movement of upper incisors is not an easy operation but even the comparatively small amount in this case is adequate when compared with the alternative of a tilting action which would move the apex in the opposite direction. Although some growth took place in this patient, the vertical growth was less than in the previous case and we should not have achieved the necessary overbite reduction without the use of fixed appliances, nor could we have brought about the very satisfactory incisor relationship.

Long dental bases

The extraction of teeth is the treatment for crowding thereof and in an ideal world this would be the only reason why teeth should be extracted. Where the dental bases are long and there is an absence of crowding in the ante-molar region, the postnormal occlusion of the posterior teeth would normally be treated by moving these teeth distally into a Class I relationship with their antagonists. In many otherwise uncrowded mouths, it becomes apparent that there will not be sufficient space for the third molars to erupt normally and in these cases the extraction of second molars, either in the upper or both arches, will relieve this crowding. It is frankly admitted that this is to some extent an excuse since in these cases the distal movement of the upper posterior teeth is quicker and easier. In moving the upper buccal teeth distally, clearly

some point of anchorage is required. Formerly this was often the lower arch using inter-maxillary traction and there may be a few cases where this is still indicated either alone or in combination with the more usual solution of extra-oral traction. If inter-maxillary traction is used this will of course have a reciprocal affect and tend to bring about a proclination of the lower incisors. I have already indicated those few cases where this is permissible.

Florence is an example of this type of treatment. It will be seen from Figure 10.11B that her dental arches are well aligned, apart from minimal crowding in the lower canine region. This was confirmed in the lateral skull radiograph, except that there was a marked lack of space for the third molars in this 11-year-old girl. The posterior occlusion was postnormal but only to the extent of half the width of a cusp. In practice, these cases where the occusion is only half a unit postnormal respond well to the use of extra-oral traction. The overjet was increased to 11 mm with the overbite increased and virtually complete onto the palate. An interesting feature, to be seen in the lateral skull tracing of Florence in Figure 10.11C is that the skeletal pattern is mildly Class III. The increased overjet has been produced by a retroclination of the lower incisors and marked proclination of the upper incisors.

It was decided to extract $\underline{7/7}$ only. With the benefit of hind-sight it might have been better to extract all four second molars since the position of the lower third molars was favourable for their eruption and this might have been sufficient to prevent the slight increase in crowding which occurred in the lower arch. An upper removable appliance of the type shown in Figure 10.12 was then used to move the buccal segments distally into normal relationship. When this had been achieved, further removable appliances were fitted, reinforced by extra-oral anchorage, to retract firstly the upper canines while reducing the overbite, and finally to move the upper incisors lingually. A pure tilting action was adequate for the last tooth movement since the teeth were excessively proclined and moreover, where the malocclusion occurs in a mild Class III skeletal pattern, some forward movement of the upper incisors apices is actually beneficial, provided this

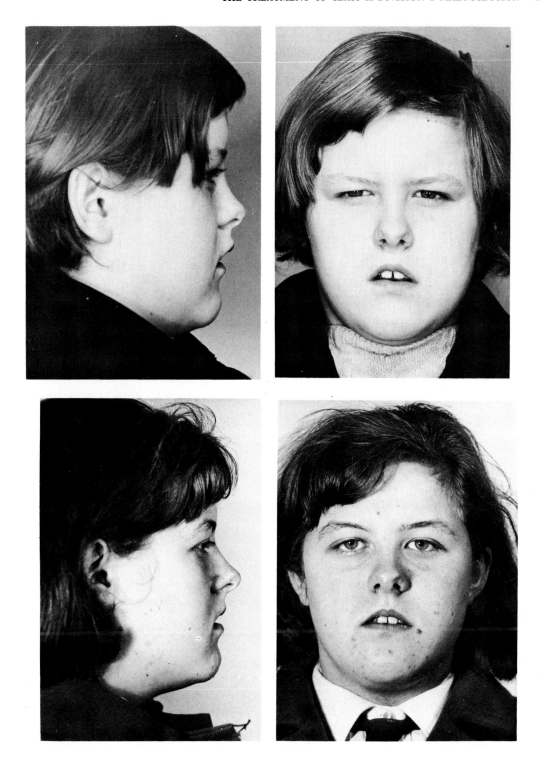

A

Fig. 10.11 Florence. A, Photographs before and after treatment. B, Study models before treatment, at end of retention and $5\frac{1}{2}$ years later. C, Tracings before treatment superimposed on those at end of retention. D, Tracings at end of retention superimposed on those $5\frac{1}{2}$ years later (B, C and D overleaf).

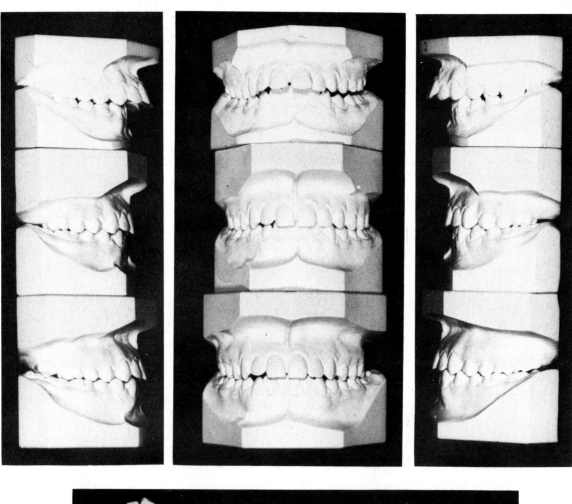

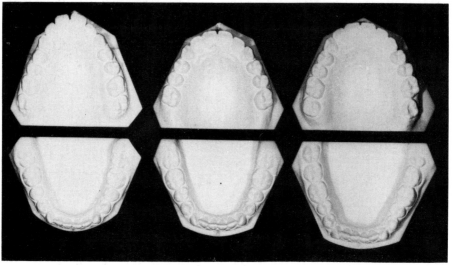

B

Fig. 10.11 (*cont'd*)

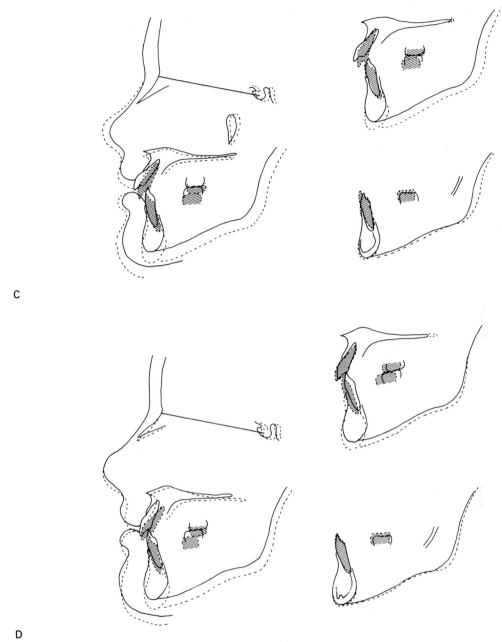

C

D

Fig. 10.11 (*cont'd*)

is not so extreme as to cause apical resorption by contact of the incisal apices against the labial plate of bone.

The result of treatment, and the condition 5 years later, can be seen in Figure 10.11. The superimposed tracings in Figure 10.11C show the picture somewhat more clearly. When superimposed upon the line SN with N registered the whole maxilla appears to have moved posteriorly. This is in fact an illusion brought about by the substantial growth in length of the line SN. It is not the maxilla which has gone backwards but the

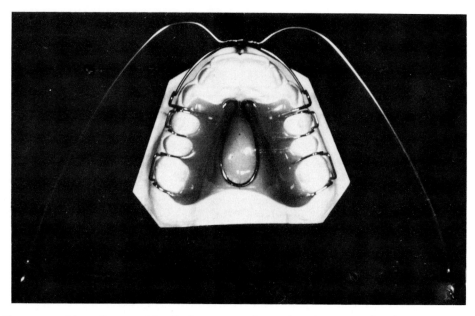

Fig. 10.12 Upper removable appliance used for distal movement of upper buccal segments of teeth.

nasion which has has come forwards. Similarly, in this superimposition, the mandibular symphysis appears to have grown almost directly downwards and while mandibular growth in this case was not particularly favourable, it will be seen, when the tracings are superimposed on the palatal outline, that the symphysis has in fact come forwards slightly relative to the maxilla. This of course helps the reduction of the postnormality and of the overjet but it will also be noted that there has been substantial vertical growth of the face. Vertival growth seems at least as important as antero-posterior growth in successful treatment with distal movement of upper buccal segments. Although orthodontic treatment had done nothing to change the normal growth pattern, nevertheless it is possible to divert the path of eruption of teeth within this growth pattern and extra-oral traction should not be used in the patient who has finished growing.

As already mentioned in considering theoretical treatment, the extraction of teeth is normally only indicated where the dentition is crowded. On the other hand the distal movement of buccal segments is prolonged and requires a co-operative and actively growing patient. There is a small proportion of patients in whom it is justifiable to extract upper first premolars only, as an alternative to extra-oral traction. These cases should be carefully selected and if only upper extractions are proposed, the operator should ensure that the lower arch is really uncrowded. One so frequently sees cases where the extractions have been confined to the upper arch, only for the patient to return at the age of 18 with a crowded lower labial segment for which treatment is desired but not easily provided. In this small minority of uncrowded cases, the extraction of the upper first premolar is followed by retraction of canines, reduction of overbite and of the overjet. If the latter is corrected by a tilting action, the inter-incisal angle at the end of treatment will be increased as will the overbite. In these cases there is a strong tendency to have residual spacing in the upper labial segment and/or crowding of the lower labial segment; this point is discussed in some detail in the next chapter where a similar situation arises with Class II Division 2 malocclusion.

Functional appliances

The type of case just described, with long dental bases and an absence of crowding, is that which responds best to the use of functional appliances.

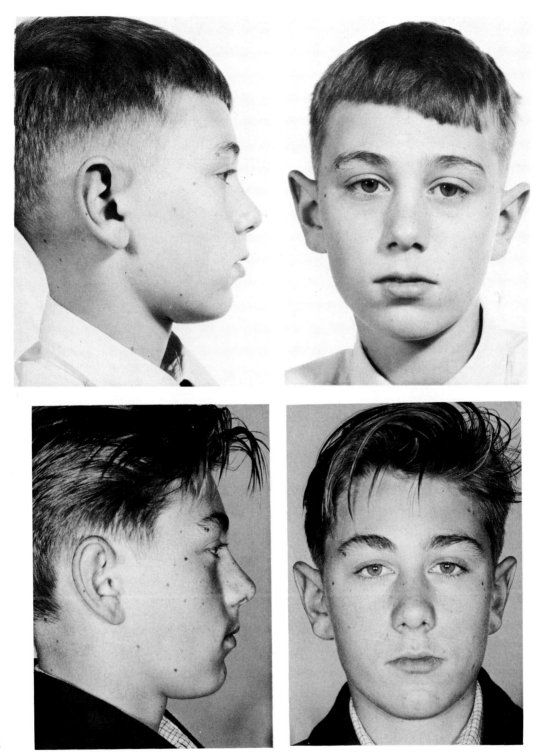

A

Fig. 10.13 Paul. A, Photographs before and after treatment. B, Study models before treatment, at the end of retention and 4 years later. C, Tracings before treatment superimposed on those at the end of retention. D, Tracings at the end of retention superimposed on those 4 years later (B, C and D overleaf).

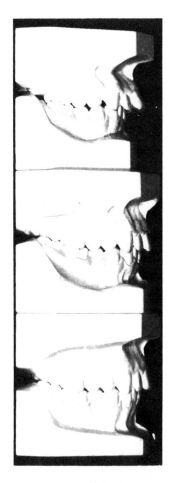
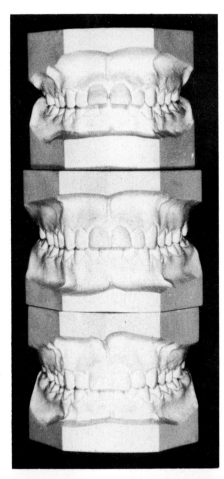
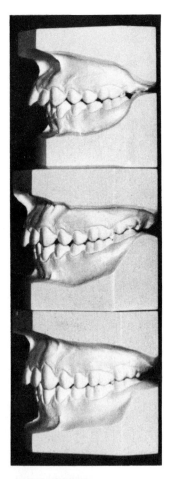
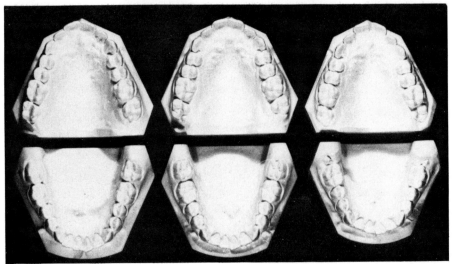

B

Fig. 10.13 (*cont'd*)

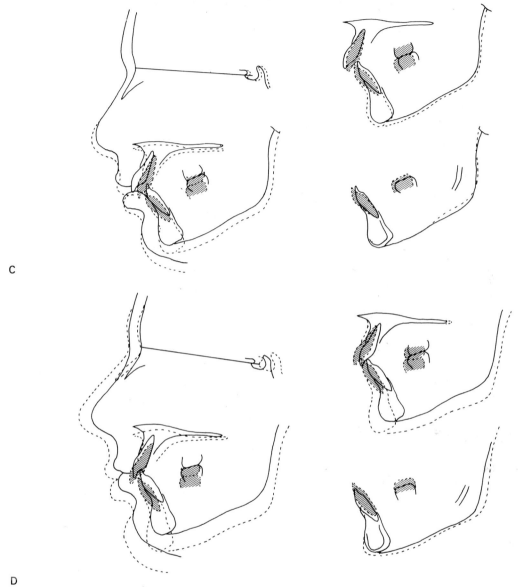

C

D

Fig. 10.13 (cont'd)

Although these have little or no effect on the skeletal pattern, they can provide a method of achieving very satisfactory results.

The most important features in selecting patients for treatment with functional appliances are therefore:

1. Long dental bases and an absence of antemolar crowding. Second molars may be extracted if this is indicated.

2. A co-operative patient and a confident operator. A lack of confidence in the operator will be transmitted to the patient at least subconsciously.

3. Many authors advocate the use of functional appliances in the mixed dentition or even earlier. They are most effective in a rapidly growing patient — indeed they are contra-indicated where growth has ccased. The best time would seem therefore to be at or just before puberty and this

agrees with my own experience. The desire for early treatment possibly arises from a desire to leave time for other methods if this one fails.

Paul (Fig. 10.13), is an example of a patient treated with an Andresen appliance. Treatment commenced at 11 years 6 months and took 1 year 5 months to complete. There was substantial vertical growth of the face during this period, although growth in the antero-posterior dimension was not particularly favourable (Fig. 10.13C). The upper molars were not actually moved distally, but rather their normal forward movement was prevented, while the lower molars grew forward beneath them. The small amount of proclination of the lower incisors was apparently stable. It will be seen from Figure 10.13D that considerable facial growth took place after the end of active treatment. This was presumably the pubertal growth spurt, and theoretically treatment was a little early. However, this late growth may well have aided stability, especially of the lower incisors. Growth in this case was exceptionally favourable and did much to ensure the good result.

There is no doubt that excellent results can be achieved with functional appliances, although it is doubtful whether the more elaborate types have any advantage over the conventional Andresen appliance and most of them are more difficult to wear and more liable to damage. In fact many operators find their results disappointing. A high standard of co-operation is necessary, together with favourable growth. They would seem to work most satisfactorily in patients with long dental bases whose skeletal and soft tissue patterns are not grossly abnormal. Clearly some abnormality of these must be present otherwise the patient would not have a malocclusion. A wise rule in using these appliances is to set a time limit of 6 months and if at the end of that time no discernible improvement has occurred then a more conventional form of treatment should be instituted.

Retention

Retention of all treated malocclusions is a subject of controversy. A colleague has expressed the opinion that 'when you've got a nice result you don't like to let go', and there is much truth in this statement. Generally speaking, if the result is unstable at the end of treatment, then no amount of retention will turn it into a stable one. There is a small proportion of patients in whom permanent retention, perhaps by wearing a suitable appliance at night in bed, is indicated as the lesser of two evils. Otherwise retention should not be continued to an excessive extent. If the interincisal angle is reasonably normal, or alternatively if the height of the lower lip is sufficient to act as a permanent retainer against the labial surface of the upper incisors, then the case is unlikely to relapse and retention should be minimal. A Hawley retainer worn for perhaps 2 months full-time, followed by a further 2 or 3 months nocturnally, should be quite adequate. Indeed recent work by Wood at the Eastman Dental Hospital, would cast doubt on the usefulness of any retention.

The one exception to the above statements may occur when considerable rapid overbite reduction has been achieved. This will cause a downward and backward rotation of the mandible due to the further development of the buccal teeth, and an essentially 'over-opened' situation. In such a case, fairly prolonged retention is indicated. In the growing patient this will allow the face to grow sufficiently to accommodate the new vertical dimension, while there is evidence that over a long period the over-erupted teeth will tend to depress into the bone so as to correct, to some extent, the over-opening.

SUGGESTED READING

Ahlgren J, Laurin C 1976 Late results of activator-treatment: A cephalometric study. British Journal of Orthodontics 3: 181–7

Bennett T G, Tulloch J F C, Vig K W L, Webb W G 1975 Overjet stability after treatment of Class II Division 1 malocclusion. British Journal of Orthodontics 2: 239–46

Bernstein L, Ulbrich R W, Gianelly A A 1977 Orthopedics versus orthodontics in Class II treatment: An implant study. American Journal of Orthodontics 72: 549–58

Björk A 1947 The face in profile. Svensk Tandlakare Tidskrift 40 Suppl. 5B

Edwards J G 1976 A study of the anterior position of the

palate as it relates to orthodontic therapy. American Journal of Orthodontics 69: 249–73

Graber T M, Neumann B 1977 Removable Orthodontic Appliances. Saunders, Philadelphia

Jakobsson S O 1967 Cephalometric evaluation of treatment effect on Class II Division 1 malocclusions. American Journal of Orthodontics 53: 446–57

James G A 1963 Cephalometric analysis of 100 Angle Class II Division 1 malocclusions with special reference to the cranial base. Transactions of the British Society for the Study of Orthodontics 39–50

Melsen B 1978 The effect of cervical anchorage during and after treatment studied by the implant method. American Journal of Orthodontics 73: 526–40

Melsen B, Enemark H 1969 Effect of cervical anchorage studied by the implant method. Transaction of the European Orthodontic society 435–47

Mills J R E 1966 The long-term results of the proclination of lower incisors. British Dental Journal 120: 355–64

Mills J R E 1978 The effect of orthodontic treatment on the skeletal pattern. British Journal of Orthodontics 5: 133–43

Parkhouse R C 1969 A cephalometric appraisal of cases of Angle's Class II Division 1 malocclusion treated by the Andresen appliance. Dental Practitioner 19: 425–34

Ricketts R M 1952 A study of changes in temporomandibular relationship with the treatment of Class II malocclusion (Angle). American Journal of Orthodontics 38: 918–33

Ten Hoeve A, Mulie R M 1976 The effect of antero-posterior repositioning on the palatal cortex, as studied with laminagraphy. Journal of Clinical Orthodontics 10: 804–22

Weislander L 1975 Early or late cervical traction therapy in Class II malocclusion in the mixed dentition. American Journal of Orthodontics 67: 432–9

Weislander L, Buck D L 1974 Physiological recovery after cervical traction therapy. American Journal of Orthodontics 66: 294–301

Wood C M 1983 The effect of retention on the relapse of Class II Division 1 cases. British Journal of Orthodontics 10: 198–202

11

The treatment of Class II Division 2 malocclusion

DEFINITION

According to Edward Angle, Class II malocclusion is the condition where the lower first molars occlude in a postnormal relation to the uppers by the width of one premolar. Division 2 includes only those cases where the upper central incisors are retroclined. The British Standard classification of incisor relationships defines Division 2 in the following words: 'The upper central incisors are retroclined. The overjet is usually minimal but may be increased'. Essentially therefore the condition is one in which the posterior teeth will probably be in portnormal relationship, but, more important, the upper central incisors will be retroclined from their normal angle, with an increase in overbite, but without an increase in overjet. The upper lateral incisors may be proclined as shown in Figure 11.1B and indeed they often are, but this is not an essential part of the condition. This type of overbite, often very deep, is referred to in the German speaking countries as 'deckbiss'; literally 'coverbite'.

Class II Division 2 patients have a typical facial appearance. The lips are held in contact, unlike the typical Class II Division 1 malocclusion. There is a prominent chin with the dento-alveolar structure set back within the face. While this can be attractive in the younger individual, it is less so in late middle age.

AETIOLOGY

Skeletal pattern

Several authors have shown that the average skeletal discrepancy in this type of malocclusion is somewhat less severe than in Class II Division 1 malocclusion (Fig.11.1A and C). This is probably because, on a severe Class II skeletal pattern, the upper incisors would tend to rest outside the lower lip and therefore give rise to a Class II Division 1 malocclusion. In fact, however, the typical Division 2 malocclusion can occur on any type of skeletal pattern from a severe Class II to a mild Class III, although the more extreme variants are rare.

In the vertical dimension, Class II Division 2 is traditionally associated with a reduced lower facial height. It can be shown statistically that there is an inverse relation between the depth of overbite and the lower facial height, but this correlation is not a high one. The reduced lower facial height and small maxillo-mandibular planes angle is found in a minority of cases, although when it is present the malocclusion is usually severe and overbite reduction is likely to be particularly difficult. It would seem that this condition when present is produced by a forward and upward rotation of the mandible (Fig. 11.2). Figure 11.2A shows the lateral skull tracings of a boy at the age of 8 years superimposed on a tracing of a later radiograph taken 8 years later. This superimposition is on the base of skull, and it would appear that the face is growing in an orderly fashion, with the lower border of the mandible becoming slightly more horizontal. Turning to Figure 11.2B, the tracings have been superimposed on structures in the mandible as described in Chapter 1. It will be seen that on this basis there is a marked rotation of the rest of the skull during growth. This is of course a relative matter and it will be more logical to say that the mandible has rotated forwards and upwards

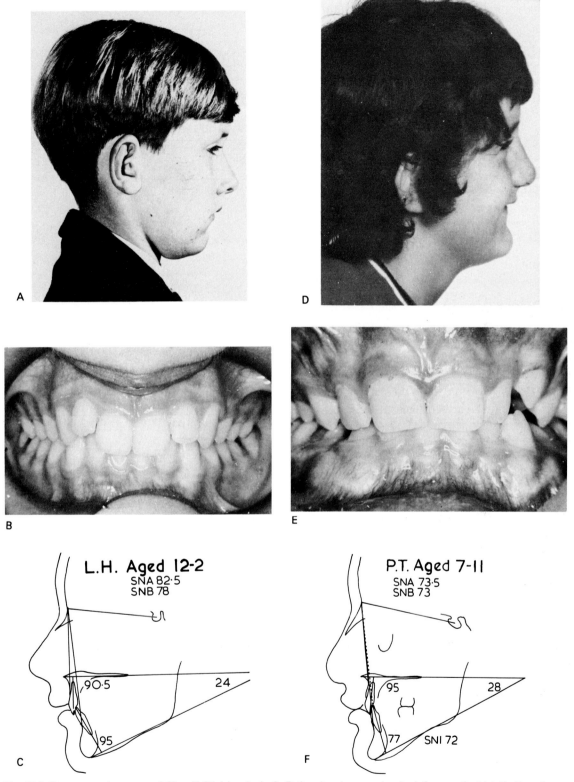

Fig. 11.1 Two contrasting types of Class II Division 2. A–C, Patient in whom, under the influence of a high lip line, the upper incisors have retroclined to compensate for a Class II skeletal pattern. D-F, The lip line was high and the lower lip hyperactive in facial expression. Both upper and lower incisiors are severely retroclined on a Class I skeletal pattern.

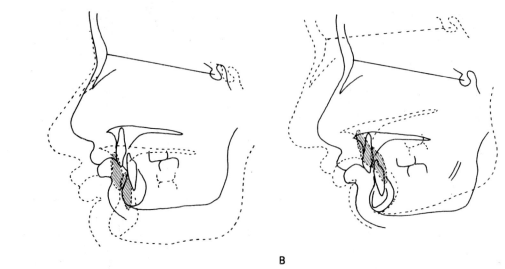

A   B

Fig. 11.2 Tracing of lateral skull radiograph of a boy with a severe Class II Division 2 malocclusion at ages 8 years and 16 years. A, Tracings superimposed on the line SN. Note the apparently regular growth pattern. B, On Björk structures in the mandible. Note the marked forward rotation, with compensatory deposition and resorption of bone in the mandible.

during growth, with the skull remaining stationary. Although the lower incisors actually procline relative to the internal bone of of the mandible (Fig. 11.2B), they appear to retrocline relative to the upper jaw and indeed relative to the newly recontoured mandible outline (Fig. 11.2A).

Soft tissues

The most important single factor in bringing about this retroclination of the upper central incisors is the lower lip. It is an almost invariable finding in Class II Division 2 malocclusion that the level of the lower lip is high relative to the upper incisors. In the presence of a Class II skeletal pattern the upper incisors will erupt at more or less the average angle to their base. Where the lip line is low relative to these upper incisors, they will continue to erupt at this angle with an overjet which exactly reflects the degree of skeletal abnormality. If, however, the lip line is high, the upper teeth will not be stable in this position and will either procline, to lie outside the lower lip, or retrocline to lie inside it. In the latter case, the arrangement of the central incisors will be typical of Class II Division 2. The question of whether the incisors lie inside or outside the lip depends to some extent on the degree of skeletal abnor-

mality and in border-line cases, may be almost a matter of chance. Several cases have been reported of identical twins where the dentitions also are identical apart from the central incisors. In one twin they have come to lie outside the lower lip and in the other inside it. We occasionally also see a case where one central incisor is proclined and the other retroclined with the lip lying in between. Not infrequently, the lateral incisors, being shorter, come to lie on the lower lip, as shown in Figure 11.1B although this is not invariable and with a higher lip line they may also be retroclined and parallel to the central incisors (Fig. 11.1E).

A small proportion of Class II Division 2 malocclusions develop in connection with the type of hyperactive lower lip which has already been described in Chapter 3. This activity of the lower lip in expressive behaviour is well known to produce a retroclination and retro-position of the lower incisors, but if the lip line is low it will not affect the upper incisors. If we have a high lip line associated with this hyperactive lip, it will retrocline both upper and lower incisors (Fig. 11.1D to F). This produces a very severe type of Class II Division 2 malocclusion which is difficult to treat but which is in fact often found on a Class I or even mild Class III skeletal base.

It has long been realised that most patients with

this type of malocclusion have an increased inter-occlusal clearance and that in closing from the rest position, the mandible moves upwards and backwards instead of closing by a simple hinge action. This was thought to indicate an 'over-closure' with a posterior displacement of the condylar head in the glenoid fossa. Research, notably by Ricketts, has shown that this is not the case. In occlusion the condylar head occupies a normal position in the glenoid fossa and it is the rest position which is abnormal. These individuals have a habitual rest position with the condylar head displaced downwards and forwards on to the articular eminence. The reason for this is not clear. It seems probable that it is dictated by the need to bring the incisor teeth into a more functional relationship.

Dental factors

In a normal incisal relationship, the incisal edges of the lower incisors occlude onto the cingula of the upper incisors thus preventing further eruption. This is a reciprocal activity also maintaining the upper incisors in their correct position. It would seem that in many cases of Class II Division 2 malocclusion a failure of this mechanism is at least a contributory factor in producing the very deep overbite. One reason for this is the high inter-incisal angle produced by the retroclination of the upper incisors.

It has been shown by Robertson and Hilton (1965) that the crown of the central incisor is sometimes abnormally thin labio-lingually, so that there is a lack of properly contoured cingulum. In other individuals there may be an angulation between the long axis of crown and root so that, with the root at its normal angle to the base, the crown is somewhat retroclined and more likely to lie inside the lower lip. Both these conditions have been described in Class II Division 2 malocclusion but they are certainly not present in every case, and would appear to be rare.

Class II Division 2 is not therefore a single clinical entity but is the product of many different factors, not all acting in a given case. The most constant factor is a high lower lip line.

In Figure 11.1A to C we see a boy who has a moderate Class II skeletal pattern with an otherwise well proportioned face. The lower lip line is slightly higher than average, perhaps associated with a slightly reduced maxillo-mandibular planes angle. This has enabled nature to compensate for the Class II skeletal pattern, by retroclining the upper central incisors, until they come into contact with the lower incisors, which lie at a reasonably normal angle to their base. So far as central incisors are concerned, nature has done its best. However, the molar relationship is also Class II, again reflecting the skeletal discrepancy. This means that the upper first premolar occludes between the lower canine and first premolar in the position which should be occupied by the upper canine. He has therefore essentially six upper incisor teeth where there should be four and since there is no increase in overjet, 'something has to give'. In this case lateral incisors have proclined out of the arch and come to lie outside the lower lip. Figure 11.1D to F shows another patient with a Class I or mild Class III skeletal pattern. His lower lip line is high and as previously described, is hyperactive in expression. This causes a retroclination of both upper and lower incisors and therefore a very high inter-incisal angle. This lingual tilting of the teeth causes an increase in overbite which may be somewhat exacerbated by some over-eruption of the incisor teeth due to their lack of occlusal antagonists. In this case, the high lip line has also retroclined the upper lateral incisors. Since the molars here again reflect the skeletal pattern and are therefore in Class I relationship, we do not have the problem of 'too many upper incisors'. Figure 11.2 illustrates yet another type of case. Due to the forward and upward rotation of the mandible, the lower facial height is very much reduced. The lower lip here is of normal length but since the chin is too close to the nose, the lip line is also unduly high and in occlusion the lips appear over-competent. This high lip line again has the affect of retroclining the incisor teeth, and the deep overbite is made even worse by the small lower facial height. This would be a particularly difficult case to treat.

TREATMENT

Class II Division 2 malocclusion has over the years acquired for itself a bad reputation so far as treatment is concerned. In many cases an ideal incisal relationship has been achieved only to relapse, and it would seem that this relapse can take place some years after the end of treatment.

Treatment planning

This follows the procedures used so far, commencing with the lower incisors. The labio-lingual position of the lower incisors should usually be accepted and if crowding is present, this will be treated by the extraction of teeth in the lower buccal segments. Crowding is then relieved by distal movement of the lower canines and alignment of the incisor teeth. However, it will be recalled that in considering Class II Division 1 malocclusion, it was suggested that some proclination of lower incisors was possible where the incisal edge was 'trapped' behind the cingula of the upper incisors or the anterior part of the palate. Such a 'trapping' is not uncommon in the more severe type of Class II Division 2. The problem here again is knowing how far the lower incisors may be proclined in such a case without later relapse and crowding. An upper anterior bite plane, which reduces the overbite and allows the lower incisors to find their position of balance, may be of value in these severe cases, and here treatment may even be started, exceptionally, in the early mixed dentition. Figure 11.3A shows the lateral skull tracings before treatment of a patient whose upper incisal edges were traumatising the gingival margins around the lower incisors at the age of 8 years. An upper bite plane was fitted to reduce the overbite and this was worn as a retainer until premolars could be extracted. Treatment was completed with upper removable appliances only and the result some 4 years out of retention is seen in Figure 11.3B. It will be noted that the lower incisors have spontaneously proclined through 12.5°.

In Class II Division 2 there is, therefore, an exception to the general rule in a minority of cases. In general the labio-lingual position of the lower incisors should be maintained. In very severe cases, where the incisal edges of the lower incisors are trapped behind the cingula of the uppers, limited proclination of the lower incisors, associated with the overbite reduction, may be

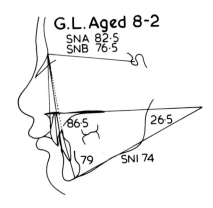

A

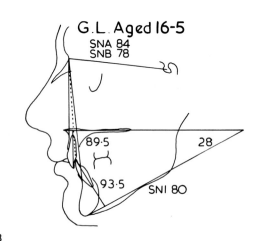

B

Fig. 11.3 A, Tracing of patient who, at the age of 8 years had upper central incisors traumatising the lower gingival margin. B, At age of 16½ years, 4 years after discarding an upper bite plane.

acceptable. This will have the effect of bringing the lower incisal edges on to the upper cingula. In adopting this line of treatment it may be necessary to accept some crowding of the lower incisors at a later stage.

Having therefore, in the mind's eyes, aligned the lower arch, attention is now turned to the upper dental arch. In the milder type of case, epitomised in Figure 11.1A to C, the position of the central incisors, although retroclined, is neither traumatic nor aesthetically objectionable and can be accepted. As a rough guide, if the angle between the long axes of the upper central incisors and the maxillary plane is not less than about 95°, their position should be accepted apart from correction of any rotations. This has the advantage that since the teeth have not been moved they will not relapse. The problem is therefore, to align the remaining upper anterior teeth with the central incisors. This will involve accepting some increase in overbite. If the upper canines are retracted into a normal relationship with the lower canines because of this increased overbite, there will be too much space for the upper anterior teeth and this space (often between the lateral incisor and canine) can be difficult to close. The upper canines should, therefore, be retracted empirically, until there is sufficient room to align the remaining teeth. These canines and the upper lateral incisors are then aligned with the central incisors. Unfortunately, the typically proclined upper lateral incisors have a strong tendency to relapse. This is probably because the lower lip does not control them and they therefore return to their natural angle to the maxilla, while the upper central incisors remain somewhat retroclined under lip pressure. Prolonged retention is a partial answer and if the upper lateral incisors can be placed in a position where the lower lip will control them, so much the better. It will be appreciated that if spaces are not to be left in the upper arch then the lower buccal segments will have to be placed in a slightly postnormal relation to the upper buccal segments. When treatment is complete this relationship should be carefully checked to ensure that there is no occlusal trauma or interference both in the intercuspal position and during lateral excursion.

If during this treatment an anterior bite plane is used, despite the fact that no appliance therapy has been used on the upper incisors, natural growth will often produce some improvement in incisal relationship. This can be seen in Figure 11.4 where the patient was treated during the period of puberty.

The more severe type of case (Fig. 11.1D to F) presents rather more of a problem. In these cases usually both upper and lower incisors are retroclined with a high inter-incisal angle and an excessively deep overbite which may well be traumatic. Not infrequently, it is associated with a small lower facial height and evidence of a forward rotation of the mandible during growth. Paradoxically such a case is usually on a Class I or even a mild Class III skeletal pattern. The aim in these cases should be to produce a reasonable approximation to normal occlusion.

The three factors which have been shown to be associated with the Class II Division 2 type of deep overbite are a small lower facial height, a high inter-incisal angle and a high lower lip line. If these three factors could be eliminated, clearly we would have a good chance of a stable result. The small lower facial height is probably unchangeable at least in the long term. It is quite possible to increase the lower facial height, for example by use of a bite plane, with a downwards and backwards rotation of the mandible. This will be discussed in detail in a later chapter, for the moment suffice it to say that it has a strong tendency to return to its original position, apart from the effect of any growth over the intervening period. This leaves the other two alternatives, attempting to achieve a better inter-incisal relationship and raising the upper incisors relative to the lower lip. Intrusion of the upper incisors with a suitable fixed appliance may be attempted but is difficult to achieve. It is however very much easier to hold the upper incisors in their original position, thus eliminating the normal downward eruption of these teeth. Since the rest of the face continues to grow, the lower lip is carried down away from the effect of the upper incisors.

This is illustrated in Figure 11.6. It will be noted here that there has been minimal increase in the lower facial height and indeed upward and forward rotation has continued during treatment, although the upper face has continued to grow. Nevertheless, the inter-incisal angle has been improved by a slight proclination of the lower incisors and substantial palatal movement of the upper incisor apex. Moreover, the incisors have been held at their original level so that the lip line is relatively lower in the later radiograph. The tracings in Figure 11.6C and D show another point which is not uncommon in Class II Division 2 malocclusions. Due to the forward rotation of the mandible, the dental bases tend to become rather more Class III. Advantage can sometimes be taken of this, together with overbite reduction to position the incisal edges of the lower incisors on a more stable part of the upper incisal cingulum without unduly proclining these lower teeth.

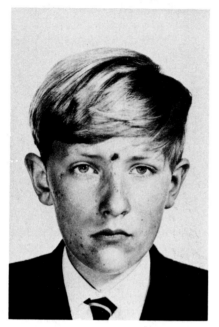
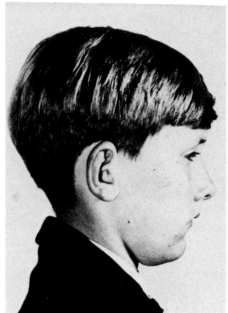
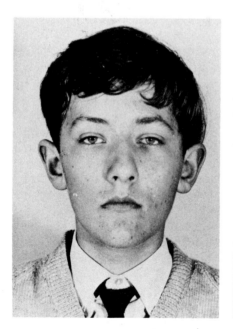
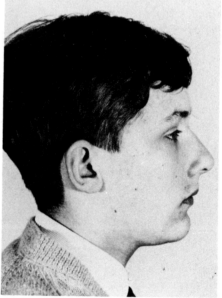

A

Fig. 11.4 Laurence. Mild Class II Division 2 malocclusion on moderate Class II skeletal pattern, treated with extraction of 7/7 and removable appliances. A, Photographs before and immediately after treatment. B (opposite), Models before and at end of treatment, also 5 years out of retention. C (overleaf), Tracing at end of treatment superimposed on initial tracing. Note favourable growth causing improvement of incisal relations. D, Tracing 5 years out of retention superimposed on the end of treatment.

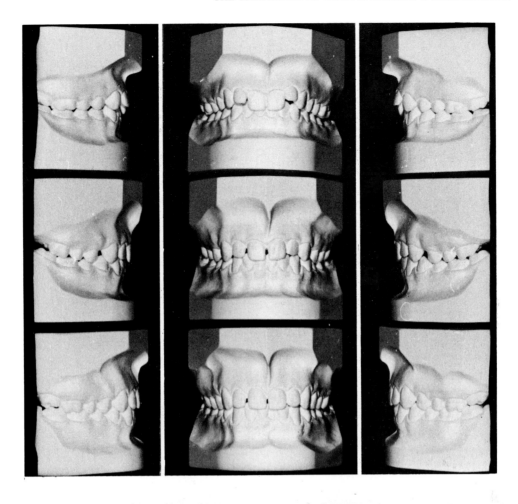

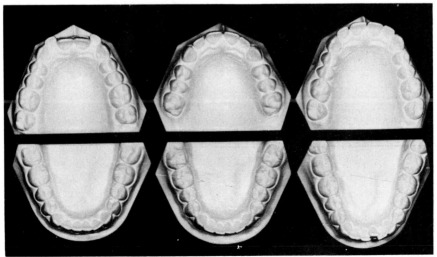

B

Fig. 11.4 (*cont'd*)

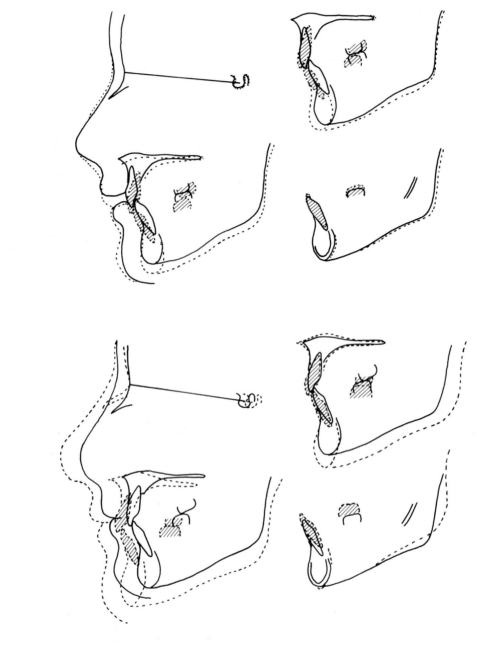

C

D

Fig. 11.4 (*cont'd*)

Practical treatment

The practical treatment of Class II Division 2 malocclusion follows the same basic principles as in Class II Division 1. In the absence of crowding, treatment should be by distal movement of the upper buccal segments, although if crowding is present in the post-molar region, the extraction of upper second molars may be considered, on the same lines as in the previous chapter. Laurence (Fig. 11.4), is such a case. The posterior occlusion was here Class II and there was a typical, although

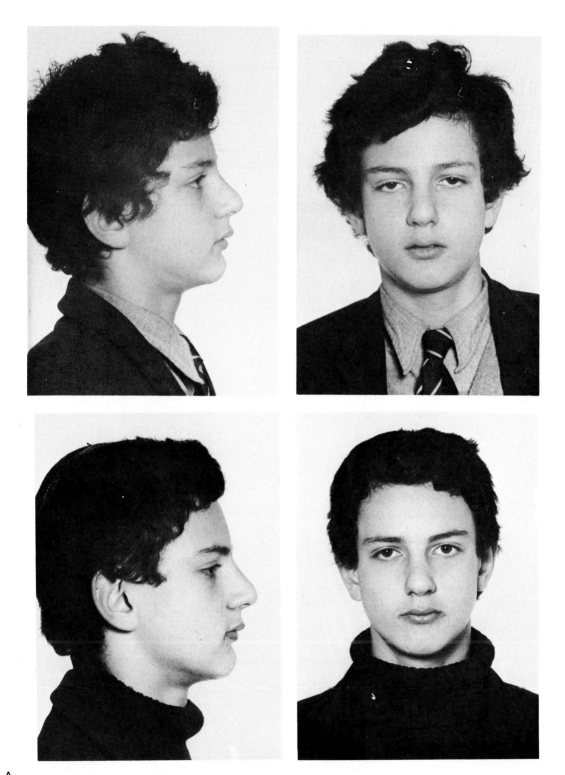

A

Fig. 11.5 Alan. Moderate Class II Division 2 malocclusion, treated by extraction of second premolars and removable appliances. A, Photographs before and at end of treatment. B, Models before treatment, at end of retention and 2 years thereafter. C, Tracing at end of retention, superimposed on original tracing. D, Tracings at end of retention and 2 years later, superimposed (B, C and D overleaf).

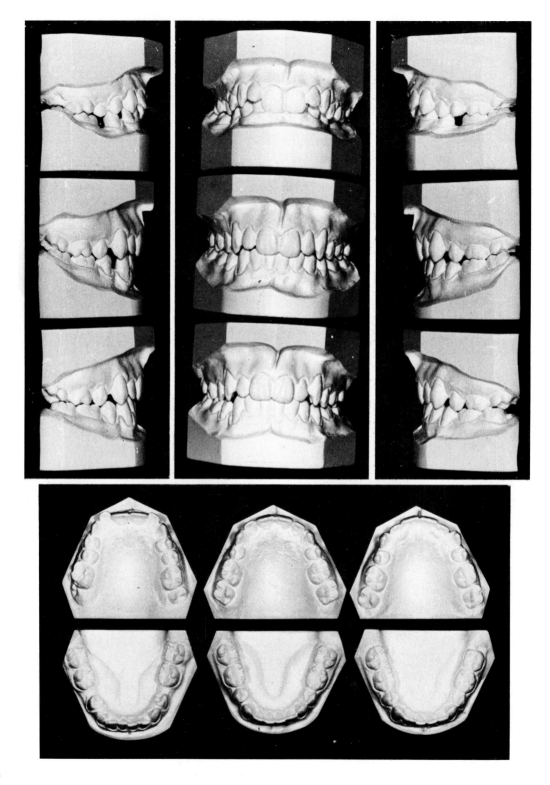

B

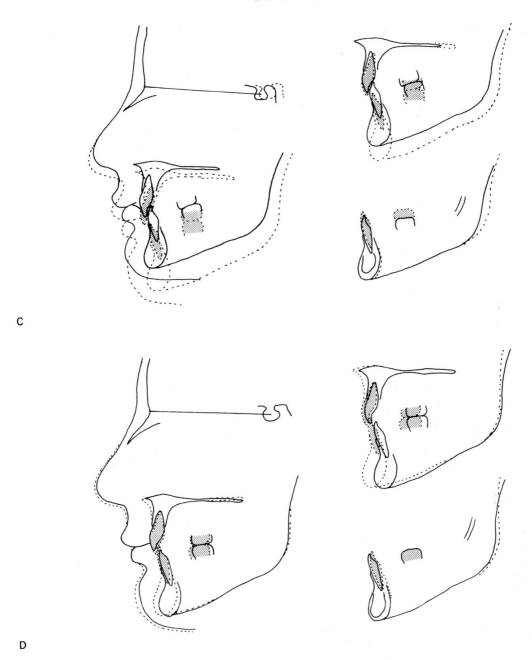

C

D

Fig. 11.5 (cont'd)

fairly mild, incisal relationship. He is in fact the boy shown in Figures 11.1A to C. Radiographic examination showed that although there was an absence of crowding in the ante-molar region, there was a lack of space for the developing upper third molars. The upper second molars were therefore extracted, thus facilitating the distal movement of the upper buccal segments of teeth with a removable appliance, into a Class I relationship and this was followed by subsequent appliances to retract the upper canines and finally to align the labial segment with retroclination of

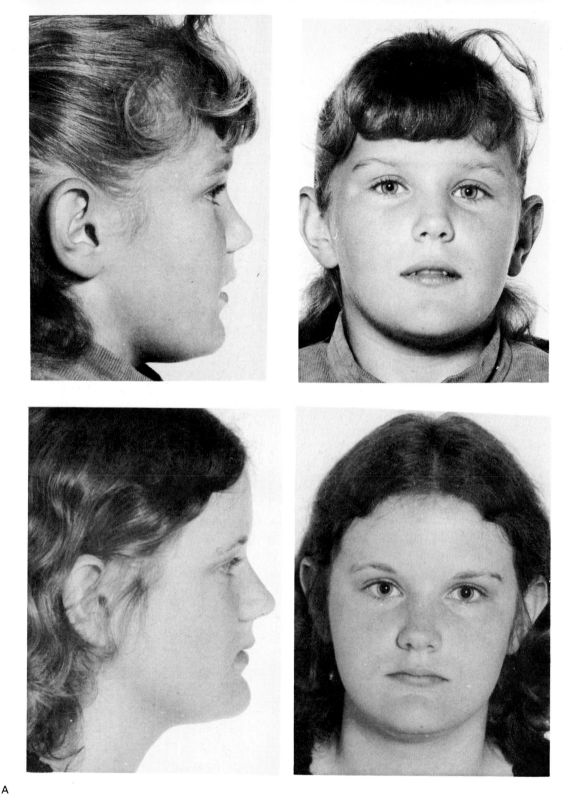

A

Fig. 11.6 Trina. Severe Class II Division 2 malocclusion associated with forward rotation of the mandible and small anterior lower facial height. Treated by extraction of first premolars and upper and lower edgewise appliance. A, Photographs before treatment and at end of retention. B (opposite), Models before treatment, end of retention and 2 years thereafter. C (overleaf), Tracing at end of retention superimposed on initial tracing. D, Tracing 2 years out of retention, superimposed on that taken at end of retention.

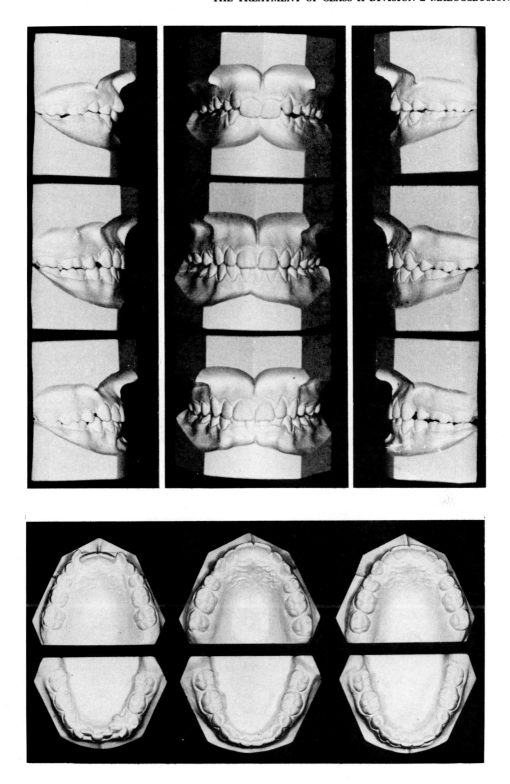

B

Fig. 11.6 (*cont'd*)

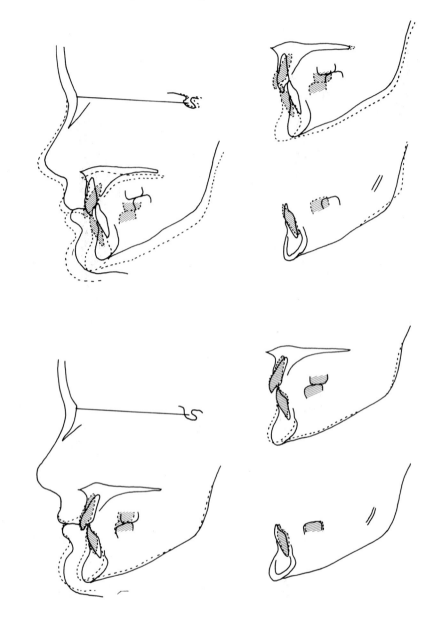

C

D

Fig. 11.6 (*cont'd*)

<u>2/2</u>. In this case the upper buccal segments were somewhat over-retracted into an ideal occlusion, and it will be noted in Figure 11.4B that the end of treatment, since the overbite was still somewhat increased, there was slight spacing distal to the upper canines. Five years out of retention, this spacing had almost closed but a slight crowding has appeared in the lower labial segment. This might have been prevented had a mildly post-

normal occlusion of the posterior teeth been accepted. Nevertheless, it is a good result and owes a great deal to the favourable growth which took place during treatment. It can be seen in Figure 11.4C that the mandible has grown downwards and forward relative to the maxilla and has spontaneously proclined the upper incisors to a more acceptable relationship than the original, a process which continued after the end of the treatment (Fig. 11.4E). This shows the importance of treating patients during the active growth which normally takes place around the age of puberty. It will be noted that 8/8 have erupted to replaced 7/7 and extraction of the partially erupted 8/8 was arranged at this visit.

Where crowding is present in the ante-molar region, extractions in this region will be necessary. A case of this type is shown in Figure 11.5. He had a moderate Class II Division 2 malocclusion with reasonably good facial proportions apart from a Class II skeletal pattern. Upper second premolars were extracted, since 5/5 were congenitally absent and crowding was not severe. An upper removable appliance was fitted to retract the upper canines, until sufficient space was made for the upper lateral incisors to be aligned with the central incisors. It was decided to accept the position of the latter teeth. This removable appliance carried an anterior bite plane to reduce the overbite to a slight extent in the hope that favourable growth would take place. The upper lateral incisors were then brought into the line of the arch with a second removable appliance and the final result was retained for some 12 months. No treatment was carried out in the lower arch, and the space was allowed to close spontaneously. This arch was of course kept under close observation and an appliance would have been inserted had this been necessary. It will be seen from Figure 11.5C that growth had taken place during this period in a rather unfavourable, downward direction, together with considerable backwards rotation of the mandible resulting from use of the bite plane. Although it had been decided to accept the position of the upper central incisors, at 96° to the maxillary plane they are about the limit of the acceptable range. During the ensuing period this backwards rotation relapsed. Growth was slight but favourable. As a result of these two factors, the symphyseal region came forward, causing a slight but useful proclination of the upper incisors.

This boy was treated entirely with removable appliances, and the result should be compared with that in the case of Trina in Figure 11.6. There are many reasons why removable appliances may be used for individual patients but in a case of this severity it must be accepted that the result will be less than perfect. On the other hand, it represents a considerable improvement on the original condition. This kind of decision is one which will often face the orthodontist. The type of appliance used on Trina requires a high degree of orthodontic skill and a committed and co-operative patient, with excellent oral hygiene. In the absence of any of these, a simpler line of treatment may be indicated.

These two cases illustrate a simple and effective line of treatment for a comparatively mild malocclusion. While the result is not ideal, it is atraumatic and aesthetically acceptable. The more severe type of Class II Division 2 malocclusion presents rather greater problems and involves more complicated treatment. It is almost always associated with short dental bases which will require the extraction of teeth. It is usually better to treat this type of case with fully banded appliances from an early stage. A practical problem may well be that the overbite is so deep that it is impossible to put brackets on the lower incisors, since these would be bitten off by the upper incisors. In such a case the upper canines may be retracted with a removable appliance carrying an anterior bite plane which will take the teeth out of occlusion and allow the lower arch to be banded, while also assisting in the reduction of the overbite. Alternatively, the upper incisors may be proclined so that they can no longer damage the lower brackets. When the overbite has been adequately reduced the upper arch may be banded and upper and lower incisors depressed simultaneously. A case of this type is shown in Figure 11.6, where the above plan was adopted. After the preliminary use of aligning arches, upper and lower Edgewise appliances were fitted to reduce the overbite and improve the inter-incisal angle. In the lower arch all the teeth were banded, including the second molars, giving additional anchorage in an effort to intrude the lower incisors into the bone. In the upper arch the appliance was used with a torque force to move the upper incisor apices palatally, this appliance is illustrated in Figure 13.6 and with the addition of a high-pull headgear, to intrude the upper incisors into the bone. It is noticeably easier to move upper incisor apices in this type of case than in Class II Division 1 malocclusion. Since the lower incisors were initially 'trapped' behind the cingulum of the uppers, it was felt that a small amount of lower incisor proclination would be acceptable. It will be noted from Figure 11.6 that despite strenuous efforts the incisors were not intruded to any great extent but they remained stationary while a small amount of growth took place and this, together with the change of angulation, enabled the operator to achieve a reasonably normal inter-incisal relationship which remained stable. In this type of case a mere alignment of the incisors on the original position of the upper central incisors would not be acceptable aesthetically and might well cause trauma by the incisal edges to the opposing soft tissues. It will be noticed that in this girl, as in many severe Class II Division 2 malocclusions, the skeletal pattern was initially Class I and tended to become Class III during the period of observation. This was due to a continuing forward rotation of the mandible. If untreated, the lower incisors would have retroclined further, increasing the inter-incisal angle and probably the overbite, as in the case shown in Figure 11.2. By moving the upper incisors away from the influence of the lower lip and changing their angulation, it was possible to take advantage of the forward rotation and consequent forward movement of the lower incisor region, to produce a stable inter-incisal relationship.

Functional appliances

Most of the standard functional appliances have modifications for use in the treatment of Class II Division 2 malocclusion. In those based on the Andresen appliance the central incisors are traditionally first proclined, thus producing a Class II Division 1 malocclusion, which is treated as such. The proclined upper incisors have a strong tendency to relapse during the initial period while the patient is becoming familiar with the appliance, and an upper retainer must be worn during the daytime to prevent this. With the Fraenkel appliance wires are built in to the framework to produce this proclination during treatment.

My own practice is rather different. The central incisors are not proclined, but the working bite is taken with the mandible lowered, and protruded to the smallest extent possible. This involves

rather more opening of the bite than would be used in treating Class II Division 1 malocclusion.

A case treated in this way is illustrated in Figure 11.7. Stella had long dental bases, and the vertical relation of the jaws was not typical, the lower facial height being slightly increased. This combination is rare in Class II Division 2, which may explain why functional appliances are used less than in Class II Division 1. They do not work well in crowded mouths, and generally are not very successful in reducing the overbite, especially where this is associated with a small lower facial height.

An interesting feature of this case was the late relapse of the incisor relation. There was a slight relapse, chiefly rotational of 2/2 shortly after the end of treatment, but 5 years later the angulation of the upper central incisors was unchanged. In the period between 5 and 14 years out of retention the central incisors retroclined, with their apices moving forward into contact with the labial plate of bone. This very late change is difficult to explain although, as previously mentioned, it is a feature of this type of malocclusion. It will be noted that the posterior occlusion did not relapse.

Retention

With its notorious tendency to relapse, there has always been a tendency to retain this type of malocclusion for an unduly long time. It is important to realise that no amount of retention will prevent a grossly unstable incisor position from relapsing. At the same time it may be that a slightly unstable result, if held for some period, will become stable because of natural vertical growth of the lower face. This applies for two reasons. In the first place the overbite reduction may have been produced by a backward and downward rotation of the mandible (Fig. 11.5C) and if this vertical relationship is maintained the face may grow sufficiently to accommodate the 'over-opened denture'. Secondly, if the position of the upper incisal edge can be retained, the growth downwards and forwards of the face may carry the lower lip downwards relative to the upper incisal crown. Where rotations of teeth, especially of the upper lateral incisors, are found in association with Class II Division 2, retention may be indi-

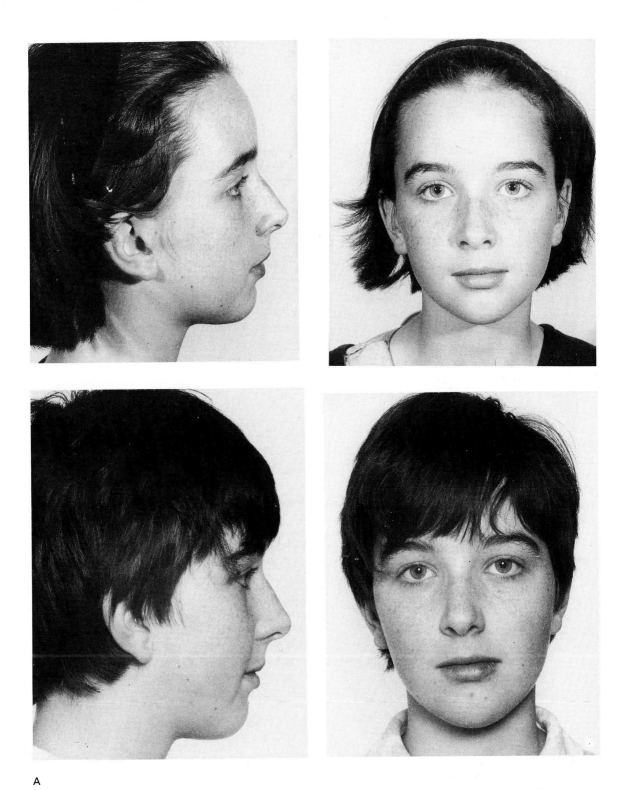

A

Fig. 11.7 Stella. A, Before and after treatment with Andresen activator. B, Study models before treatment, at end of retention and 14 years later; note mild relapse. C, Tracing before treatment superimposed on end of retention. D, End of retention on situation 5 years later. E, 5 years out of retention superimposed on 14 years. Note change in incisal position in E (B, C, D and E overleaf).

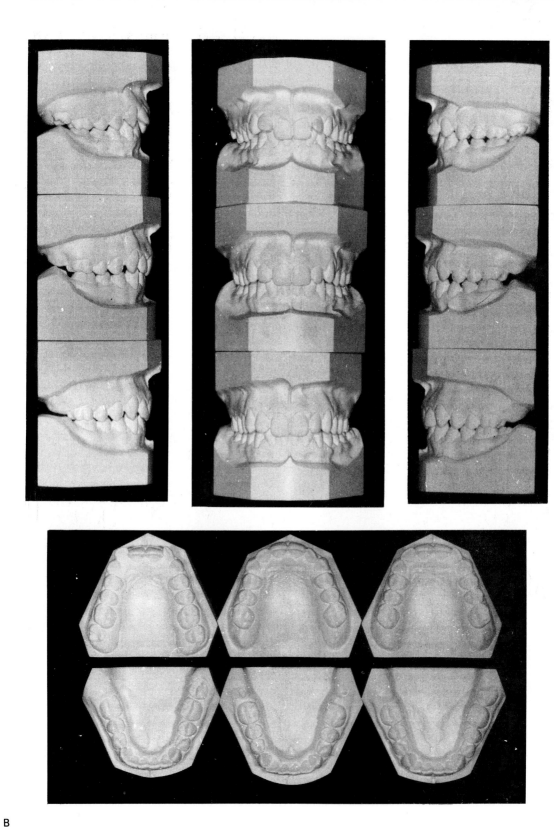

B

Fig. 11.7 (*cont'd*)

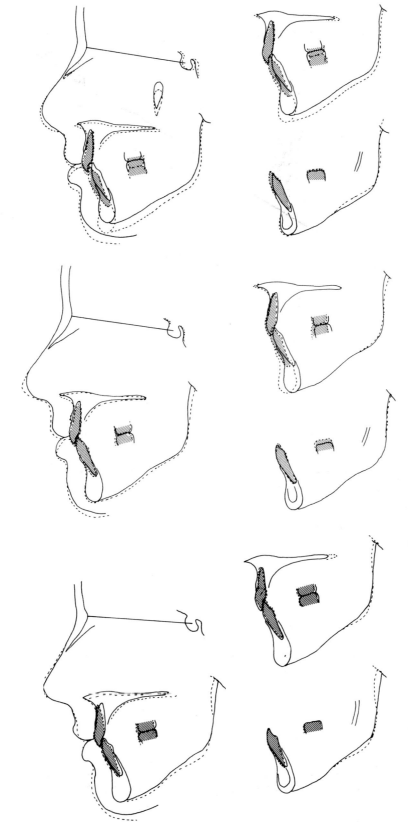

C

D

E

Fig. 11.7 (*cont'd*)

cated as for any rotated teeth. Pericision may help to reduce the risk of rotational relapse but will not prevent their proclination if this is otherwise likely. Prolonged retention is therefore sometimes indicated, but this should never exceed 12 months.

There is a very small proportion of cases where the overbite is traumatically deep and treatment is carried out after growth has ceased. In these cases the only possibility of preventing relapse is by the fitting of a permanent retainer. This would take the form of a metal appliance with an anterior bite plane. Suitable clasps will be required for retention and in addition some mechanism is necessary to prevent the upper central incisors from proclining, and the bite plane being bitten into the anterior part of the palate. This usually takes the form of small spurs passing over the contact point between adjacent incisors. It should be regarded as a last resort since the disadvantage in terms of 'gum-stripping' are obvious and also because patients usually fail to persevere, and tend to discard the retainer after at most a few years. In the adult or late adolescent a surgical approach is to be preferred, as described in Chapter 16. While each case must be judged on its merits, the general line of treatment would be to procline the upper incisors and then move the anterior bone segment posteriorly, while the lower incisor segment is 'set down', and the lower jaw advanced, with reduction of the chin point if this becomes unduly prominent. Such cases are not always stable, and particular care should be taken not to increase the lower facial height during surgery.

SUGGESTED READING

Fletcher G G T 1975 The retroclined upper incisor. British Journal of Orthodontics 2: 207–16

Hitchcock H P 1976 The cephalometric distinction of Class II Division 2 malocclusion. American Journal of Orthodontics 69: 447–54

Houston W J B 1967 A cephalometric analysis of Angle Class II Division 2 malocclusion in the mixed dentition. Transactions of the British Society for the Study of Orthodontics 46–50

Leech H L 1957 The treatment of Angle's Class II Division 1 and Class II Division 2 in identical twins. Transactions of the British Society for the Study of Orthodontics 60–7

Leech H L 1961 Angle's Class II Division 1 and Class II Division 2. Transactions of the British Society for the Study of Orthodontics 45–7

Mills J R E 1973 The problem of overbite in Class II Division 2 malocclusion. British Journal of Orthodontics 1: 34–48

Nicol W A 1963 The lower lip and the upper incisor teeth in Angle's Class II Division 2 malocclusion. Transactions of the British Society for the Study of Orthodontics 81–4

Ricketts R M 1952 A study of the changes in temporo-mandibular relations associated with the treatment of Class II malocclusion (Angle). American Journal of Orthodontics 38: 918–33

Robertson N R E, Hilton R 1965 A feature of the upper central incisors in Class II Division 2. Angle Orthodontist 35: 51–3

Smeets H J L 1962 A roentgenocephalometric study of the skeletal morphology of Class II Division 2 malocclusion in adult cases. Transactions of the European Orthodontic Society 247–59

12

The treatment of Class III malocclusion

As usual, Angle defined his Class III malocclusion on the basis of molar relation, Class III malocclusion being that where the mesio-buccal cusp of the lower first permanent molar occludes anteriorly to the buccal cusp of the upper second premolar. Such cases are rare and probably constitute less than 3 per cent of the population. The British Standard definition of incisor relationship defines the class as 'The lower incisor edges lie anterior to the cingulum plateau of the upper incisors. The overjet is reduced or reversed'. It therefore includes all those cases with a reduced overjet and overbite. In practice, the majority of Class III malocclusions have an anterior crossbite, with the lower incisors occluding labially to the uppers.

AETIOLOGY

Skeletal pattern

Class III malocclusion almost always occurs on a Class III skeletal pattern. This is illustrated by the histogram shown in Figure 12.1A. The angle ANB is represented above the line for a sample of Class III malocclusions, while the histogram below the horizontal line is the same angle for a group of unselected patients. Although there is, of course, individual variation, very few of the Class III cases fall within the normal range. Björk (1947) and Hopkin (1962) have shown that this is often due to a mandible which is large relative to the size of the maxilla, although other factors, notably in the base of skull, may be important. Class III is not the reciprocal of Class II malocclusion. In the latter the dental bases are usually of comparable size, whereas in Class III the discrepancy frequently lies in the jaws themselves.

The vertical relationship of the skeletal bases is of considerable interest in Class III cases although its importance has probably been exaggerated in the past. One often hears statements that there are two types of Class III malocclusion, those with a high mandibular angle and those with a low mandibular angle. This is certainly a gross over-simplification. The histograms in Figure 12.1B represent the same samples as in Figure 12.1A but this time indicate the maxillo-mandibular planes angles. It will be seen that the Class III sample has rather more extreme cases but nevertheless the vast majority of patients fall within the normal range. The extreme cases are noticeable because they present very considerable problems in treatment, but they constitute the exceptions.

A lateral relationship of the dental bases is probably more important in Class III malocclusion than elsewhere. It is common to find that the lower arch is wider than the upper causing a posterior buccal crossbite. As previously explained this may be a genuine discrepancy in width or may reflect the antero-posterior skeletal discrepancy with the prenormal occlusion causing a wider part of the lower arch to be opposite a given part of the upper, as explained in Chapter 3.

Soft tissue pattern

The soft tissues do little to contribute to the Class III malocclusion and indeed their tendency is to compensate for the skeletal discrepancy. The lower incisors are almost always retroclined and in fact are on average about 10° more retroclined than the random sample. There is some tendency for proclination of the upper incisors in some cases but this is much more variable. This is not

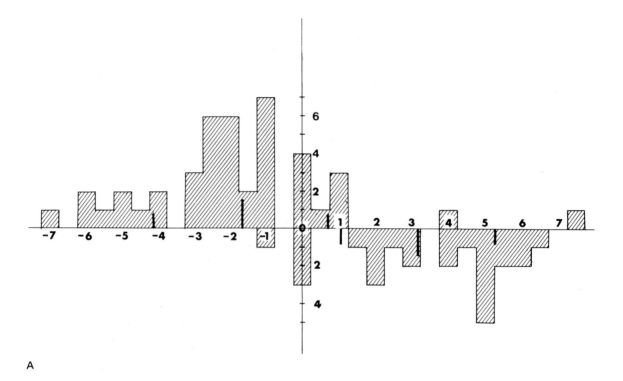

A

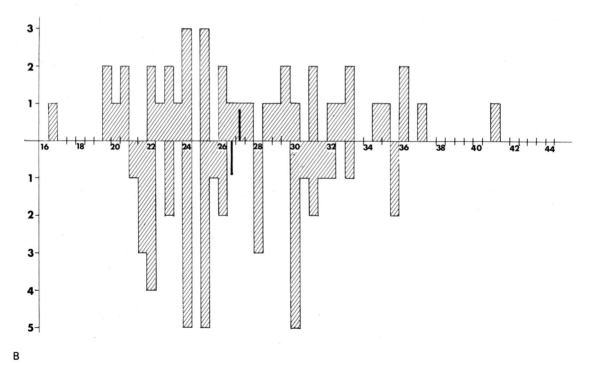

B

Fig. 12.1 A, Histogram to compare the angle ANB in a group of patients with Class III incisor relations (above the horizontal line) with a random group (below the line). B, The maxillo-mandibular planes angle of the same two samples.

perhaps, the advantage it may seem because a patient requiring treatment usually has a reverse overjet despite this compensation. In other words the skeletal pattern is worse than the dental pattern and if the latter is corrected by a tilting of the incisor teeth, they may end up very tilted indeed.

Dental pattern

As already indicated, the lower incisors are usually retroclined and the uppers sometimes proclined. Crowding can of course occur in any mouth but it is common in Class III cases to find this more severe in the upper than in the lower arch.

Path of closure

Many textbooks describe a type of Class III malocclusion which is variously referred to 'pseudo-Class III' or 'postural Class III'. It is suggested that these patients have a normal skeletal pattern and that the abnormality is produced by a tilting of the teeth. Such cases undoubtedly exist and their treatment is comparatively easy. The theory then goes on to say that these cases may be diagnosed by the fact that the patient can achieve an edge-to-edge incisor relationship. Most patients who have a reverse overjet and a reasonably deep overbite can achieve this edge-to-edge relationship and some of them may be very difficult indeed to treat. The skeletal assessment is far more valuable in indicating the prognosis.

An interesting, but unimportant aspect of this type of case is illustrated in Figure 12.2. The tracing with the solid outline is taken from a patient with a fairly severe Class III skeletal pattern and a deep overbite. Another tracing of the mandible was then made on a second piece of tracing paper and superimposed on the first, being attached to it by means of a single drawing pin through the condylar head. By rotating the second tracing around the drawing pin the picture illustrated by the dotted outline was produced. That is the incisors became edge-to-edge, with the mandibular condyle still in its normal position in the fossa. In order to move the tracing from the edge-to-edge to the occlusal position, the lower incisors have to pass 'through' the upper incisor

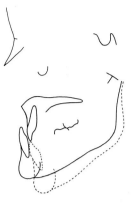

Fig. 12.2 Tracing of patient with a Class III malocclusion and deep overbite, solid outline in occlusion. The broken outline has been produced by rotating a second superimposed tracing of the mandible around a drawing pin through the condylar head region.

and this is clearly impossible in life. It would seem therefore that in these cases with a deep overbite the forward displacement of the mandible in occlusion is more apparent than real. From the edge-to-edge position the patient has to displace the mandible forward in order to avoid the upper incisors but the condyle returns to its normal position in the glenoid fossa as occlusion is reached. Where a deep overbite is present the condylar head is not displaced forward on the eminentia articularis when the teeth are in occlusion, although there is some forward displacement where the overbite is minimal.

It has been suggested that the type of deep overbite seen in Figure 12.2 is the result of 'over-closure'. It is usually assumed that this over-closure can be corrected if the incisor relationship is corrected. This again is an oversimplification. It would seem that this type of Class III malocclusion is associated with an extreme forward rotation of the mandible during growth, very similar to that sometimes in Class II Division 2 malocclusion. Bryant (1980) has shown that if the upper incisor relationship is corrected the forward rotation usually continues but the centre of rotation is moved from the premolar region to the point of contact of the incisors. Some increase in lower facial height may occur during treatment (as it does in many types of malocclusion) but the original pattern is usually re-established after treatment is completed. She showed a few cases in whom there appeared to be an increase in lower facial height which was more permanent but such a result is unpredictable and uncommon.

TREATMENT

In considering the treatment of Class III malocclusion I am proposing to refer to only those cases with a reverse overjet. The type of case with a decreased but positive overjet will be illustrated in Chapter 13.

In planning the treatment and assessing the prognosis for Class III malocclusion two factors are important: the degree of skeletal discrepancy and the amount of overbite present. The latter frequently but not invariably reflects the vertical relationship of the skeletal bases. It is proposed therefore to divide treatment into these categories.

CASES WITH NORMAL OR INCREASED OVERBITE

Skeletal pattern normal or very mild Class III

In this type of case the dental arches are of comparable size and the incisors at a normal angle to their bases. Occasionally the lower incisors may even be proclined or the uppers retroclined. The patient can achieve an edge-to-edge relationship from which he displaces forward into occlusion. Such a case is illustrated in Figure 12.3 for Sandra. It will be seen both from her photograph and from the tracing that her skeletal pattern is normal or even mildly Class II. The lower dental arch is well aligned but the upper arch is slightly crowded with labial displacement of one upper canine and the opposite second premolar. Both upper and lower incisors are proclined, producing a bimaxillary proclination which was racial in origin, but this incisor proclination was more marked in the lower jaw.

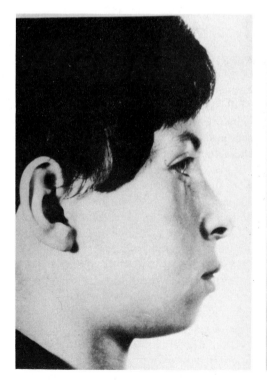 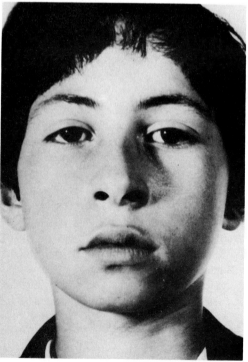

A

Fig. 12.3 Sandra I. Class III incisor relationship in Class I skeletal pattern. A, Photographs before treatment. B (opposite), Study models before and after treatment and 4 years later. C (overleaf), Tracing before treatment superimposed on that after treatment. D, Tracing after treatment superimposed on that 4 years later.

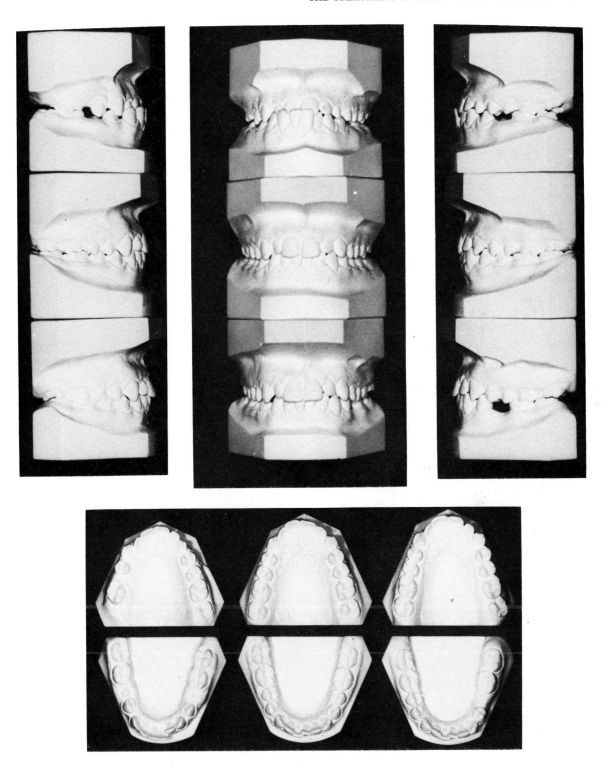

B

Fig. 12.3 (cont'd)

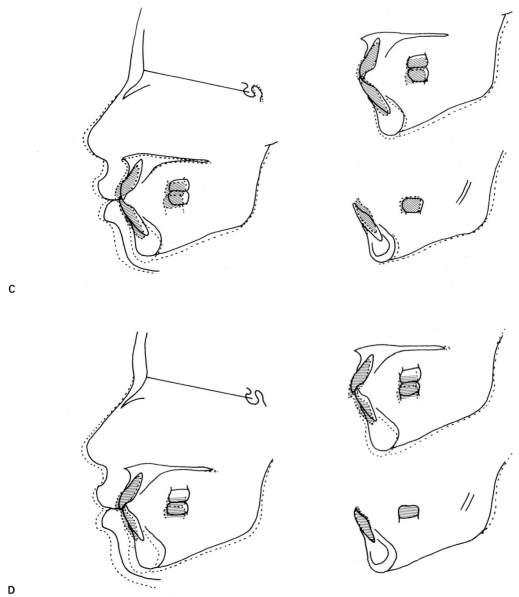

C

D

Fig. 12.3 (*cont'd*)

The first decision to be made is concerning the need for extractions. If there is a genuine inherent crowding then the only satisfactory treatment is by extraction of teeth. On the other hand the treatment of the upper arch frequently involves a mild antero-posterior expansion which may accommodate teeth which at first sight appear to be crowded. The key therefore lies in the lower arch. If this is not crowded then every effort should be made to avoid extractions in the upper arch or to delay such extractions until the incisor relationship has been corrected. In Sandra's case only three incisors were occluding lingually to the lowers and these were corrected without undue difficulty with an upper removable appliance of the type shown in Figure 12.4. Suitable teeth are clasped (it is necessary to give some thought to this and usually the clasps should be on first

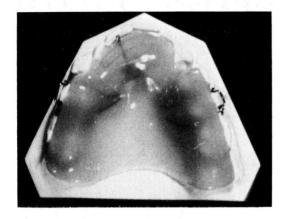

A

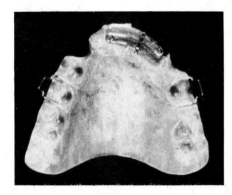

B

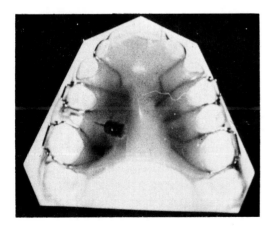

C

Fig. 12.4 Removable appliances used in treatment of Sandra. A, First appliance, for proclination of upper incisors. B, Fitting surface of first appliance to show spring. C, Second appliance with screw to open space for 5/.

premolars or second deciduous molars rather than the first molars). A doubly recurved cantilever spring is then activated to move the upper incisors labially. There is often some controversy as to whether it is necessary to place bite blocks over the posterior teeth as has been done in Sandra's case. It is certainly possible in most cases to correct the incisor relationship without this, although difficulties may be encountered where the overbite is very deep. Nevertheless, I feel that if a thin acrylic capping of the posterior teeth, equal to one thickness of wax, is constructed and then trimmed in the mouth so as just to eliminate the overbite of the incisors, the patient will immediately close in the edge-to-edge relationship. The forward movement of the upper incisors is then minimal and the lower incisors are not working in the reverse direction every time the patient occludes. As indicated, this is not essential but it would seem a logical step to facilitate the correction of the incisors.

When the incisors had been corrected it was apparent that there was now insufficient room for the upper right second premolar. A second removable appliance was made with a screw to re-open the space for this tooth which was achieved without difficulty, giving the result seen in Figure 12.3.

This type of Class III occlusion which is found on a normal skeletal pattern is easy to treat and the result is usually quite stable as shown in the lowest models in Figure 12.3 which were taken 4 years out of retention, although unfortunately /5 had been lost due to caries. Although Sandra was treated in the complete permanent dentition, this is one of the few cases where an equally good, and even perhaps easier, result is achieved by treating in the mixed dentition as soon as all four permanent incisors have fully erupted in both jaws.

Mild to moderate Class III skeletal pattern

This type of case, with a fairly deep overbite is probably the most common type of Class III malocclusion. The patient can achieve an edge-to-edge incisor relationship and it is easy to confuse this type with the previous ones often with disappointing results. Such a case is shown in Figure 12.5. Her name was also Sandra but there the

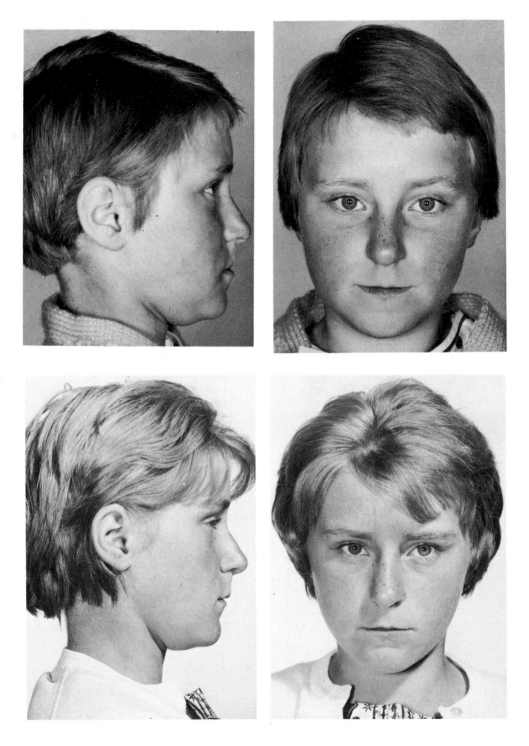

A

Fig. 12.5 Sandra II. Class III malocclusion on moderate Class III skeletal pattern. A, Photographs before and after treatment; compare the profile with Sandra I in Fig. 12.3B (opposite), Study models before treatment, after correction of incisors and 5 years out of retention. C, (overleaf) Tracing before treatment superimposed on that after treatment. D, Tracing after treatment superimposed on that 5 years later. Note increased severity of Class III skeletal pattern.

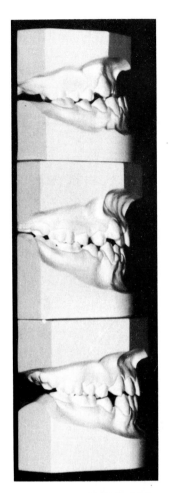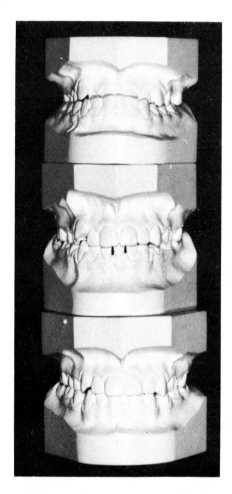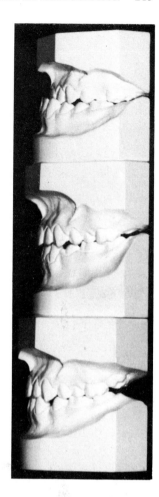

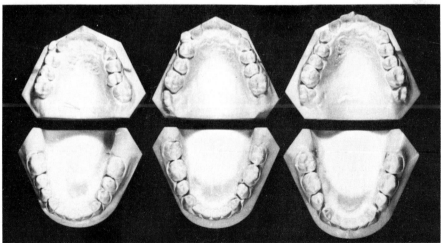

B

Fig. 12.5 (*cont'd*)

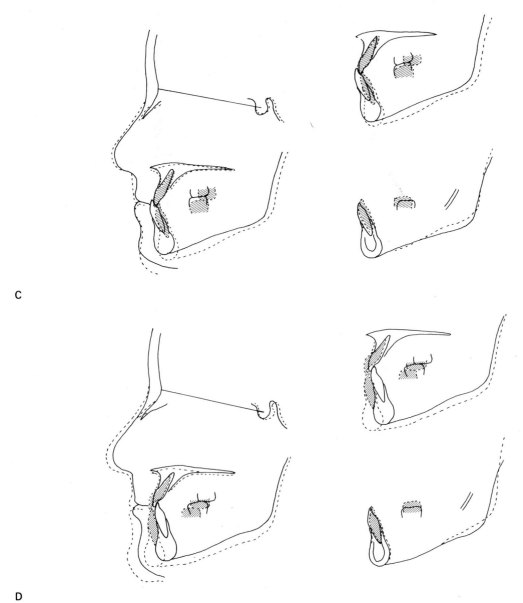

C

D

Fig. 12.5 (*cont'd*)

resemblance ends. She could achieve an edge-to-edge relationship of her incisors without difficulty but looking at the lateral skull tracing in Figure 12.5C it will be seen that she has a marked Class III skeletal pattern with a small lower facial height. The upper incisors are somewhat proclined and the lowers are retroclined at least relative to the maxillary plane. The difference in skeletal patterns can be seen by examining photo-

graphs of the two Sandras in Figure 12.3 and 12.5.

The effect of trying to treat this type of case by proclining the upper incisors alone is illustrated in Figure 12.6. Both the patients shown in this figure had a Class III incisor relationship on a moderate Class III skeletal pattern with a deep overbite. In both cases the angulation of the incisors had tended to compensate for the Class III

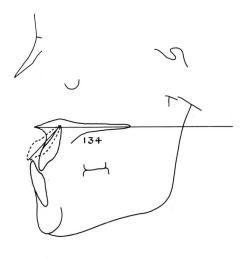

A

as the upper incisors were proclined, they gradually achieved an edge-to-edge relationship with the lower incisors when in centric occlusion, with an absence of both overbite and overjet. Further attempts to procline the upper incisors produced no apparent result and it would be seen from the tracing that, as the upper incisors had been proclined to a quite unacceptable degree, the lower incisors had also spontaneously proclined. It is difficult to know the reason for this but it is not an uncommon finding if this type of treatment is attempted in the wrong case.

In Figure 12.8A we see the patient in Figure 12.6B and in his case the lip morphology was

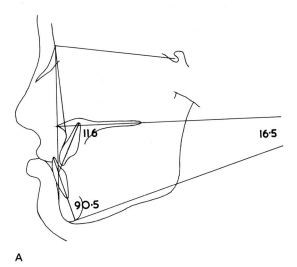

A

B

Fig. 12.6 Tracings of two difference patients with moderate Class III skeletal pattern. The broken outline indicates the final position necessary to correct the incisors by proclination of upper incisors only.

skeletal pattern and both patients could achieve edge-to-edge relationship without difficulty. Nevertheless, it will be seen that if we were to try to correct the condition merely by proclining the upper incisors, they would have to be proclined to an angle something over a 130° and such a position would clearly be extremely traumatic. In fact it is not quite as simple as this. One of two things may happen. Figure 12.7 shows the patient in Figure 12.6A. It will be seen from the facial outline that he had full and rather flaccid lips and

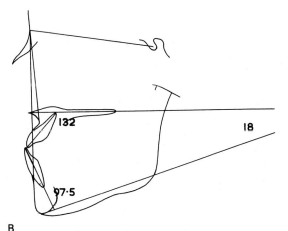

B

Fig. 12.7 The patient shown in Fig. 12.6A, before treatment and after an attempt at treatment by proclination of the upper incisors.

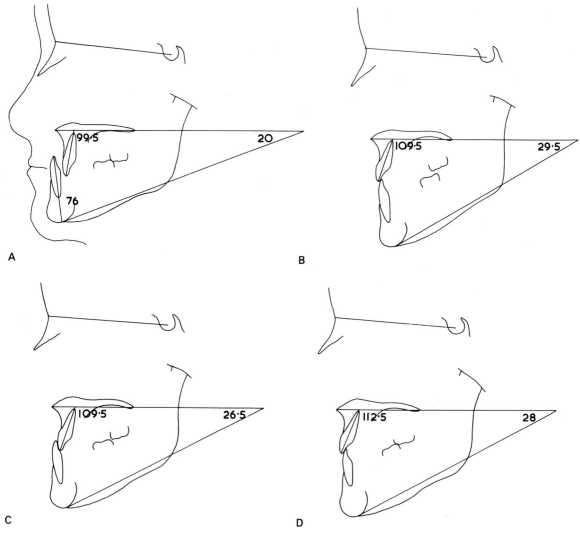

Fig. 12.8 The patient shown in Fig. 12.6B. A, Before treatment, B, reconstruction from description in patient's notes of corrected incisor relation with 'posterior open bite'. C, The actual radiograph taken on the day when the above entry was made. D, Following successful treatment involving retroclination of lower incisors.

somewhat different. The lips were firm with a more marked contraction which did not allow the lower incisors to procline with the uppers. As will be seen in Figure 12.8B, the incisors were proclined over the bite but at this stage there was an apparent posterior open bite. Such an entry was made in the patient's records and this type of result can occasionally be corrected by fitting an upper anterior bite plane. In the present case this did not work. It was, however, interesting that where the patient's record stated that the incisor

relationship was normal, a lateral skull radiograph taken on the same day produced the picture shown in Figure 12.8C, that is with the incisors still in Class III relationship. This was the only way in which the patient could bring the posterior teeth into occlusion. As will be seen in the lower right tracing this patient, and incidentally the one in Figure 12.7D was successfully treated by extractions in the lower arch and retroclination of the lower incisors.

This indicates the policy which should be

followed in these moderately severe Class III malocclusions. In considering the treatment of other forms of malocclusion, I have suggested that the labio-lingual position of the lower incisors should be regarded as the datum from which to commence treatment planning. This is only slightly modified in Class III malocclusions. If the upper and lower incisors are in contact, albeit with a reversed overjet, then this combination of teeth lies within a narrow zone of balance between the soft tissues labially and lingually. If the teeth are displaced from this position of balance they will tend to return to their original position but it is of course possible to exchange the position of upper and lower incisors, and a slight overall lingual movement can be achieved especially if lower first premolars have been extracted. In the case of Sandra II the lower first premolars have been extracted and Class III inter-maxillary traction used to correct the incisor relationship (Fig. 12.9). Since no tooth alignment was required at this stage in the upper arch an upper lingual arch was fitted with hooks on the buccal aspect of the upper molar bands. Elastics were worn from this to a free-sliding lower labial arch. It is convenient if this arch is attached to the incisor teeth and for this purpose Begg brackets have much to recommend them since they allow free tilting of the lower incisors. The whole upper dental arch was therefore balanced against the lower anterior teeth and this caused a retroclination of the latter. If slight anterior movement of the upper arch were produced, this would be all to the good. Many variants of this are possible: if there is an excessive amount of space in the lower arch lower intra-maxillary traction may be used either instead of or in addition to, the inter-maxillary traction. If the upper arch requires alignment a fully banded appliance may be employed and there is no reason why edgewise brackets should not be used in the upper arch even though Begg brackets are used in the lower.

Patients with Class III malocclusion frequently have large mandibles and therefore this is one of the few cases where premolars may be extracted in uncrowded mouths. The resultant space does not close readily and it is necessary to use appliances to bring this about. At the same time it is eminently desirable that the lower labial

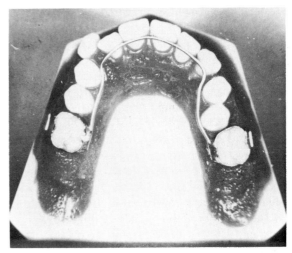

A

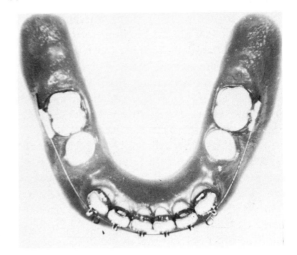

B

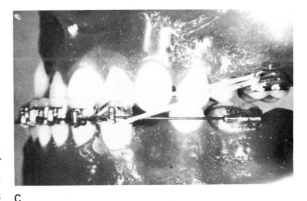

C

Fig. 12.9 Fixed appliances used in first stage of treatment of Sandra II. A, Upper lingual arch. B, Lower free-sliding arch-wire. C, Class III intermaxillary traction.

segment should not be supported by the posterior teeth, in order to keep these incisors in the most lingual possible position. It is therefore recommended that a small space should be left between a lower canine and second premolar. This should only be large enough to be self-cleansing but it should be borne in mind that, as in this girl's case, it may not close spontaneously. It will be noted that here again no attempt was made to relieve the crowding of the upper canine until the incisor relationship had been corrected. This produced some increase in space and the upper teeth were aligned with distal movement of the upper molars as shown in the lower models of Figure 12.5. In treating Class III malocclusions the overbite is all too easily reduced. A positive overbite is necessary to retain the corrected incisor relationship. If it is desired to move the upper buccal segments distally, thought should be given to the effect on the overbite and, in general, the use of cervical anchorage alone should be avoided.

It has already been pointed out that the initial labio-lingual position of the combined upper and lower incisors is comparatively stable. Although the position of the teeth can be reversed, if they are moved far from the position of balance they will tend to return to their original place. In the case of Sandra I, the upper incisors were proclined over the bite so that the combined teeth were somewhat too far labially placed. They tended to move lingually with retroclination of both upper and lower incisors and this would in turn increase the overbite and also the stability. In the case of Sandra II, the lower incisors were retroclined with minimal proclination of the uppers so that the final position was rather too far towards the lingual. Such teeth tend to relapse labially and as they move labially the overbite tends to reduce. In extreme cases this can mean that the overbite disappears completely and the upper incisors relapse inside the lowers. Furthermore it will be noticed in both these cases that the mandible grew forward relative to the maxilla: the skeletal pattern became more Class III. This may happen in all types of patients but is particularly marked in Class III malocclusion and is again liable to give rise to relapse. The prognosis in these cases should therefore always be guarded and if there is doubt

about the severity of the skeletal pattern one should be pessimistic.

Severe skeletal discrepancy

The borderline between the moderate Class III case which may be treated orthodontically and the severe one which may not, is not easy to define. As a rough guide an ANB angle beyond $-3°$ should be regarded with considerable foreboding, as should any patient with a deep overbite who is unable to achieve an edge-to-edge incisor relation. Further growth is difficult to assess and even the patient within these guidelines may still relapse. The severe type of Class III malocclusion is associated with an unacceptable facial appearance and the treatment of these cases should be surgical. This is dealt with in detail in Chapter 16 and illustrated there in Figure 16.3. While major facial surgery should never be minimised, the treatment of mandibular prognathism associated with a deep overbite is usually extremely satisfactory and in competent hands this is a safe and not very complicated operation. Improvement in facial appearance is extremely pleasing to the patient.

Cases with reduced overbite

The problem in those patients where the overbite is initially reduced is one of stability — the common problem in treatment of Class III cases. If the incisors are initially in a Class III relation on a Class III skeletal pattern they will have an inherent tendency to go back to that position. If their relationship can be corrected, the teeth left in labio-lingual balance, and with a good overbite, then this overbite will act as a permanent retainer and prevent relapse. During the correction of the reverse overjet, there is usually a loss of overbite so that if this is initially reduced it may well end up completely absent and there is nothing to prevent the relapse.

Mild skeletal discrepancy

Where the skeletal pattern is normal or the discrepancy mild, the incisor relationship will either show a small positive overjet or be

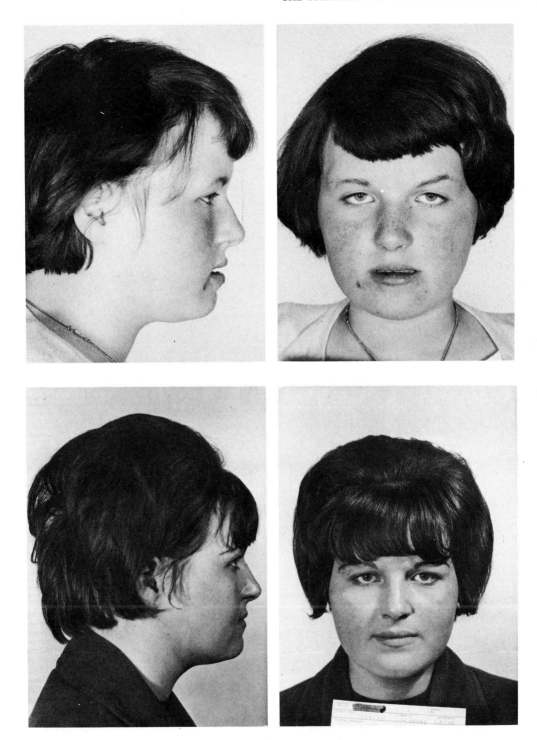

A

Fig. 12.10 Theresa: Class III malocclusion with reduced overbite although with normal or reduced lower facial height. A, Photographs before and after treatment. B, Study models before treatment, at end of retention and 4 years later. C, Superimposed tracings before and at end of treatment. D, Superimposed tracings at end of treatment and 4 years later (B, C and D overleaf).

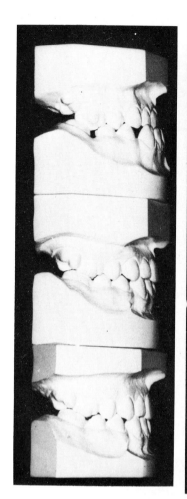
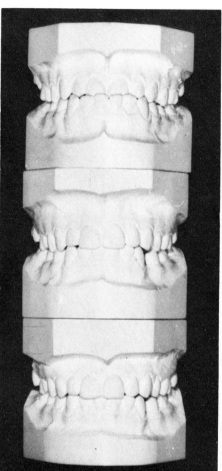
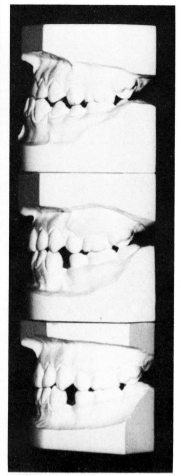
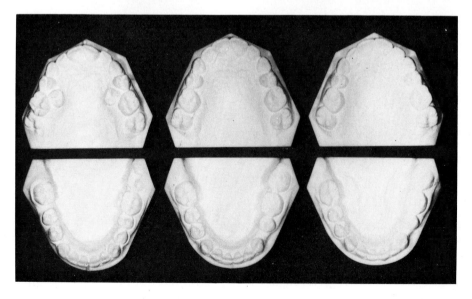

B

Fig. 12.10 (*cont'd*)

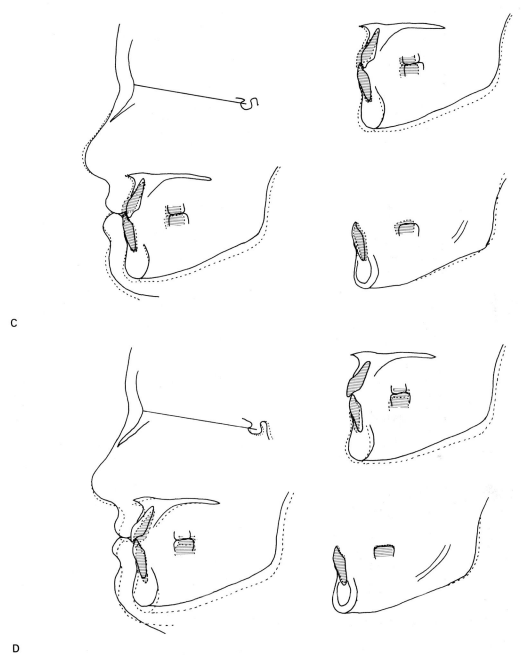

C

D

Fig. 12.10 (*cont'd*)

completely edge-to-edge with a lack of both over-bite and overjet. In such cases the incisor position should be accepted and the problem becomes merely one of aligning the teeth. In this type of case there is usually a basal discrepancy in arch size so that it is associated with a tendency, to a greater or lesser extent, to a posterior crossbite. If the lower dental arch is well aligned and the posterior teeth in Class I relationship then inevitably there will be crowding in the upper arch in the absence of a normal overbite and overjet. This is not easy to treat and will be dealt with in more detail when considering the general problem of crossbite in Chapter 13.

Moderate skeletal discrepancy

This would usually be associated with a reverse overjet and with a somewhat reduced overbite. Such a case has an indifferent prognosis but treatment may be possible provided the antero-posterior skeletal discrepancy is not too severe and, perhaps more especially, provided the vertical skeletal patterns is within normal limits. Such a case is shown for Theresa in Figure 12.10. She had a reversed overjet with a slightly reduced overbite but it will be seen both from her photograph and the lateral skull tracing that the lower facial height is not increased: indeed it was somewhat low. In these cases the incisor relationship can be corrected either by proclining the upper teeth or retroclining the lowers depending on the degree of antero-posterior skeletal discrepancy. The important feature of such treatment is that bands should be used on the teeth to be moved and an appliance fitted which will tend to extrude these teeth from their sockets.

In the case of Theresa the skeletal discrepancy was comparatively mild and it was felt that treatment could be confined to the upper arch. There was some crowding in the lower left buccal segment but on the right side the first molar had been lost. The upper second premolars were palatally excluded and these teeth were therefore extracted together with the lower left first premolar. Treatment was confined to the upper arch and was carried out by means of a modified twin wire arch (Fig. 12.11). Bands with appropriate brackets were selected for the first molars and four incisors and the twin wire arch was somewhat modified in that the normal twin wires were replaced by a piece of multistrand wire in end tubes. Stops were constructed by squeezing the anterior end of the end tube and a piece of coil spring added between this stop and the buccal tubes on the molar bands (Fig. 12.11A). This was compressed in the mouth and would therefore have the effect of moving the incisors labially with the molars as anchor teeth (Fig. 12.11B). In addition the archwire was so angled that the multistrand wire lay below the brackets, approxi-

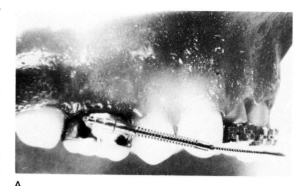

A

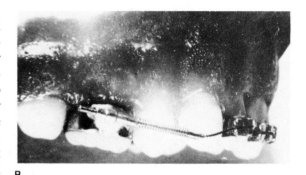

B

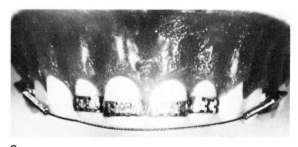

C

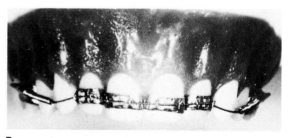

D

Fig. 12.11 Modified twin wire arch used to procline and mildly extrude upper incisors. A, Lateral view, to show coil which when the archwire is tied in will tend to procline anterior teeth. B, Lateral view with the appliance tied in and the coil compressed. C, Anterior view to show passive position of multistrand wire. D, Archwire tied in: note the extrusive effect of multistrand wire.

mately level with the incisal edges of the incisor teeth (Fig. 12.11C). When it was tied into the brackets it therefore tended to extrude these teeth which was of course the movement required (Fig. 12.11D). The twin wire is particularly suitable for this purpose because of the long flexible arm which is available to produce a gentle extruding force on the teeth. Had the skeletal pattern been more severe, a lower banded appliance would have been fitted to move the lower incisors lingually in addition to the labial movement of the uppers and this would also have used a fine wire lying above the brackets of the lower teeth so as to cause some extrusion of these teeth. Using this technique, it is usually· possible to maintain the overbite which exists before treatment commences, although one should not expect to increase this overbite permanently.

In Theresa's case no treatment was carried out in the lower arch and the result there is acceptable rather than excellent. Fortunately, as can be seen from the superimposed tracings, growth in Theresa's case was favourable and the result remained stable.

Severe skeletal discrepancy

The type of case which falls into this category might almost be described as a syndrome. A typical case is shown in Figure 12.12. The skeletal discrepancy is in the vertical rather than in the antero-posterior dimension. The gonial angle is high with a large lower facial height and a reduced overbite or even a frank open bite. Although from examination of the models it will appear that there is a severe skeletal discrepancy, very frequently the ANB angle is not grossly abnormal because the whole dental area is steeply inclined, including both the occlusal and maxillary planes.

This type of case presents a major problem. In the case of Veronica in Figure 12.12, the solution was to align the teeth and relieve the crowding without making any attempt to correct the incisor relationship. This is often acceptable. A Class III incisor relationship with a deep overbite is extremely ugly, but where there is an absence of overbite, so that the upper incisors are visible from the anterior view, the reverse overjet is much less noticeable. Any attempt to correct this ortho-

dontically is doomed to failure and while in a proportion of cases surgery may be indicated, such an approach is much more difficult than in the cases with deep overbite and very much more prone to relapse after operation. Fortunately, this type of Class III malocclusion, associated with the 'long face syndrome' is very rare.

'ORTHOPAEDIC' TREATMENT

The chin cap

A number of methods have been used in Class III malocclusion in the hope of correcting the skeletal pattern or preventing it from becoming more marked. Probably the earliest of these was the chin cap; a cup-shaped device fitting the chin and attached by elastic material to a head cap. It was used by Angle and probably much earlier, and has found favour with a few orthodontists to the present day. If it is successful, it is surprising that it is not more widely used.

The effect has been studied by Thilander (1963), Lee Graber (1977) and in a modified form by Bennett (1968). There seems general agreement that its principal effect is to retrocline the lower incisors and to rotate the mandible downwards and backwards, thus lengthening the face and making the chin-point less prominent. Graber, in his very thorough investigation, showed shortening of the vertical ramus an interesting finding, contrasting with the lengthening found by several authors in the treatment of Class II Division 1 malocclusion.

Unfortunately, none of these authors has followed the results for an appreciable time after treatment.

Functional appliances

Most, if not all, of the well-known functional appliances have versions for the treatment of Class III malocclusion, from Andresen onwards. The fact that these are not widely used tells its own story. The most popular is, perhaps, the Fraenkel F.R.3 appliance, which protagonists of this technique claim to be successful. It is essentially an inverted F.R.1 appliance; that is it has a lip-pad anterior to the upper alveolus and a labial bow

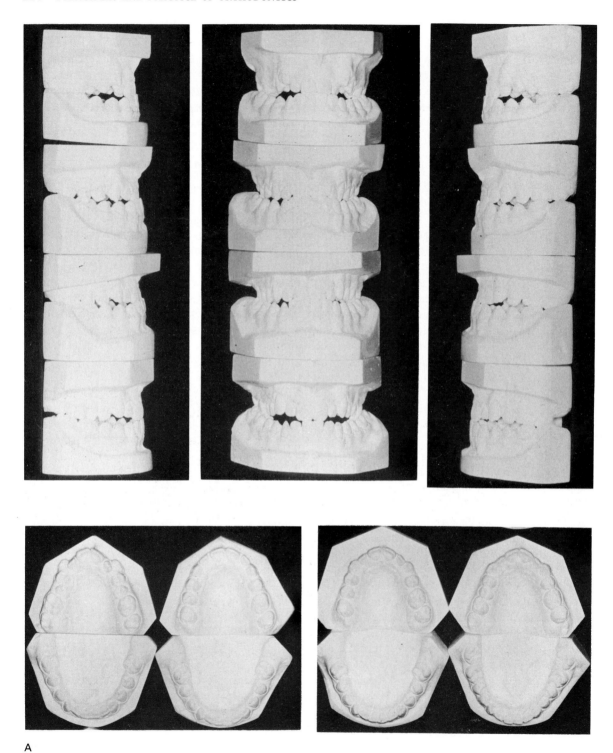

A

Fig. 12.12 Veronica: Class III malocclusion with discrepancy in jaw size, steep mandibular angle and large lower facial height. A, Study models before treatment, after alignment of upper arch and 4 years later. B (opposite), Superimposed tracings before treatment and 1 year out of retention.

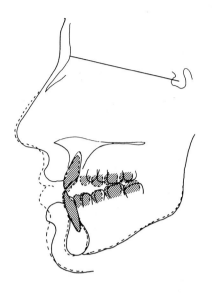

around the lower incisors. Dr Fraenkel claims that it causes anterior growth of the maxilla, but it seems more probable that its effect is largely, if not completely, dento-alveolar. It is difficult to tolerate and probably has no advantages over a simple fixed appliance such as that illustrated in Figure 12.9.

Extra-oral traction

The idea of anterior extra-oral traction, from a face-mask, was popularised some years ago by Delaire, in France. The face-mask is commercially available and is, on the whole, well tolerated by patients. Figure 12.13 describes the treatment of Heather, who had a Class III malocclusion with a mild bilateral crossbite. The latter was treated with rapid maxillary expansion as described in Chapter 14, and the appliance shown in Figure 12.14 was then fitted. The edgewise appliance

B

Fig. 12.12 (*cont'd*)

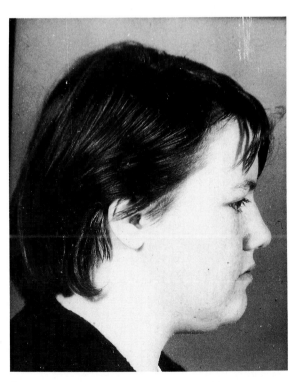

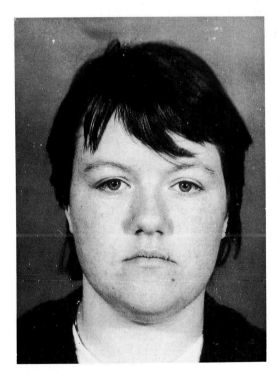

A

Fig. 12.13 Heather. A, Before treatment. B, Study models; before treatment, at end of treatment with final appliance in place, and 6 months later. C, Superimposed tracings before and after treatment (B and C overleaf).

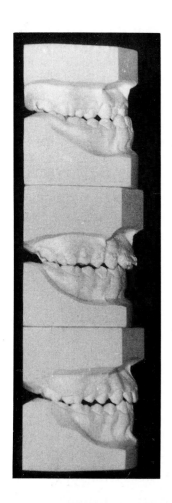
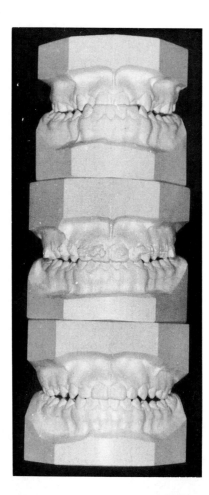
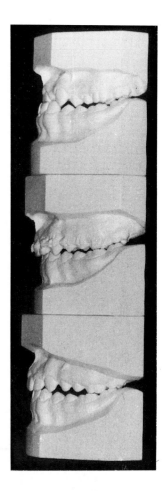
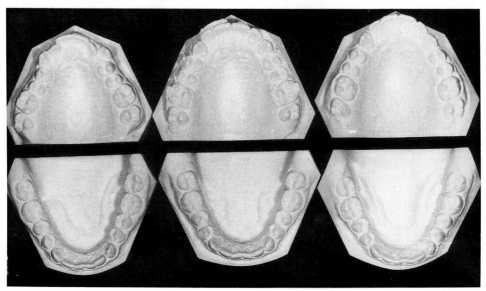

B

Fig. 12.13 (*cont'd*)

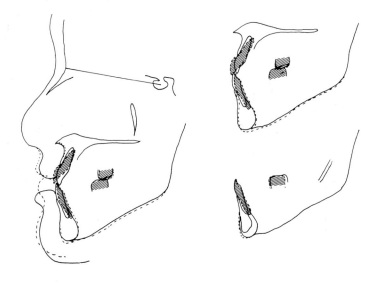

C

Fig. 12.13 (*cont'd*)

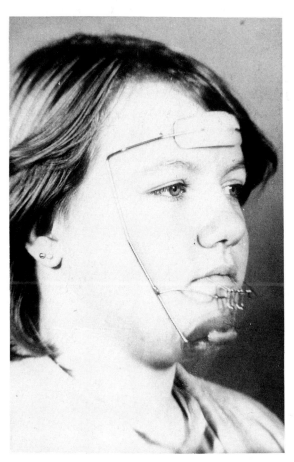

A

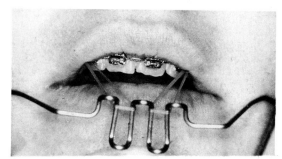

B

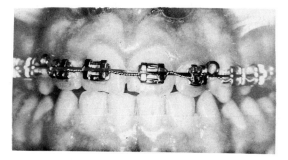

C

Fig. 12.14 Face mask for anterior traction. A, Heather wearing mask. B, Close-up, extra-oral view. C, Edgewise appliance. Note loops to which elastics are attached.

heavy rectangular arch, adjusted with root torque to minimise labial tilting of the incisors, in the hope of encouraging forward growth of the whole maxilla. Any such effect is probably small, and in Heather's case the correction of the anterior crossbite has been essentially due to tooth movement. After only 6 months follow-up there is a tendency to relapse of the posterior crossbite, although the incisal correction has been maintained.

Retention

As I have already indicated, stability is the problem in the treatment of Class III malocclusion. In this prolonged retention does not help in any way. A positive overbite may provide a form of permanent retention for the corrected incisor relationship, but if this is not the case then no amount of artificial retention short of permanent retention, will succeed. The problem is particularly exacerbated by the tendency of the skeletal pattern to worsen as a result of normal growth. Nothing short of surgery can prevent this.

On the other hand, the permanent retention provided by the incisor occlusion can be very effective if the overbite is adequate. It may have the effect of holding the upper incisors in a position somewhat labially of their true position of balance. If this is the case they not infrequently remain slightly mobile for up to 12 months following the completion of treatment. In my own experience such mobility has invariably disappeared in the long run without any harm to the teeth. Leech (1966) has reported a case where excessive root resorption took place following such treatment. Such a possibility should always be borne in mind although I have not personally encountered this phenomenon.

SUGGESTED READING

Björk A 1947 The face in profile. Svensk Tandlakare Tidskrift 40 Suppl. 5B

Bryant P M F 1981 Mandibular rotation and Class III molacclusion. British Journal of Orthodontics, 18: 61–76

Graber L W 1977 Chin cap therapy for mandibular prognathism. American Journal of Orthodontics 72: 23–41

Hopkin G B 1962 A roentgenographic cephalometric analysis of treatment and growth changes in a series of cases of mesiocclusion. Transactions of the British Society for the Study of Orthodontics 130–48

Hopper J 1955 Preliminary investigation of mandibular guidance in postural Class III cases. Transactions of the British Society for the Study of Orthodontics 112–6

Joffe B M 1965 Cephalometric analysis of mandibular prognathism. Journal of the Dental Association of South Africa 20: 145–56, 173–80 and 212–9

Leech H L 1966 in discussion to paper by Mills, J.R.E. (1966) Transactions of the British Society for the Study of Orthodontics 37

Mills J R E 1966 An assessment of Class III malocclusion. Dental Practitioner 16: 452–65 and Transactions of the British Society for the Study of Orthodontics, 22–37

Thilander B 1965 Chin-cap treatment for Angle Class III malocclusion. Transactions of the European Orthodontic Society 311–27

13

Problems of overbite

The relation between the dental arches in the vertical dimension is essentially a differential one between the levels of anterior and posterior teeth in one or both arches. Occasionally, an individual tooth or a small group of teeth may fail to develop to the normal occlusal level in any part of the mouth, usually due to the ankylosis of the tooth or teeth affected. In the present chapter, however, it is proposed to deal with those cases in which the anterior teeth have produced either a reduced or an increased vertical overbite.

REDUCED ANTERIOR OVERBITE

In ideal occlusion the upper incisors overlap approximately one third to half of the height of the lower incisors. Where the overjet is increased it will usually be found that the lower incisors occlude either with a more lingual part of the cingulum of the upper incisors or with the hard palate, depending on the degree of overjet. If this is not the case, that is if the lower incisors are not in contact with either the upper teeth or the hard palate when the posterior teeth are in occlusion, then the overbite is stated to be incomplete. Thus a patient may have an incomplete overbite even though the overbite is in fact increased from the normal because of the increase in overjet. If, when viewed from the front, there is a gap between upper and lower incisors in the vertical dimension, although the posterior teeth are in occlusion, then the patient is said to have an open bite. This can exist irrespective of the amount of overjet.

Aetiology

Skeletal factors

It has been shown by a number of authors that there is a fairly high correlation between the overbite and the anterior lower facial height. This correlation exists not only in cases of frank open bite but even where the overbite is incomplete. It would seem therefore that a vertical skeletal factor has an affect in producing a decreased overbite. This is often associated with a steep lower border of the mandible and in extreme cases, such as that shown in Figure 13.1, the open bite may extend back into the premolar region and even involve the first molar, leaving the patient occluding only on the most posterior teeth in the mouth. In such a case, it will be found that the linear distance from the incisal edge of upper or lower incisors to their respective bases is increased beyond the normal level, although the alveoli are abnormally thin, giving the impression, in a lateral radiograph, that the teeth are placed on the end of a 'stalk' of bone. A logical explanation would seem to be that the teeth have the potential to erupt up to a certain level. If at that level they have no antagonist, then they will continue to erupt further with more alveolar bone deposited. There is, however, a limit to this additional vertical development and if the inter-maxillary space is too great for it to be bridged by such a procedure, then an open bite or an incomplete overbite, will result. The type of case shown in Figure 13.1 is of course exceptional but it would seem probable that this factor occurs to a limited extent as a contributory cause of incomplete overbite in many patients.

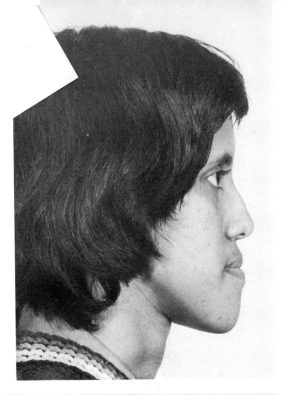
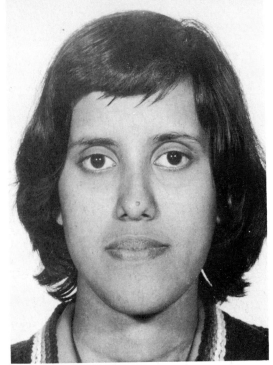

A

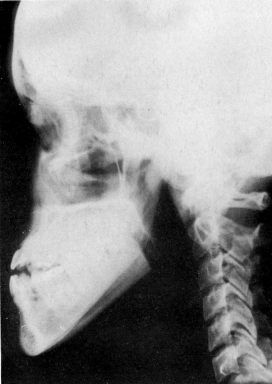

B

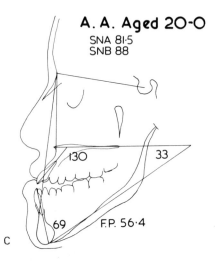

A. A. Aged 20·0

SNA 81·5
SNB 88

130   33

69   F.P. 56·4

C

D

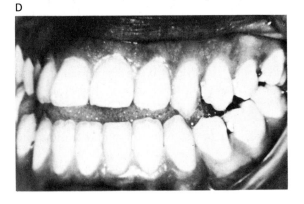

Fig. 13.1 Patient with anterior open bite associated with increased facial height and steep mandibular angle. A, Photographs. B, Lateral skull radiograph. C, Tracing of lateral skull radiograph. D, Intra-oral photograph to show open bite extending to molar region.

Soft tissue factors

There is some controversy about the importance of soft tissues, notably the tongue, in the aetiology of anterior open bite. If an incomplete overbite exists, then the tongue will rest in this space and will be thrust through it during swallowing, in order to produce an anterior oral seal as detailed in Chapter 3. It may be that in a small proportion of cases, the tongue is actually the cause of the anterior open bite, either due to its abnormally large size or to some lack of control over the movement of the tongue, producing the so-called endogenous tongue thrust. Such cases are certainly very rare and for practical purposes may be ignored. They are somewhat more common in children of negroid ancastry.

Dental factors

These do not play a great part in the aetiology of anterior open bite, except, as indicated above, insofar that the teeth may achieve their full eruptive potential without meeting their antagonists. Very occasionally in an otherwise normal dentition, a small group of teeth will fail to erupt to the occlusal level, although they are apparently normal in other respects. This would seem to be a localised failure of alveolar development and can occur in the anterior region but is more frequently seen among the posterior teeth (Fig. 13.2).

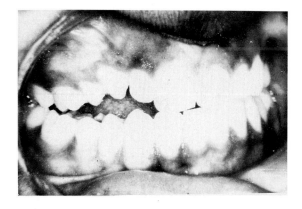

Fig. 13.2 Localised open bite in right buccal segment. There is no obvious cause for this except a failure of local development of the alveolus.

Habits

As already indicated in Chapter 4 a persistent digit sucking habit will almost invariably produce an incomplete and often a frank open bite.

Treatment

Treatment of an anterior open bite is usually disappointing. If an open bite is seen in a younger child, it will usually be found that this has disappeared by the time the child is fully grown (Worms and others, 1971), but if an appliance is inserted at the appropriate stage, it is possible to take the credit for something which nature has produced. An open bite produced by a digit sucking habit will resolve spontaneously once the habit has been discontinued. In children under the age of 8 years, Bowden has shown that the overjet will correct itself in approximately 12 months, while it may well take 3 years for the overbite to re-establish. Where the open bite has been produced by the digit, the tongue will fill the space at rest and it may be that the presence of the tongue retards the re-establishment of a normal overbite. It does not however, other things being equal, prevent it.

The conventional method of closing an anterior open bite is to use a banded appliance with a large elastic band crossed and recrossed between the anterior teeth so as to produce an extruding force on these teeth. This may help to increase an overbite slightly, but is unlikely to have any dramatic affect unless the condition is resolving spontaneously. Where the open bite is due to skeletal factors such a practice can produce looseness of the teeth without appreciably decreasing the open bite. The type of open bite which is associated with skeletal abnormality, as shown in Figure 13.1 does not respond to conventional orthodontic treatment. It may be treated surgically, and in fact was so treated in this case, but relapse is rather common, to a greater or lesser extent, in this type of case.

INCREASED OVERBITE

A deep or increased overbite is more common than the reverse condition and happily responds more readily to treatment, although difficulties may be encountered at times. This condition was formerly called 'close bite' but in term is now out of favour.

Aetiology

Skeletal factors

Just as an increased lower facial height and mandibular angle may be associated with a reduced overbite, so a decreased lower facial height and low mandibular angle may be associated with a deep overbite. The relationship is, however, less close. Where the lower facial height is reduced, the incisors will tend to erupt towards their full potential and to migrate towards a predetermined distance from their bases. Clearly they cannot do this if they occlude in the normal relationship, since the cingulum of the upper incisor obstructs the lower incisor and vice versa. Depending on the soft tissue pattern, a number of possibilities occur, of which a selection is shown in Figure 3.3. The reduced lower facial height is often associated with a forward rotation of the mandible during growth and this forward rotation will tend to cause the mandibular symphysis, and with it the lower incisors, to tilt lingually. This may well take the lower incisors away from the cingula of the upper incisors and permit further development into either a Class II Division 1 or Class II Division 2 incisor relationship. Examples of these have been shown in the appropriate chapters.

An antero-posterior discrepancy in the skeletal pattern may also have an affect in producing a deep overbite. If the anterior teeth do not erupt into a normal relationship, they may not meet their antagonists and may therefore continue to develop to a limited extent beyond their normal level, thus producing a deep overbite, in a Class II or a Class III malocclusion. This would obviously be more severe where the lower facial height is reduced and very much less severe where it is increased.

Soft tissue factors

Any abnormal posture or behaviour of the lips which prevents the teeth from occluding in their normal relationship may, as in the case of the skeletal pattern, allow the teeth to develop beyond their normal level and tend to produce an increase overbite. A high lip line acting on the labial surface of the incisors or a hyperactive lip will have the affect of moving the teeth lingually and this again will produce a deep overbite as already explained in Chapter 10.

Dental factors

On a Class I skeletal pattern the overbite is directly related to the inter-incisal angle. Where both upper and lower incisors are retroclined, as indicated in Chapter 10, the overbite will be increased. This can be brought about by a simple geometric construction as shown in Figure 13.3, and in such cases the distance of the incisal edges from their respective bases, is usually within normal limits: the teeth have not 'over-erupted'. Similarly, if the inter-incisal angle is low, with a bimaxillary proclination, the overbite is correspondingly reduced. There is quite a high correlation between the height of the lower lip line and the inter-incisal angle and it would seem that this relation is one of cause and effect.

Treatment

The treatment of deep overbite has been considered in some detail in previous chapters and it is not proposed here to do more than summarise the points made in those contexts. Basically, the overbite may be reduced by one of two methods.

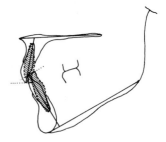

Fig. 13.3 A normal incisor relationship is shown by the solid outline. The effect of tilting upper and lower incisors lingually (broken outline) produces a high inter-incisal angle and deep overbite. Note that the incisal edges have not increased their distance from their respective bases (dotted line).

An upper anterior bite plane may be fitted on which the lower incisors impinge. This holds the posterior teeth out of occlusion. It does not normally depress the lower incisors into the bone, although it may retard their eruption, while the posterior teeth erupt more rapidly than usual into occlusion. This reduces the overbite and also increases the lower facial height with some backward rotation of the mandible. Some authorities consider this to be undesirable and prone to relapse, and it is in many ways similar to the fitting of a denture in which the vertical dimension has been unintentionally increased. There is however one important difference. The orthodontic patient is usually a child who is growing. Success may therefore well be achieved if growth is sufficient to accommodate this 'over-opened denture'. Even in an adult a slight to moderate overbite decrease may be produced with an anterior bite plane in favourable cases. While the denture will initially be over-opened, there is some evidence that if the condition is retained, then the teeth will gradually depress into the bone so that the original vertical dimension is restored, with both anterior and posterior teeth moving together.

The response to bite-opening procedures varies very much between patients. In some cases the overbite will reduce very rapidly with the use of a bite plane, and this is often accompanied by an increase in overjet due to the downwards and backwards rotation of the mandible. At the other extreme, some cases prove extremely resistant. This is particularly true in patients who have a small lower facial height and the appearance of a forward mandibular rotation during growth.

Overbite reduction may be carried out with fixed appliances because such appliances have been chosen for other reasons. In most cases the effect will be concentrated in the lower jaw, especially where the lower dental arch exhibits an increased curve of von Spee. In certain cases, especially of Class II Division 2, it may be desirable to 'depress' the upper incisors also.

In some cases a comparatively simple fixed appliance will be adequate, and the Ricketts 'utility arch' shown in Figure 13.4 is such a simple appliance. The archwire fits into tubes on the molar bands and in this position the anterior segment lies well below the brackets on the

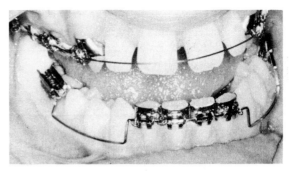

Fig. 13.4 The Ricketts 'utility arch' for 'depression' of lower incisors. Note the reciprocal force will elevate the molars and tip them distally.

anterior teeth. When lifted and tied into the brackets on the incisors, it will exert a depressing force on these incisors. This will be most effective if a fine wire, of hard resilient material, is used. Care is, however, necessary in the use of this appliance. In the hands of its originator it is used in conjunction with sectional arches on the posterior teeth, which stabilise the first molars. In the absence of these the appliance is liable to elevate the molars and tip them distally.

With suitably designed appliances, a small amount of active depression of the incisor teeth may be achieved but an archwire used for this purpose will have an 'equal and opposite reaction' on the anchor teeth. It should be remembered that teeth have been designed to withstand stress in a vertical direction and equally they have been designed to erupt. It is not therefore surprising that the effect of such arch-wires is to encourage further development of the posterior teeth much as with a bite plane although possibly to a somewhat lesser extent. It is usually found that any depression of the incisor teeth into the bone quickly relapses to the original level of these teeth. Nevertheless, the teeth have been held to their original level, whereas without treatment they would have, as part of general growth, erupted further. There is therefore a relative depression compared with the untreated condition. If a round archwire is fitted and made active in such a way as to depress the incisors, it will usually have the affect of proclining them. The labial side of the root, just below the crown, will come closely into contact with the alveolar crest, while the apex of the root will tend to move into contact with the lingual plate of bone. It will then apparently become jammed across the alveolus and any depressing will certainly become impossible. This affect may be overcome by using an appliance which controls the axial inclination of the teeth, either an edgewise wire or some attachment such as the Begg spurs, so that the tooth is moved along what Levason has called the 'corridor of bone'.

Where overbite reduction is particularly difficult, a number of devices may be used which are combined in Figure 13.5. This lower arch is designed to achieve the maximum intrusion of the lower incisors. The second molars have thus been banded to increase the anchorage. Loops have been introduced into the archwire between the incisors and canine to increase its flexibility and to concentrate all the effort on to these four teeth. If necessary, the lower canines may be depressed later with a subsequent archwire. Finally rectangular wire has been used to control the angulation of the teeth and to move them, as already stated, down the 'corridor' of cancellous bone.

If an archwire will tend to elevate the posterior teeth rather than depress the anterior teeth it would seem logical to move the anchorage outside the mouth. This has been achieved by the use of a high-pull headgear hooked on to the archwire in the incisor region as indicated in Figure 13.6. It is not known to what extent this does produce actual intrusion of the upper anterior teeth but such an appliance should not of course be used without a full archwire to control the teeth against proclination and such an archwire will inevitably be active and will therefore have some reciprocal effect on the molars. High-pull headgear, placing an intrusive force on the incisors, is prone to cause apical resorption of the teeth if excessive forces are employed. Such forces should not exceed 70 g.

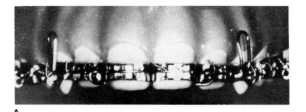

A

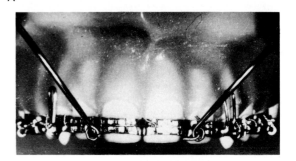

B

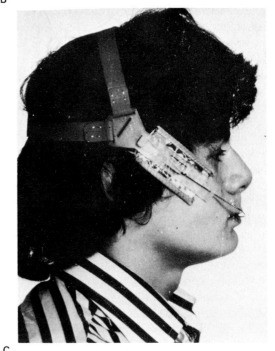

C

Fig. 13.6 High-pull headgear attached to anterior part of upper archwire. A, Intra-oral view of arch-wire. B, The same with hooks from head cap attached. C, Extra-oral view.

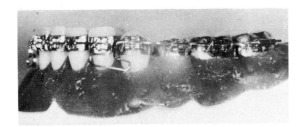

Fig. 13.5 Lower rectangular archwire to depress lower incisor teeth.

From the above description, it may seem that overbite reduction is at best a chancy business. Whatever one does there is a tendency to cause a backward rotation of the mandible and to produce an over-opened denture. Nevertheless, in practice

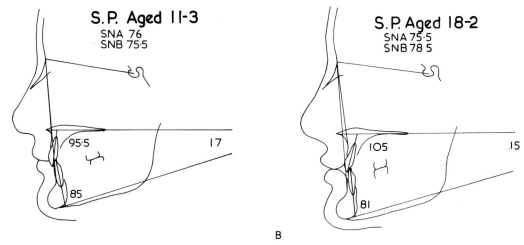

Fig. 13.7 Class II Division 2 patient with deep overbite, before treatment and 5 years out of retention. Note that orthodontic treatment with considerable forward growth of the mandible has produced a stable result on a Class III skeletal base.

this seems to be of little importance and overbite reduction can be achieved, with varying degrees of ease, in almost all patients. As with all malocclusions, having achieved the result it is necessary to prevent it from relapsing. The solution here would seem to lie in producing an ideal incisor relationship or the nearest which can be achieved to this ideal. That is, the lower incisal edge should occlude on the cingulum plateau of the upper incisor with the upper and lower incisors at approximately a normal angle to their bases and to each other. If this is achieved, it is unlikely that the overbite will relapse even in the presence of further forward rotation of the mandible. An example of this is shown in Figure 11.6. This is

not the only stable interincisal position. On a Class III skeletal pattern it is possible to achieve stability with retroclined lower incisors, and the upper incisors at their normal angle, so that the incisal third of the cingulum occludes against the labial surface of the lower incisor as shown in Figure 13.7, again preventing any further development and allowing any further rotation of the mandible to take place about the incisors.

The prognosis for the reduction of deep overbites is therefore much more favourable than for the correction of open bites. This is especially true in the young growing child and while some relapse frequently occurs from the final condition, this is not usually sufficient to cause any embarrassment.

SUGGESTED READING

Atherton J D 1964 The influence of the face height upon the incisor occlusion and the lip posture. Transactions of the British Society for the Study of Orthodontics 87–91

Bowden B D 1966 A longitudinal study of the effects of digit and dummy sucking. American Journal of Orthodontics 52: 887–901

Cousins A J P, Brown W A B, Harkness E M 1969 An investigation into the effect of the maxillary bite plate on the height of the lower incisor teeth. Transactions of the British Society for the Study of Orthodontics 55: 105–10

Menezes D M 1975 Comparative analysis of changes resulting from bite plane therapy and Begg treatment. Angle Orthodontist 45: 259–66

Parker C D 1964 A comparative study of intermaxillary spaces with treated and untreated occlusions. Transactions of the British Society for the Study of Orthodontics 16–34

Richardson A 1967 A cephalometric investigation of skeletal factors in anterior open bite and deep overbite. Transactions of the European Orthodontic Society 159–71

Richardson A 1970 Dento-alveolar factors in anterior open bite and deep overbite. Dental Practitioner 21: 53–7

Worms F W, Meskin L H, Isaacson R J 1971 Open-bite. American Journal of Orthodontics 59: 589–95

14

The treatment of crossbite

The British Standard Glossary of Dental Terms defines crossbite as follows:

> 1. A transverse discrepancy in tooth relationship. In a buccal crossbite, the lower arch is wider than the upper so that the buccal cusps of the lower occlude lateral to the buccal cusps of the upper teeth. Where the lower buccal teeth occlude lingually to the upper buccal teeth there is a lingual crossbite or scissors bite. A crossbite may be unilateral or bilateral and may involve varying numbers of teeth.
> 2. Also used to describe reverse overjet of one or more incisor teeth.

The second definition has of course already been covered in considering Class III malocclusion and in this chapter it is proposed to confine attention to the first.

There has in the past been considerable confusion about terminology, one man's buccal crossbite being another man's lingual. The British Standard would seem to solve this problem by following the convention used by Angle for antero-posterior classification, that is that we should describe the lower teeth relative to the upper rather than vice versa. The two types of crossbite are shown in Figure 14.1A and B.

AETIOLOGY

Skeletal pattern

It would seem that the majority of crossbites are to a greater or lesser extent a result of a discrepancy in width of dental bases. This may occur in one of two ways. Quite simply it may be that the upper dental arch is narrower than the lower producing a buccal crossbite such as is shown in Figure 14.1A, or the lower dental base may be narrower than the upper, producing the reverse, lingual type of crossbite, as in Figure 14.1B. A

gross antero-posterior skeletal discrepancy can however also cause a crossbite as shown in Figure 14.2. This patient had a very marked Class III skeletal pattern (Fig. 14.2C) but if the lower

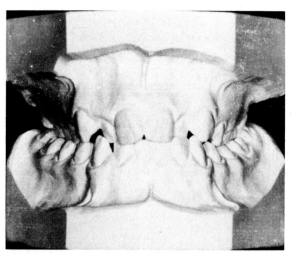

A

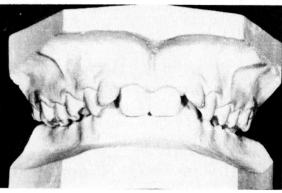

B

Fig. 14.1 Study models showing examples of: A, buccal crossbite; B, lingual crossbite.

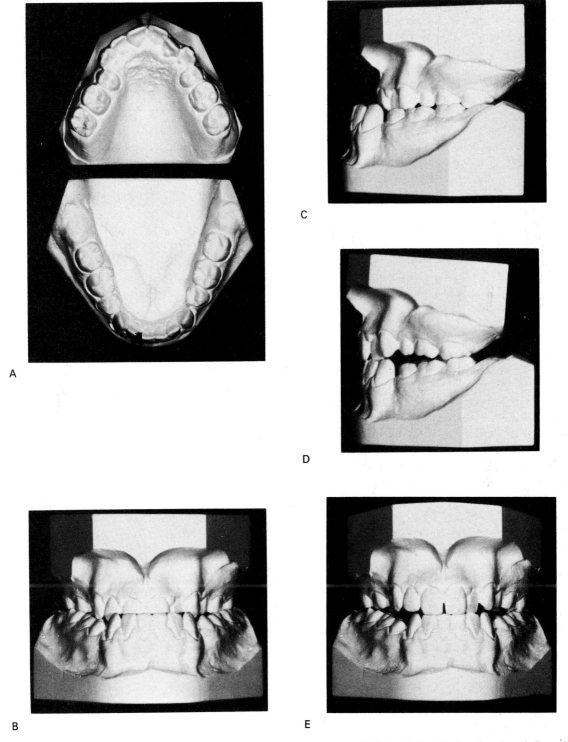

Fig. 14.2 Buccal crossbite associated with marked Class III skeletal pattern. A, Occlusal view. B, Anterior view. C, Lateral view. D, The lower arch has been moved distally to produce a normal antero-posterior relation. E, The crossbite then largely disappears.

dental arch in the form of the plaster model, is moved distally (Fig. 14.2D) then the crossbite will effectively disappear (Fig. 14.2E). This treatment was in fact carried out surgically and to produce a good occlusion; only minimal expansion of the upper arch was required. Crossbites are not infrequently coincident with an antero-posterior discrepancy with the Class III malocclusion producing a buccal, and severe Class II skeletal discrepancies producing a lingual crossbite.

Soft tissue pattern

The effect of the soft tissues in producing crossbites is rather more problematical. It has been suggested that a buccal crossbite may be caused by a low tongue position so that the tongue does not support the upper buccal segments against the pressures from the cheeks, and these teeth therefore develop rather more vertically than is desirable, into the crossbite. Such a low tongue position is often seen in a patient with an increased lower facial height but this does not necessarily indicate that the relationship is one of cause and affect. Linder-Aronson has suggested that this effect may be produced as a result of mouth-breathing. He examined a group of patients from an ear, nose and throat clinic in whom the nasal passages were completely occluded and found that this was associated with a tendency to crossbite. He suggested that this was due to the resultant mouth-breathing and consequent inability of the patient to position the tongue high in the dental arch. It is emphasised that his patients were extreme cases. Genuine mouth-breathing is a rare phenomenon and is always associated with an inability to breathe through the nose, either temporary or permanent. Linder-Aronson also suggested that following elimination of the nasal obstruction, usually by removal of adenoid tissue, a more normal growth pattern was reintroduced. A buccal crossbite is sometimes associated with digit-sucking, but this is by no means always the case. Presumably this results from displacement of the tongue from the upper arch, the presence or absence of the crossbite depending on details of the digit and tongue position.

It has similarly been suggested that the lingual type of crossbite may be the result of a high tongue position. Since the tongue is firmly attached in the lower arch it is difficult to visualise how such a position could arise and it is rather difficult to take this suggestion very seriously.

Dental effects

Not surprisingly a discrepancy in width of the dental bases is seldom exactly such as to produce a crossbite of one cusp width. It not infrequently happens that the posterior teeth erupt, due to the skeletal discrepancy, so that the lower teeth meet the uppers in more or less a cusp-to-cusp relationship bucco-lingually. In this case one of two things may happen. The teeth may be deflected and tilt in the appropriate direction so as to produce a full bilateral crossbite. This may not involve necessarily all the teeth in the segment and it is not uncommon to find that the crossbite is confined to perhaps the premolars, especially in the lingual type. Alternatively, the cuspal interference may cause the individual to diplace the mandible to the one side. This produces an apparent unilateral crossbite with the remaining teeth erupting into this relationship. If the patient can be persuaded to open the mouth and relax completely, and the mandible is then gently closed, it will be found that the unilateral crossbite becomes in fact a bucco-lingual cusp-to-cusp relationships as shown in Figure 3.15. Although this crossbite appears to be asymmetrical, it is in fact a mild form of bilateral crossbite and usually responds well to treatment by expansion of the narrower dental arch bilaterally.

Some care is necessary in diagnosing this type of unilateral crossbite. Some malocclusions of this type are due to a genuine asymmetry either by tilting of the teeth or by an asymmetry of the dental base. Where a basal asymmetry is present, it is not uncommon to find that there is in addition, some degree of mandibular displacement to the affected side on closing. If there is a genuine mandibular asymmetry, it is advisable to obsesrve this for a period without carrying out treatment, in order to eliminate the possibility that it is a progressive condition. Once treatment has been instituted, it is very difficult to check this factor.

TREATMENT

It is usually considered that the teeth lie in a position of balance between the soft tissue forces acting upon them. If this is the case then in a bilateral buccal crossbite, the upper teeth are in a position of balance and if they are moved buccally by expansion, the soft tissues of the cheeks will have more affect than that of the tongue and the teeth will relapse. This is not infrequently the case and extensive expansion to correct a severe buccal crossbite is contraindicated since the teeth are likely to return more or less to their original position. It is doubtful whether a bilateral crossbite with no mandibular displacement is any disadvantage to the individual and it can usually be accepted. However, there are certain other factors involved. The upper cheek teeth may be held in a somewhat lingual position by the cuspal lock against the lower posterior teeth, and equally it may be possible by expansion to place them in a position where the cuspal lock will retain them slightly more buccally, while the lower cheek teeth move a little lingually so as to produce a position close to that of balance. Unfortunately, as the upper posterior teeth tilt buccally, those surfaces of the teeth which should provide the cuspal lock become rather more horizontal and there is certainly a limit to the amount of expansion which can be held in this way. Treatment should therefore only be attempted in mild cases of crossbite and this applies particularly to those unilateral crossbites which are associated with a mandibular displacement to the affected side. Such a displacement should always be eliminated if possible and as already stated, these cases respond well to expansion.

There are two basic ways of achieving such an expansion. The conventional method is by means of a fixed or removable appliance exerting gentle pressures on the teeth so as to move them through the bone into a normal relationship. Frequently this is by buccal movement of the upper cheek teeth but a useful reciprocal movement may be achieved by banding the upper and lower posterior teeth and arranging for elastics to be worn from a suitable attachment on the lingual of the upper teeth to the buccal of the lower. This moves the teeth reciprocally and will often

produce a stable result although it is of course best suited to localised crossbites.

The alternative is rapid maxillary expansion. This was apparently first described by Angell in the middle of the last century but has achieved a new popularity fairly recently. The type of appliance shown in Figure 14.3, usually ascribed to Biedermann is one of several methods of producing this movement. The first premolars and first molars are banded on each side and a screw known as a Hyrax screw, is attached to these bands by soldering. It will be noted that the appliance touches only these four teeth. The name Hyrax, although the name of an animal, is derived from the phrase 'hygienic rapid expansion'. This appliance is constructed as seen in the figure with the screw lying almost horizontally across the palate. It must not lie in the vault of the palate or it will cause ulceration of the mucosa. When it is cemented in the mouth the patient is instructed to turn the screw twice per day. This is of course very much more frequent than the normal rate of turning for screw appliances. There seems no doubt that it has the effect of springing open the inter-maxillary suture and actually moving the two parts of the maxilla apart. This is confirmed, not only by radiographic evidence, but by the appearance of a diastema between the two central incisors (Fig. 14.3) and by the fact that other teeth such as the second premolars move with the banded teeth. The procedure is not painful although patients sometimes describe a feeling of numbness and without prompting some individuals have spoken of 'something seeming to give way'. The median diastema closes spontaneously in a few weeks (Fig. 14.3D). The technique appears to be trouble-free and apart from other possible advantages, it moves the teeth rapidly. There is of course some tilting movement of the teeth through the bone in addition to the opening of the suture and this is shown by the fact that the median diastema is always substantially narrower than the actual expansion of the screw. It would seem from several authors work that something between 25 and 50 per cent of the expansion will later relapse but clearly this depends on such factors as cuspal lock and the amount of expansion achieved.

A case treated by this technique is shown in

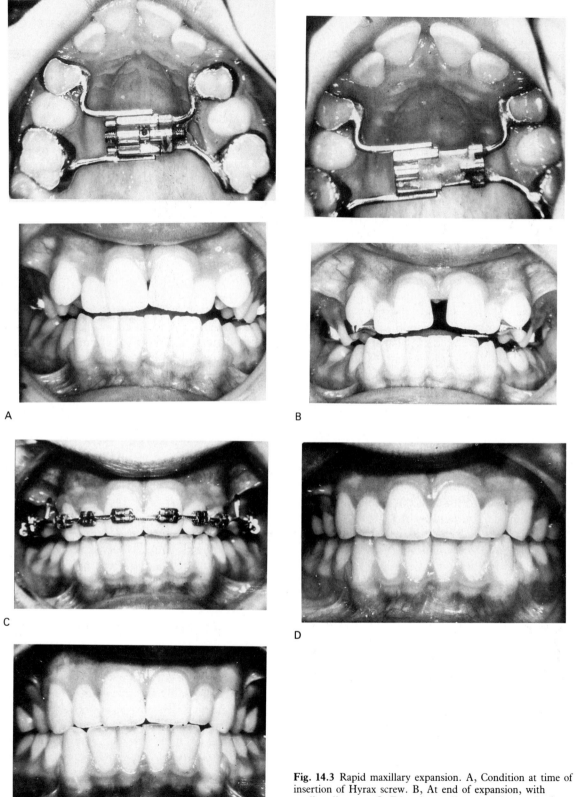

Fig. 14.3 Rapid maxillary expansion. A, Condition at time of insertion of Hyrax screw. B, At end of expansion, with median diastema. C, Edgewise appliance to align teeth after extraction of 4/4. D, At end of treatment. E, One year out of retention; note slight relapse.

A

B

C

D

E

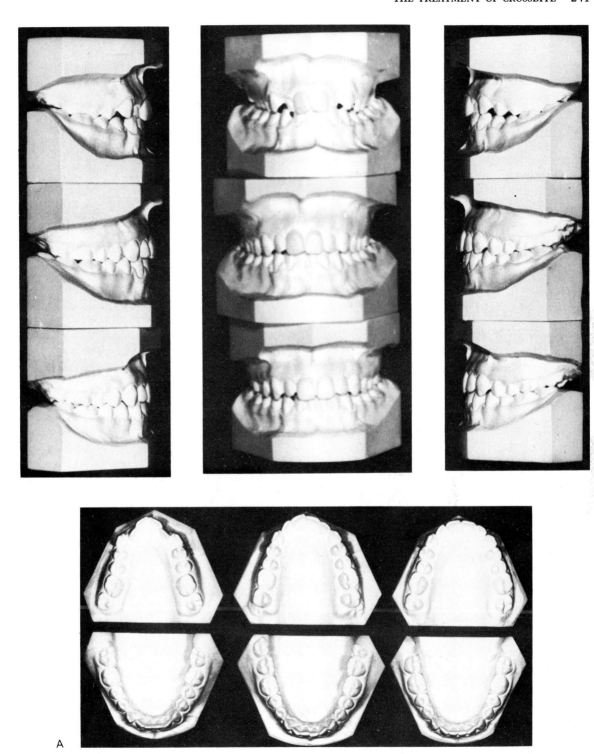

Fig. 14.4 Lesley. Bilateral mild crossbite treated by rapid maxillary expansion. A, Study models before the treatment, at end of retention and 7 years thereafter. B, Superimposed tracings, before and after treatment. C, Superimposed tracings at end of retention and 7 years later. D, Intra-oral photographs taken 7 years out of retention (B, C and D overleaf).

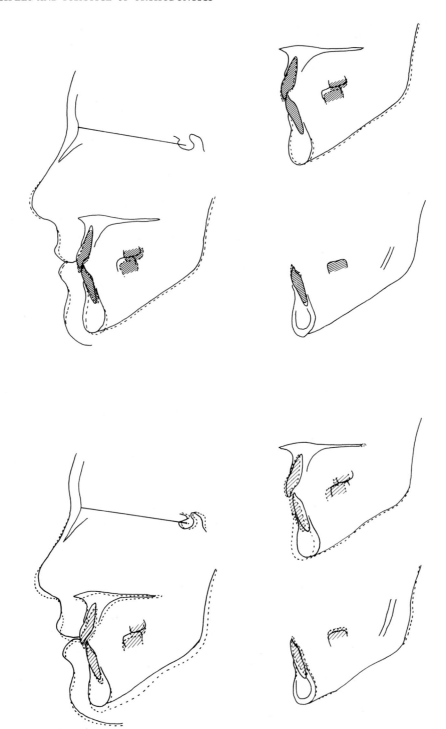

B

C

Fig. 14.4 (*cont'd*)

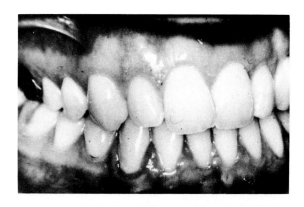

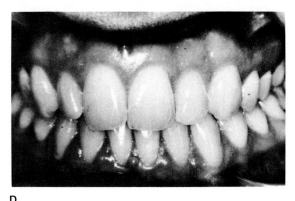

D

Fig. 14.4 (*cont'd*)

Figure 14.4. Lesley first came to see us shortly after her thirteenth birthday. she had a well aligned lower arch, with all teeth as far as the second molars erupted, but the upper dental base seemed somewhat smaller than the lower, so that there was a rather mild crossbite of the posterior teeth. The overbite and overjet were reduced on the central incisors with 2/2 tending to occlude lingually to the lowers. She was treated with the Biedermann type of appliance using a Hyrax screw and somewhat unusually encountered a little discomfort in the earlier stages of treatment. The appliance also caused a marked speech abnormality, which again is unusual. When the required degree of expansion had been achieved, in about 1 month, the appliance was removed. On the same visit bands were selected and an impression taken for an upper lingual arch to act as a retention appliance, and the original appliance was reinserted. This rapid expansion relapses very rapidly in the early stages and the appliance must not be

left out for more than an hour or so. The palatal arch was fitted at the next visit. This type of retaining palatal arch must be worn for about 12 months following rapid expansion, although during this period, of course, other parts of the treatment may be carried out. It was noted at this stage that the upper lateral incisors had spontaneously moved over the bite. I have seen this occur occasionally in the treatment of these patients. Biedermann (1973) has stated that, following rapid maxillary expansion, the anterior part of the dental base moves forward and that this may correct a Class III relationship. I have never personally seen this occur and recent work by Gallagher (1979) using lateral skull radiographs, did not show any forward movement of the dental base following rapid expansion in a sample of 23 cases.

The rest of Lesley's treatment was fairly conventional. Extra-oral traction was added to bring about a very small amount of distal movement of the buccal segments and a twin wire arch was then used to align and to some extent overrotate the incisors. The central incisors were pericised and a removable retainer fitted after a total of 14 months treatment. The second models in Figure 14.4 show the result at the end of retention and the final models and photographs some 7 years after the end of all retention.

Claims have also been made for rapid expansion in improving a nasal airway. It would seem from the work of Krebs using metal implants in the maxilla, that not only the teeth but also the bone of the maxilla are expanded and that in fact this bone expansion relapses less than the dental expansion. Surprisingly, no one seems to know how much the maxilla would have increased in width from normal growth and therefore the extent to which this successful expansion of the maxilla would have occurred anyway as a result of normal growth. Several authors claim that the technique is valuable in treating nasal insufficiency and certainly a very slight widening of the nasal passage is sufficient to allow normal breathing through the nose. A few oto-rhino-laryngologists tend to become somewhat overenthusiastic about this form of treatment.

Rapid expansion produces a result quickly, and may be more effective in widening the maxillary

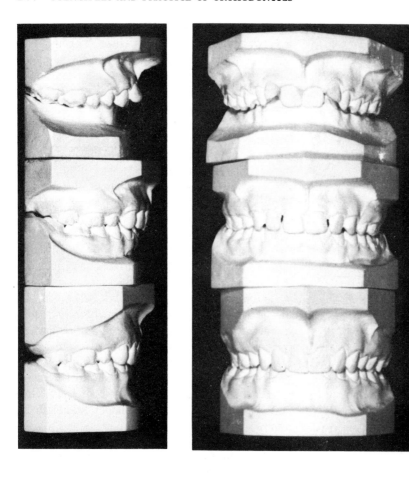
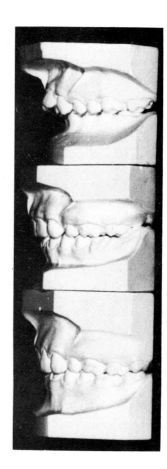
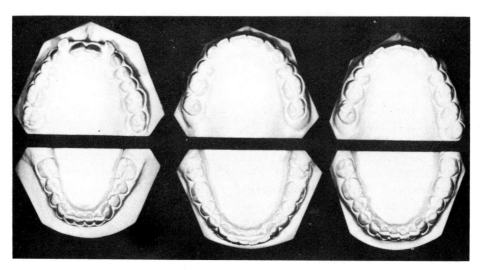

A

Fig. 14.5 Timothy. Severe Class II Division 2 malocclusion with bilateral lingual crossbite. Treated initially by bilateral expansion of lower arch. A, Study models before treatment, at end of retention and 7 years later. B (opposite), Intra-oral photographs 7 years out of retention.

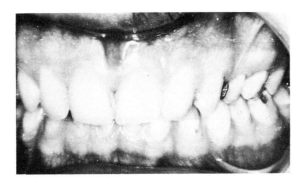

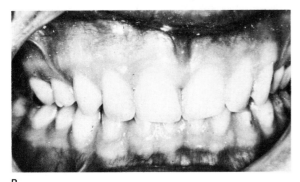

B

Fig. 14.5 (*cont'd*)

base and nasal airway. From the work of Herold it is doubtful if it is more successful in producing a stable expansion of the teeth than the quadhelix appliance illustrated in Figure 15.6B, or indeed a removable appliance with a Coffin spring.

Lingual crossbites

As already indicated, a lingual crossbite is the situation where the lower buccal cusps occlude lingually to the upper lingual cusps. In other words very little of the teeth occludes at all. Such an occlusion is sometimes called, especially in Scotland, a scissors bite. It is clearly much less efficient than the ordinary buccal crossbite, where half of the occlusal surface of upper and lower teeth are in contact. Fortunately, it responds very much better to treatment. If the lower arch is expanded bilaterally, so as to produce a cuspal occlusion, this will often be maintained to a greater or lesser extent. It has been suggested that this is because the expansion of the lower arch allows the tongue to return to its normal resting

position (although no one has explained how it gets away from that position in the first place) but it seems more probable that the secret lies in the cuspal relationship. Where the lower molars have completely escaped from the uppers, they tend to be tilted lingually, while the uppers are tilted buccally and the correction of this tilting moves the teeth into a position where the cuspal lock is effective. Be that as it may, correction of this type of crossbite is usually successful, with relapse being comparatively minor.

Timothy showed this condition to an extreme extent (Fig. 14.5). He had a severe Class II Division 2 malocclusion on a marked Class II skeletal pattern with the additional complication of the bilateral posterior lingual crossbite. This was further exacerbated by appalling oral hygiene which continued apart from occasional spurts of enthusiasm, throughout treatment. The first stage of treatment was to correct the buccal crossbite and this was carried out by Dr D. W. Williams who has described the appliance which he used (Williams, 1970). The lower appliance was used in conjunction with an upper anterior bite plane which took the posterior teeth out of occlusion so as to allow for their correction. It also had the additional advantage of reducing the overbite to some extent. The appliance used in this case was an exceptional measure to meet exceptional circumstances and various other types of appliance are available, such as the split lingual arch (Fig. 14.6). Conventional buccal arch-wires present problems, since the 'scissors-bite' will damage brackets and wire.

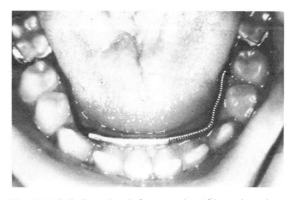

Fig. 14.6 Split lingual arch for expansion of lower buccal segments of teeth.

When the buccal occlusion had been corrected, the upper first premolars only were extracted and treatment was completed with a fully banded appliance in the lower arch but with only removable appliances in the upper. The remaining records in Figure 14.5 show the condition at the end of retention and about 7 years later. It will be noted that in this case the posterior occlusion has remained completely stable and this is by no means uncommon in this type of case.

SUGGESTED READING

Biedermann W 1973 Rapid correction of Class III malocclusion by midpalatal expansion. American Journal of Orthodontics 63: 47–55

Gallagher D P 1979 The skeletal and dental effects of rapid maxillary expansion. M.Sc. Thesis, Institute of Dental Surgery, University of London

Gray L P, Brogan W F 1972 Septal deformity, malocclusion and rapid maxillary expansion. The Orthodontist 4: 2–14

Krebs A 1964 Midpalatal suture expansion studied by the implant method over a seven year period. Transactions of the European Orthodontic Society 131–42

Linder-Aronson S 1979 Respiratory function in relation to facial morphology and the dentition. British Journal of Orthodontics 6: 59–71

Linder-Aronson S, Lindgren J 1979 The skeletal and dental effects of rapid maxillary expansion. British Journal of Orthodontics 6: 25–9

Skieller V 1964 Expansion of the mid-palatal suture by removable plates analyzed by the implant method. Transactions of the European Orthodontic Society 143–58

Timms D J 1968 An occlusal analysis of lateral maxillary expansion with midpalatal suture opening. Transactions of the British Society for the Study of Orthodontics 54: 73–9

Timms D J 1976 Long-term follow up of cases treated by rapid maxillary expansion. Transactions of the European Orthodontic Society 211–5

Williams D W 1970 A method of treating total lingual occlusion. Transactions of the British Society for the Study of Orthodontics 56: 97–8

15

Clefts of the lip and palate

Clefts of the lip and palate occur in approximately 1:700 live births in European populations. There are apparently differing incidences in various races, although completeness of reporting doubtless also varies. They are not infrequently associated with other defects and are a feature of certain well defined syndromes. Since they virtually always involve a malocclusion, their treatment requires very close co-operation between a number of clinicians. The most relevant of these are the plastic surgeon, the speech therapist and the orthodontist. The condition is best treated by a team of these three individuals who should hold combined clinics where the patient may be seen by all three specialists simultaneously, and treatment planned without the need of lengthy correspondence. Other specialists may be invited to join the clinic occasionally or may be consulted independently in cases where this is necessary. ENT surgeons, child psychiatrists, oral surgeons and of course paediatricians and paedodontists are most often consulted.

It would seem that in origin, there are two basic types of cleft. One group, often abbreviated to CL(P), include all those cases where a cleft of the lip is involved, whether this be confined to the lip or any intermediate condition up to and including a complete cleft of lip and soft and hard palates. The second group, often abbreviated CP, involves only a cleft of the posterior palate, that is the area behind the anterior palatine foramen. The genetic origin of the two types of clefts appears to differ. Clefts of the secondary palate only (CP) appear to have a lesser genetic component than the CL(P) type. Where an individual in the latter group marries a normal partner, there is a 2 per cent risk of a cleft in their offspring. This is not increased

by further family history on the affected side. With a cleft of the secondary palate only, the incidence in children of such a marriage is not great unless other members of the family are affected. If normal parents give birth to a cleft child, the risk of a similar abnormality in a further child is 1:20 for primary palate but only 1:80 for secondary palate. If an affected parent has an affected child, the incidence in further children is 1:10. The incidence does not appear to be affected by the child's rank in the family.

AETIOLOGY

The development of both primary and secondary palates has been dealt with in some detail in Chapter 1. Briefly, the primary palate which forms the upper lip and the alveolus in the anterior region as far back as the anterior palatine foramen is formed by a fusion of median and lateral nasal processes and the maxillary processes. A cleft of the primary palate is clearly due to a failure of this fusion, or according to some authorities, a failure of the penetration of the ectoderm by the mesodermal processes. Fusion normally takes place at $4\frac{1}{2}$–6 weeks. The secondary palate is in the centre line from the anterior palatine foramen to the uvula and failure of fusion here will produce a cleft of the secondary palate. Fusion in this region is from 8 to 10 weeks. A complete cleft therefore involves an interference with growth over several weeks and the detached segments are not infrequently reduced in size also. It is interesting that a cleft of the primary palate does not follow the line of fusion between premaxilla and maxilla (which bones have not commenced to calcify at this stage) and the lateral incisor may be found on either side of the cleft, or may be represented by duplicate denticles, one on each side. The exact location of the cleft of the primary palate therefore varies from an anterior position, involving the central incisor, to a very posterior position, with the canine erupting into the cleft.

This then is the mechanism of clefting but it does not explain why it should occur. It would seem that there are various possible factors involved.

Genetic factors

Undoubtedly, heredity is an important factor in the aetiology of clefts and about 25 per cent of cases produce a history of clefts if the family is traced as far back as, and including, the grand-parents. Fogh-Andersen is probably the leading authority on the statistics of clefting and he states that with CL(P) a family history is elicited in 40 per cent of cases, whereas in CP it is only elicited in about 20 per cent of cases. This is not the whole story and in cases of identical twins, where one twin has a cleft, Smith analysed 30 reported cases where in only 11 did both twins have the cleft, the remaining 19 being discordant. In the cases of cleft palate only, the proportion was even higher with 11 discordant out of 12. It would seem there-fore that the inheritance is of a tendency to clefting rather than of the cleft itself and some additional factor is necessary to precipitate the cleft. If the precipitating factor is very strong it will produce a cleft where there is no great genetic tendency. If it is very weak, it will only produce a cleft where the genetic tendency is very great. By inbreeding, it is possible to produce strains of mice which have a high tendency to clefting and these are of course used for research purposes.

Environmental factors

The factors in the maternal environment which predispose to clefts are certainly not fully known but over the past few years some factors have become clear. Cortisone, or ACTH, can be used to produce clefts in susceptible animals and might reasonably be expected to have the same effect in man. This could be the result of drug therapy or conceivably be produced naturally by stress or fear during pregnancy. Deficiencies of the so-called stress vitamins (B6 and folic acid) will also predis-pose to clefts. Peer and co-workers (1963) were able to produce clefts in 85 per cent of susceptible mice treated with cortisone acetate, reducing this to 25 per cent if B6 and folic acid were simul-taneously administered. They also found these vitamins apparently valuable when given to 156 mothers for a second pregnancy following the production of a cleft from a previous pregnancy. Anti-convulsants such as Dilantin appear to increase the risk of clefting slightly, although the Committee for the Safety of Drugs has recom-mended that it should not be withdrawn for this reason. Valium has also been accused of increasing the incidence of clefts as have, to a very slight extent, winter conception and an old mother.

Growth

It should be realised that a cleft of the lip and/or palate is not merely a failure of the segments to fuse together but is a defect of growth of the first arch. The mandible is usually smaller than average size in addition to the maxilla. Moreover, the abnormality may be associated with defects of the heart, limbs, spina bifida, etc. It is sometimes associated with hypertelorism, the face retaining some of its fetal characteristics with the eyes set wide apart.

Syndromes

Clefts, usually of the secondary palate, are a feature of a number of syndromes, some of which are inherited in a straightforward Mendelian fashion. Mandibular-facial dysostosis is a simple dominant characteristic and will therefore occur in 50 per cent of the offspring of an affected individual. Oro-facio-digital syndrome type 1 is an X-linked dominant which is lethal in the male. Fifty per cent of female children will therefore have the condition and 50 per cent of males will be aborted, the other 50 per cent of males being free of the affected gene. Type 2 of the same syndrome is a recessive gene and will therefore be most likely to occur following the marriage of close relatives. The syndrome involving CL(P) and hypospadias with ocular hypertelorism and mental retardation occurs as a simple dominant. The actual locus of this gene has been identified on chromosome 17. It produces only minor symptoms in female carriers but the males are usually not fertile. Clefts of the palate are found in Treacher-Collins syndrome, Pierre Robin syndrome and some trisomies.

Mechanical factors

It has been suggested that a delay in vertical growth of the face may cause the tongue mechanically to obstruct fusion of the posterior palate and be responsible for clefts of this type. Atherton has found this in dogs with clefts of the palate and it has been suggested as the mechanism in Pierre Robin syndrome. A deficiency of amniotic fluid with the production of fibrous bands from the fetus to the amnion is also thought to produce clefts and the deficiency of fluid may be caused by drugs or of course by amniocentesis.

CLASSIFICATION OF CLEFTS

There are several different classifications of clefts of the lip and palate in current use and the orthodontists need never feel ashamed of asking his colleagues which one they are applying. The following three are probably the most widely used.

Kernahan and Stark

This is based on embryological principles, clefts being divided into those of primary and secondary palates, in the former case unilateral or bilateral, and in both cases total or sub-total. Thus we may speak of a 'bilateral sub-total cleft of primary palate with total cleft of secondary palate'.

Veau

This classification is used on the continent and has in the past been used by orthodontists in this country although happily it is losing its popularity. It is essentially a classification of clefts of the palate. Class I involves the soft palate only, Class II the secondary palate including part of the

hard palate, Class III is a complete unilateral cleft of primary and secondary palate, while Class IV is a complete bilateral cleft. Clearly it is far from complete, for example clefts confined to the primary palate are not mentioned.

Davis and Ritchie

This again is an old established classification which is losing its popularity. In this classification Class I involves the lip only, Class II the palate only, while Class III involves both lip and palate. Class I and III are sub-divided into (i) unilateral (ii) median (which is excessively rare) and (iii) bilateral.

CLINICAL FEATURES AND TREATMENT

Clefts of the primary palate only

Lip only involved

In about 10 per cent of all clefts, the cleft is confined to the lip. The palate and alveolus are intact and at first sight one would feel that orthodontic treatment was not required. In practice it is very common to find that the incisor opposite the cleft of the lip is duplicated. There may be a supplemental central incisor or a supplemental lateral incisor and while both may erupt normally, it is not uncommon to find that one remains unerupted when the patient is first seen. Radiographic examination is therefore extremely desirable in this type of case. Again it is not uncommon to find that one of the two supplemental teeth has a deep lingual invagination and this should be borne in mind when considering which tooth to extract. A patient with this type of cleft, in this case incomplete, is seen in Figure 15.1, and the treatment involves simple lip closure with possibly some trimming at a later stage.

Cleft of the lip and alveolus

In this cases the plastic surgeon will wish to close the lip and the alveolar cleft at an early stage. The usual timing is about the third month, although a small number of surgeons believe in closing the lip as soon as possible after birth. Two conflicting

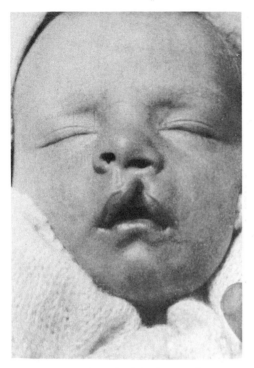

Fig. 15.1 Baby with the cleft of the lip only. The alveolus was intact but the child had a supplemental incisor.

factors are involved. It is desirable to make the child acceptable to its parents as soon as possible, but, on the other hand, surgery is easier, and therefore more successful, when the affected parts are larger.

The main portions of both dental arches are normal in these cases, and the abnormality is confined to the teeth immediately adjacent to the cleft. It should however be borne in mind that a child with a cleft of any type is just as susceptible to other forms of malocclusion as any other child, but so far as the cleft is concerned, the usual features are a displacement of the central incisor, often with rotation, and/or a lingual displacement of the permanent canine which may be in cross-bite. The lateral incisor may be represented on either side of the cleft and is usually of little value and has to be extracted.

A very mild form of cleft is shown in Figure 15.2 This patient had a cleft of the lip with little more than a notching of the alveolus. The dental arches were well formed and the general occlusion was excellent. The lateral incisor was not visible

and the upper left deciduous canine was tending to drop lingually. Radiographic examination however, showed the presence of a second central incisor, lying unerupted close to the erupted tooth. Closer inspection showed that the erupted central incisor had a lingual invagination and the unerupted tooth seemed in several respects to be superior. It was therefore decided to extract the erupted tooth, whereupon the unerupted tooth came down as seen in the second set of models. Its position was somewhat worse than the original since it was now in a traumatic relation with its antagonists, and a simple form of a fixed appliance was fitted to rotate this tooth and move it slightly labially. This was all the treatment which was required, apart from slight labial movement of /3 when it erupted and the extraction of the diminutive /2 which erupted distally to the cleft line. Treatment was complete with a small two-part chrome-cobalt denture (Fig. 15.2D) although in clefts of the primary palate only, the fitting of a bridge should be considered. The final models show that by the age of 18 years both overbite and overjet have reduced considerably and it will be seen from the superimposed tracings that the growth of the maxilla has not kept pace with the growth of the mandible. This is a common finding in clefts of the CL(P) type. Unilateral clefts involving lip and alveolus are comparatively rare, comprising only 3 per cent of all clefts.

A more severe case, although still confined to the primary palate, is illustrated in Figure 15.3, Mary had a total right-sided cleft of the lip and primary palate, seen shortly after birth in Figure 15.3A. Clefts confined to the primary palate do not usually affect the relative sizes of the jaws, but in Mary's case, although antero-posterior skeletal relations were normal or even slightly postnormal, there was a tendency to crossbite, especially on the right side. The displacement of 1/ was typical for alveolar clefts, with a diminutive lateral incisor close to the cleft on its distal side. The permanent canine was palatally displaced and unerupted, but there was adequate space for it in the arch after extraction of 2/. The canine was therefore surgically exposed, allowed to erupt, and then brought into line, using a sectional arm soldered to the Adams clasp of a removable appliance. The distal end of this arm was hooked beneath a Begg

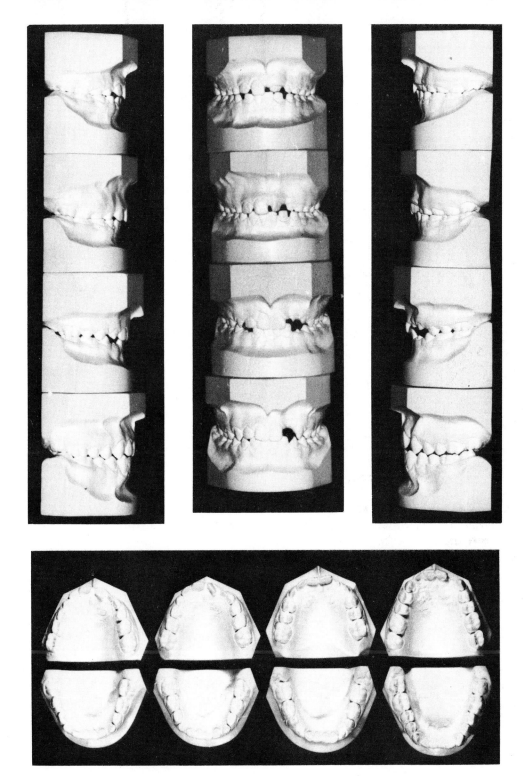

A

Fig. 15.2 Martin: Unilateral cleft of lip on left side with mild notching of alveolus. A, Study models taken when first seen; after extraction of /1 and its replacement by a supplemental tooth; at the end of treatment and 6 years later. B, Intra-oral radiograph to show unerupted supplemental /1 and invagination of erupted tooth. C, Superimposed tracings before and after treatment. D, Superimposed tracings at end of retention and 6 years later; note minimal forward growth of maxilla. E, Intra-oral photograph at age 17 years to show two-part denture (B, C, D and E overleaf).

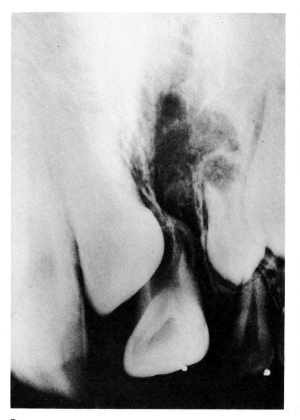

B

bracket, bonded on to the tooth, to position the tooth as shown in the second set of models.

Shortly after this the deciduous canine was extracted, the permanent canine retracted and the anterior teeth aligned and moved labially over the bite. The crossbite tendency was not treated, and this allowed the fitting of a Rochette bridge to replace 2/, rather than a denture, in a mouth where oral hygiene was a constant problem. The final records were taken at the age of 18 years. It will be seen from the superimposed tracings in Figure 15.3C that growth in this case was reasonably normal, the maxilla keeping pace with the mandible.

Bilateral clefts of the primary palate

These are rare, comprising only 2 per cent of clefts. The effects are similar to those of a unilateral cleft but of course present on both sides. Frequently, one side is worse affected than the other but if both sides have a total cleft, then the primary palate will protrude onto the face at birth, although it is usually possible to replace this by closing the lip over it and this presents a much

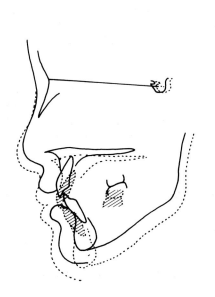

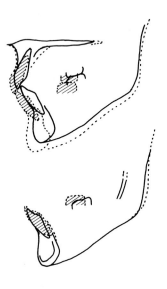

C

Fig. 15.2 (cont'd)

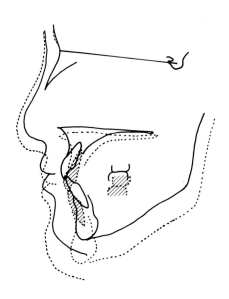

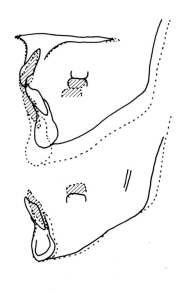

D

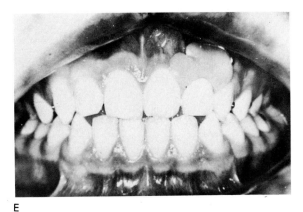

E

Fig. 15.2 (*cont'd*)

simpler problem than in the case of the complete bilateral clefts.

Clefts of the secondary palate

These comprise about 30 per cent of all clefts and are rather more common in girls than in boys in the proportion of 60:40. They are clefts of the soft or soft- plus-hard palate coming as far forward as the anterior palatine foramen. They are always median, although the septum may be attached to either side of the maxilla or detached from both.

They vary in severity from a bifid uvula to a total cleft.

In untreated clefts of this type there is often retrusion of both maxilla and mandible relative to the cranial base, but the jaws remain well related to each other. Following surgery the need for orthodontic treatment is no greater than in non-cleft individuals except that occasionally the palatal surgery can accentuate the maxillary retrusion, producing a Class III malocclusion.

Orthodontically the treatment would be that of Class III malocclusion in non-cleft individuals, bearing in mind that the abnormality is entirely in the upper jaw, with the mandible also retruded to some extent. In extreme cases surgery, as discussed later, may be indicated.

Clefts of the primary and secondary palate

Sub-total

These again are very rare, comprising only 3 per cent of all clefts. They comprise a combination of the two already described, that is a cleft of the lip and/or primary palate, together with clefting of the secondary palate but with an intermediate portion of normal palate.

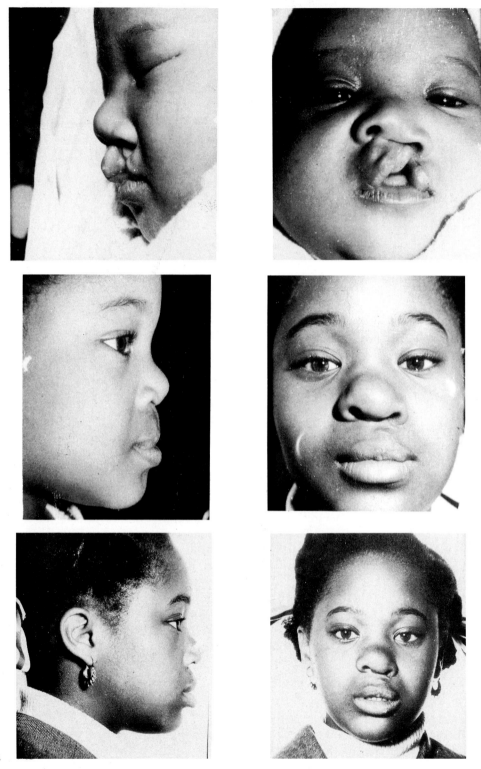

Fig. 15.3 Mary A, Photographs; at birth, and before and after orthodontic treatment. B (opposite), Models: before and after orthondontic treatment and 8 years later. C, Superimposed tracings, before treatment on end of treatment. D, Superimposed tracings, end of treatment on 8 years later (C and D overleaf).

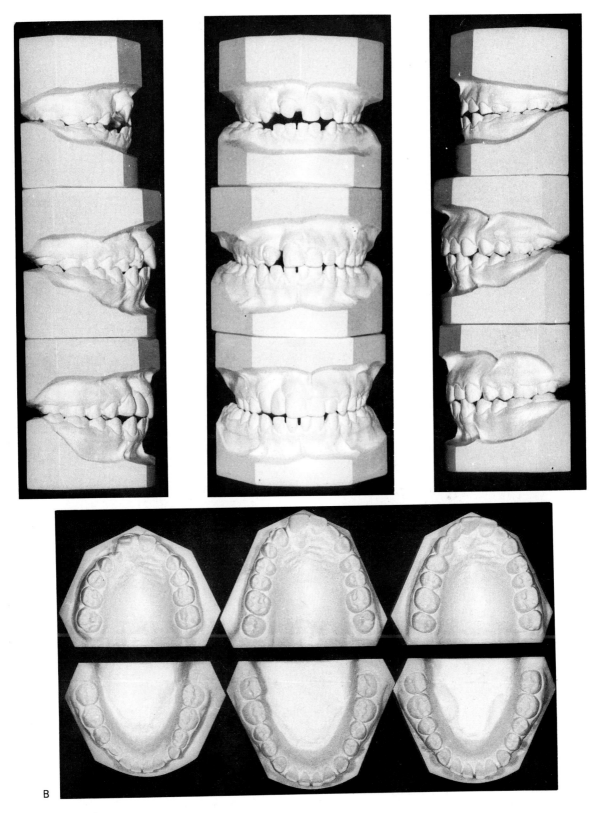

Fig. 15.3 (*cont'd*)

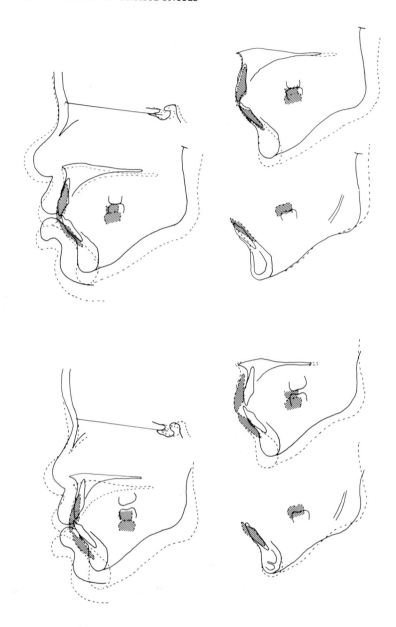

C

D

Fig. 15.3 (*cont'd*)

Total, unilateral

These are the complete unilateral clefts which extend from the lip to the uvula but involving only one side of the primary palate. They are by far the commonest type of cleft, comprising about 40 per cent of all clefts. They are twice as common in boys as in girls and twice as common on the left as on the right side. The child is born with a wide gap in the lip and the upper dental arch at this stage is usually wider than average, with the small detached fragment displaced outwards, backwards and some times upwards. The segments are not only detached from each other but are usually smaller than average, although this lack of tissue varies considerably in extent. The base of the

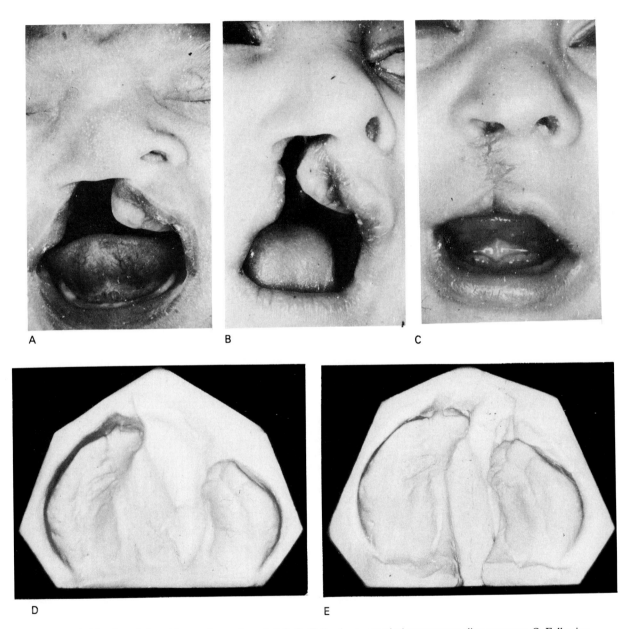

Fig. 15.4 A, New-born baby with complete unilateral cleft. B, Following presurgical treatment to align segments. C, Following surgery. D and E, Plaster models before and after presurgical treatment.

nostril (ala base) is dragged laterally so this nostril has a flattened appearance (Fig. 15.4A) and this tends to remain a typical feature throughout life. If left untreated the upper arch often remains of normal width, with reasonably normal occlusion of the posterior teeth. Sometimes it is unduly wide, with the upper buccal segment in buccal relation. Alternatively there may be some collapse of the detached segment, especially in the canine region. Following surgery there is usually some collapse of the small segment, while the incisor region and non-cleft side may also be in crossbite to a greater or lesser extent, depending on the (very variable) severity of the cleft and the excellence of the surgery. Orthodontic treatment may be carried out during four main periods, neonatally, in the complete deciduous dentition, in the mixed dentition and finally in the complete permanent dentition.

Neonatal treatment

McNeil in the 1950s introduced the idea of orthodontic treatment in the newly born cleft palate patient. His original appliance was somewhat complicated and has been considerably modified by Burston, using the type of bite-block illustrated in Figure 15.5. This has been further simplified by Elisabeth Horrocks (personal communication), who employs a simple base-plate with no bite blocks, as illustrated in Figure 15.5C. The 'wings' passing out of the mouth have been eliminated and replaced by a length of strong cord, attached through a small hole in the acrylic, as a safety line. The appliance is constructed in clear acrylic, to enable areas of pressure on the tissues to be

recognised and eliminated. In this technique the treatment should be commenced within 1 or 2 days of birth. At this stage the child is growing very rapidly and it is possible to mould the detached fragments, carrying the lip and ala base with them, into a more favourable position. An impression is taken of the upper dental arch in a suitable small tray and this is cast in artificial stone. The precise techniques vary with operators but basically the model is cut along the line of the cleft into two segments, and the smaller segment moved very slightly towards a more favourable relation with the larger one: 1–2 mm is sufficient. This usually involves moving it anteriorly and possibly slightly inwards. The two halves of the model are then reattached to the plaster base and the cleft area is plastered out.

In a proportion of cases the incisor region is rotated forwards and to the non-cleft side. This may be controlled by 'strapping' as shown in

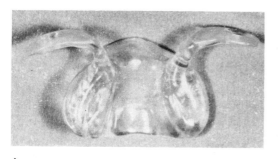

A

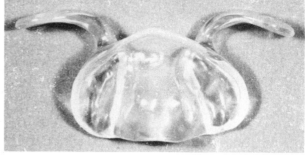

B

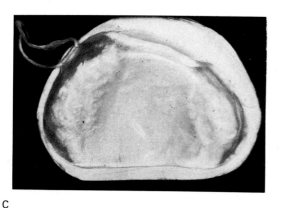

C

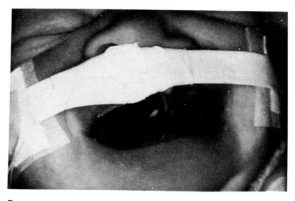

D

Fig. 15.5 A and B, Appliance for presurgical treatment (Burston). C., Presurgical appliance (Horrocks). D, Extra-oral strapping where primary palate is protrusive in unilateral or bilateral clefts.

Figure 15.5D. The cheeks are first protected by affixing Sellotape or Micropore and the actual area to be controlled is covered with Elastoplast, preferably of the non-elastic type, the centre section of which is turned in on itself, so that it is non-adhesive. The purpose of this is to gently restrain the growth forward of the prominent alveolus. It should not exert any great pressure, as this could lead to a deflected septum. Extra-oral views of a treated case are shown in Figure 15.4C. and models of a different case in Fig. 15.4D and E. The effect of these pre-surgical appliances would seem to be to move the two segments closer together and to produce a narrower cleft of the lip, with some improvement in the ala base. It is doubtful whether the individual fragments increase in size any more than they would have done in the absence of such treatment. When the maximum possible improvement has been achieved, usually by the age of about 3 months, the surgeon closes the lip and alveolus. Some operators like the child to continue to wear the orthopaedic appliance until the secondary palate is closed at the usual age of about 18 months but this later wearing of the appliance is becoming less common. At the time of the primary palate operation, some surgeons insert a bone graft across the alveolus, taking the bone usually from a rib.

It is not clear how valuable this form of presurgical dental orthopaedics is in the treatment of unilateral clefts. Huddart claims that by the age of 5 years, patients treated in this manner differ little from those treated more conventionally, while Robertson and Jolleys claimed that there is a significant difference between the two groups. Clearly any difference is comparatively slight but one would think that if the procedure makes the surgeon's work easier (as most surgeons claim that it does) then the result is likely to be somewhat better. The insertion of a bone graft at this stage would seem to interfere with normal growth of the maxilla and, again from the work of Robertson and Jolleys, would seem to have few advantages and some disadvantages.

The secondary palate is closed somewhat later. Most surgeons would undertake this operation somewhere between 12 months and 2 years, although in some countries it is left considerably later. A few surgeons believe in closing the soft palate at approximately 18 months and delaying the closure of the hard palate until anything up to 12 years. This is alleged to prevent the collapse of the hard palate which is otherwise prone to occur. Assuming that the entire secondary palate is closed, it is usual to find some lingual collapse of the smaller segment into a crossbite, and sometimes the anterior part of this smaller segment will fail to develop to the normal occlusal level. A crossbite may develop in the incisor region and also on the unaffected side, but happily both of these defects are becoming rarer with increasingly conservative surgery. It is not uncommon for the hard palate closure to break down in the region of the anterior palatine foramen to produce a small fistula, and if repeated operations are carried out to close this defect, then growth of the maxilla will be seriously impeded. Basically, orthodontic treatment will consist of expansion of the upper arch to restore occlusion, followed by alignment of the teeth. This expansion will not be stable and permanent retention will be necessary.

The deciduous dentition

The earliest stage at which expansion might be attempted is in the complete deciduous dentition and although treatment at this stage is sometimes undertaken in North America, it is not the normal practice in the United Kingdom. In expanding the segments, two procedures occur. Since the cleft is only repaired by scar tissue, this may be stretched and the bony segments moved apart. In addition, the teeth move through the bone in the normal way. Subtelny & Brodie (1954) showed that in the younger patient a larger proportion of bone expansion, compared to tooth expansion was obtained and this is probably the reason for expanding in the deciduous dentition. If such treatment is carried out it almost always has to be repeated at a later stage. Orthodontic treatment is always apt to be prolonged and starting at this age and carrying on with intervals until the age of 13 or 14 years almost guarantees that co-operation with flag.

Mixed dentition treatment

At the above stage, therefore, the patient should

merely be kept under observation to ensure that routine dental work is carried out and that nothing untoward is taking place. Appointments should be as infrequent as possible until the permanent incisors erupt. This is the first stage at which I personally undertake any treatment. Very commonly, the upper incisors erupt in a grossly rotated position and one or both of them may be inside the bite. Treatment should be confined to moving the teeth over the bite into a nontraumatic position. If the displacement is so gross as to be aesthetically distressing to the patient, then some effort should be made to rotate them and align them into a more acceptable position. Perfection should not be the goal. Treatment in all cleft palate patients seems to respond better to the use of fixed appliances and a variation of the twin wire arch (Fig. 15.6A) is useful for alignment of teeth and for their labial movement in the mixed dentition.

The permanent dentition

Further treatment is then deferred until all the permanent teeth anterior to the first molars have erupted, with the exception of any close to the line of the cleft whose eruption may be delayed. The latter not infrequently include the permanent canine on the affected side. The first line of treatment is to expand the upper arch so as to restore the occlusion. The crossbite is usually most severe in the canine region and not infrequently the first molar and almost always the second molar, are in normal bucco-lingual relation. It is advisable to carry out this expansion with forces considerably stronger than would normally be used for tooth movement. An increase in force will increase the speed at which the bony segments move by stretching of the scar tissue, but they will not increase the speed at which the teeth move through the bone. This therefore produces the maximum amount of bony rather than dental expansion. Screw appliances as used for conventional rapid maxillary expansion are not altogether satisfactory. They will produce only parallel expansion (although some modifications are available which do produce differential expansion) and in the small constricted palates often seen with clefts, it is difficult to insert a screw which will

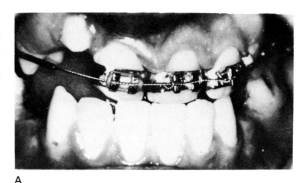

A

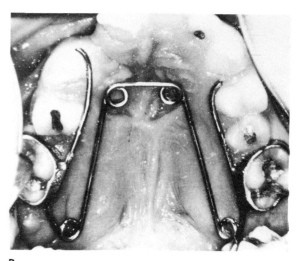

B

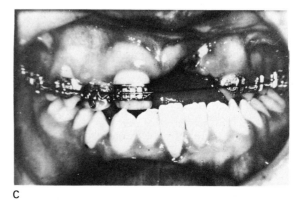

C

Fig. 15.6 Appliances used in the treatment of complete clefts. A, Modified twin arch used in mixed dentition to correct incisor displacement. B, Ricketts' 'quadhelix' used for arch expansion. C, Fully banded appliance for final alignment.

have a reasonable range. The 'quadhelix' appliance shown in Figure 15.6B works extremely well for this purpose and can be made to exert a force which is not excessive but which is adequate for the purpose.

When the desired expansion has been achieved the quadehelix should be replaced with a palatal arch and it is usually necessary to use a fully banded appliance (Fig. 15.6C) for alignment of the teeth. It is sometimes found that the anterior end of the small fragment does not erupt naturally to the occlusal level. If this is the case, the situation does not respond very well to treatment but it is usually worth while attempting to bring these teeth down into occlusion, even if they relapse to some extent. This seems in every way preferable to the alternative of an overlay denture.

A case of this type is shown in Figure 15.7. Leonard was born with a complete unilateral cleft of the left side. He thus ran true to type, since this kind of cleft is twice as common in boys as girls, and twice as common on the left side. The lip was repaired at 3 months, without presurgical orthopaedics, and the palate at 18 months. He was then kept under observation until the upper incisors erupted, later than usual, at 10 years, as shown in the uppermost set of models in Figure 15.7B. /1 was very lingually inclined, lying across the incisal edges of the lower incisors, in a traumatic position. This tooth was therefore proclined over the bite, using a removable appliance, but 2/, which was in lingual occlusion but not traumatic, was not treated at this stage. The left buccal segment was in crossbite and was also not treated at this stage.

Further orthodontic treatment was postponed until the premolars had erupted, as shown in the second set of models, at the age of 13 years. It is not uncommon for the eruption of the dentition to be delayed in cleft palate patients. Both permanent canines were grossly misplaced, the left canine erupting horizontally towards the cleft, while the right canine was lying in the palate. Both these teeth were therefore extracted. The upper arch was expanded, using the quadhelix appliance described above, followed by fully banded appliances. The final records were taken at the age of 25 years, and the superimposed tracings in Figure 15.7C and D show, here again, the continued forward growth of the mandible not matched by that of the maxilla. This has caused a slight relapse in the crossbite despite the wearing of a permanent retainer, but also some improvement in the incisal angulation.

Permanent retention is necessary with a denture. This serves three purposes. Firstly, it maintains the expansion, secondly it replaces the missing teeth and thirdly it may well serve the purpose of obturating any small fistula which is present in the height of the palate. Not only must retention be permanent, but it must also be immediate. The initial retainer, usually made of acrylic, should be inserted within 3 hours of removing the banded appliance or alternatively the bands should be replaced after taking the impression, until the retainer can be made. This first acrylic retainer allows any natural settling of the teeth to take place and is then followed by a permanent denture usually made of cobalt-chromium. Some operators advocate the fitting of bridges, usually at a later stage, and it would seem that provided the expansion is held for a prolonged period — say 5 years — then collapse is comparatively slight if the denture is replaced by a more localised bridge.

When orthodontic treatment is completed the case should normally be referred back to the plastic surgeon who may well wish to carry out some final cosmetic operations on the lip or nose. The patient must of course be warned that the denture should be worn at all times and if a lip operation is proposed, an acrylic palate with clasps on suitable teeth should be constructed since it is often impossible to wear a denture immediately following a painful lip operation.

It will be noted from the superimposed tracings in Figure 15.7C, that here again, antero-posterior growth of the maxilla has been very slight with some change in incisor angulation and in overbite. In this case the affect has been minimal and somewhat favourable.

BILATERAL CLEFTS

These form the greatest problem in both cleft palate surgery and orthodontics. They may be total or sub-total, although the latter are rare.

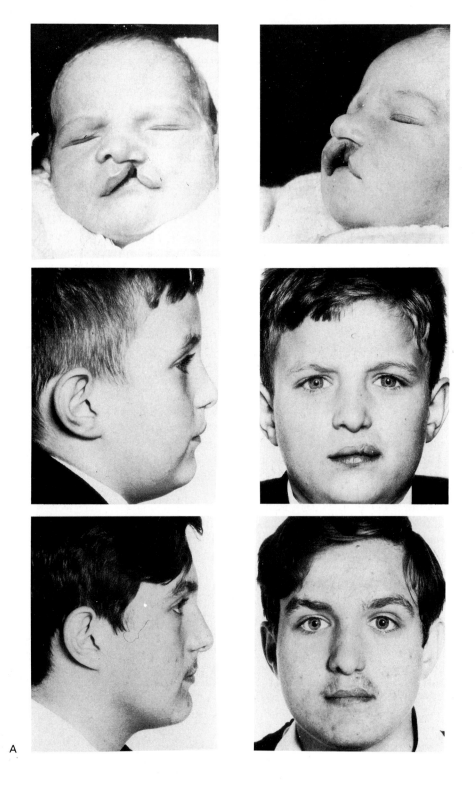

Fig. 15.7 Leonard. A, Photographs at birth, before and after orthodontic treatment. B (opposite), Models: in mixed dentition before first phase of treatment, before second phase of treatment and 8 years after end of all treatment. C, Superimposed tracings: before treatment on end of treatment, and the latter on 8 years after treatment. D, Intra-oral photograph at age 25 years (C and D overleaf).

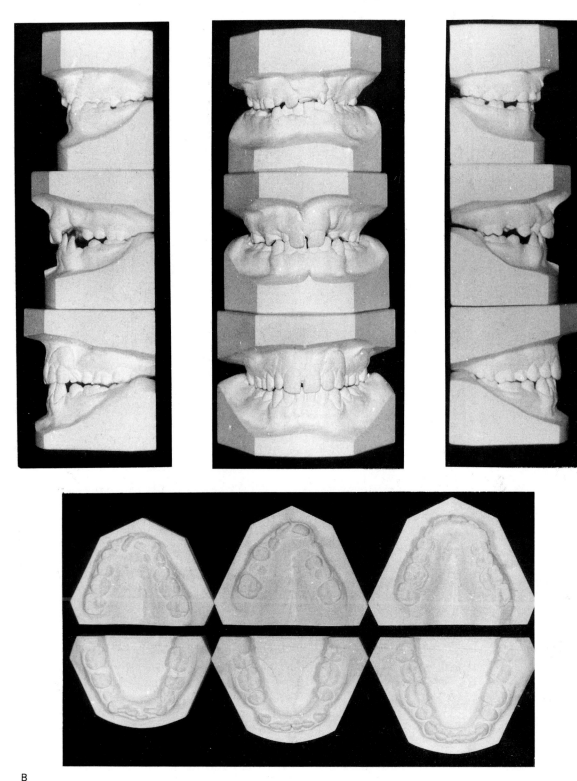

B

Fig. 15.7 (cont'd)

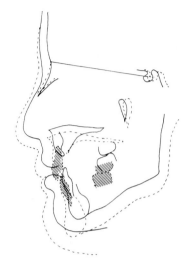

C

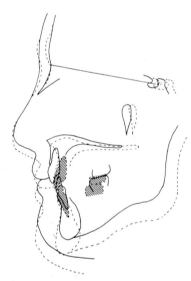

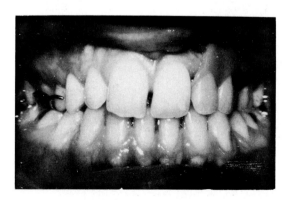

D

Fig. 15.7 (*cont'd*)

Total bilateral clefts occur in approximately 10 per cent of all clefts of the lip and palate. At birth the primary palate is completely separate from the two halves of the secondary palate and is frequently displaced forward outside the mouth. It is commonly rotated so that the alveolar crest faces more or less anteriorly and there is a lack of tissue between the tip of the nose and the vermilion border of the upper lip (Fig. 15.8A). At this stage in the newly born the posterior segments are quite often wide apart, although they may have collapsed inwards. The first problem is to close the lip, with the primary palate inside the mouth. It would seem that pre-surgical orthodontics (or

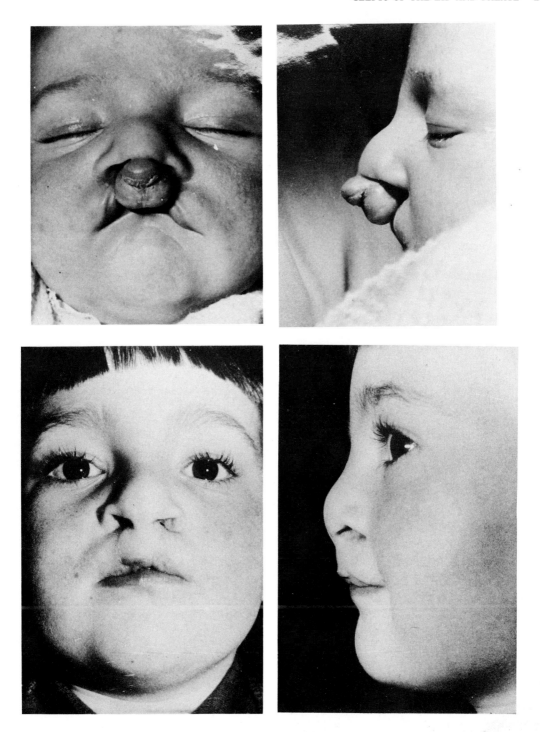

A

Fig. 15.8 David: Bilateral cleft of lip and palate. A, Photographs shortly after birth, at the age of 5 and (overleaf) 17 years, before and after lip surgery. B, Study models at beginning of orthodontic treatment, at the end of first stage and 2 years after completion of treatment. C (p. 268) Superimposed tracings, beginning of treatment on condition at age 15 years superimposed on SN at S. D, Tracings at beginning of treatment on condition at age of 15 years, superimposed on Björk's structures in mandible. E, Intra-oral photograph following treatment, with denture. 1/1 have been crowned.

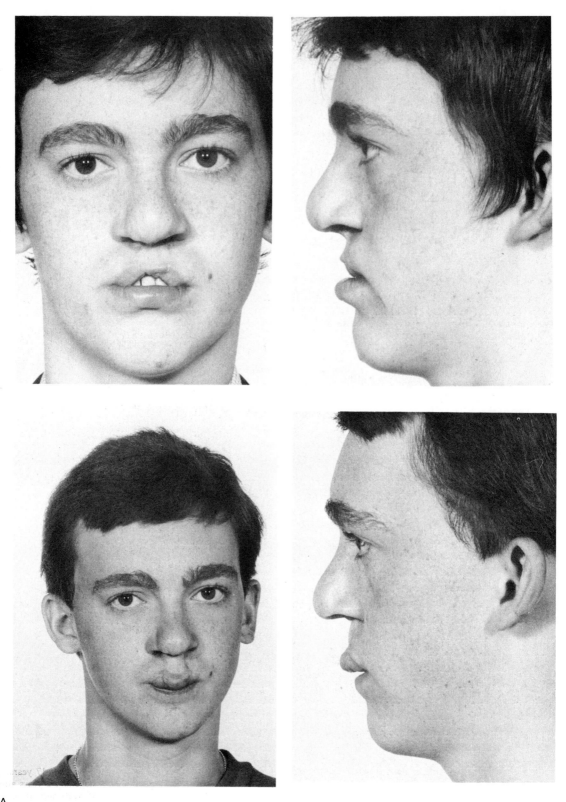

A

Fig. 15.8 (*cont'd*)

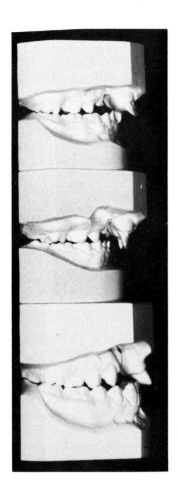
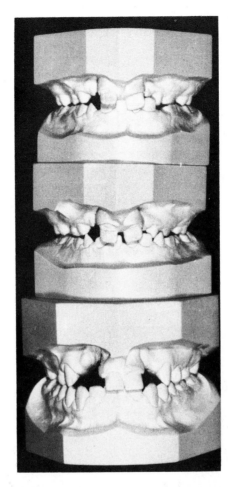
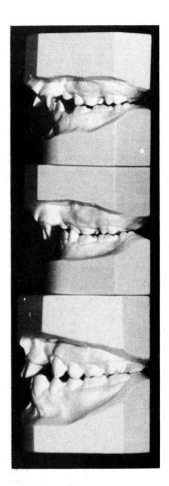

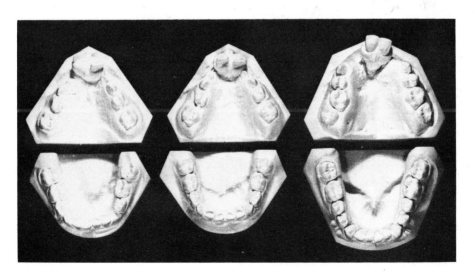

B

Fig. 15.8 (cont'd)

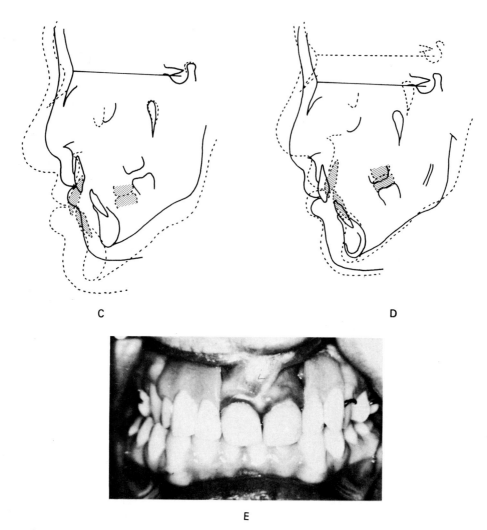

C

D

E

Fig. 15.8 (*cont'd*)

dental orthopaedics) is probably at its most valu-able in this type of case. An intra-oral plate of the type previously described is constructed, although it will not have anything to cover the primary palate. Extra-oral strapping, as described for unilateral clefts, is normally also used in cases of bilateral clefts. If this treatment is successful, closure of the lip on both sides may take place simultaneously at about the age of 3 months. If presurgical orthopaedics is not carried, out, then two alternatives present themselves to control the primary palate, depending to some extent on severity. Frequently, it is possible to close one side of the lip and this has the effect of controlling

the primary palate so that the second side may be closed a few weeks later. Some surgeons prefer to remove a wedge from the nasal septum to so as to allow the primary palate to be corrected in one operation. Although popular some years ago, this operation has fallen from favour since it is frequently found that the growth of the anterior part of the upper arch is impeded with the production of a gross Class III occlusion later in life. It is regarded by most surgeons as an act of desperation.

Here again treatment in the complete deciduous dentition is not usually indicated although by this stage, the posterior segments will probably have moved medially in a bilateral crossbite and the anterior parts of both segments may be vertically displaced out of occlusion. If early surgical treatment has been unsuccessful, it may be desired to move the primary palate inside the mouth at this stage by surgery and in that case, orthodontic treatment to expand the buccal segments may be carried out in the complete deciduous dentition. I have personally carried this out only twice.

When the patient is seen in the mixed dentition, the facial appearance is very typical (Fig. 15.8A). Due to the lack of tissue between the tip of the nose and the philtrum of the upper lip, the nose is typically tethered so that it appears very flattened with the bases of the alae displaced laterally. The incisors on the primary palate may be rotated, as in unilateral clefts, but not infrequently there is an extremely deep overbite with a Class II Division 2 type of appearance. Sometimes it is found that the incisors are inside the bite, producing a Class III incisor relationship, again with a deep overbite. At this stage treatment should, as in the unilateral clefts, be kept to a minimum and confined to aligning the anterior teeth, placing them in an atraumatic position and possibly moving them over the bite if they are in Class III relationship. The main part of the treatment is again carried out in the complete permanent dentition with bilateral expansion of the buccal teeth and alignment of the anteriors followed by the fitting of a permanent prosthesis.

David is a fairly typical example of this type of cleft. When seen in the mixed dentition, he was as shown in Figure 15.8B. The buccal segments had dropped into crossbite at their anterior end, although fortunately, they were in occlusion vertically. The primary palate was still somewhat forward of its correct position, with one upper central incisor proclined and the other retroclined. Both incisors were very hypoplastic, a not uncommon finding. The prominent incisor was unsightly and clearly liable to damage and at this stage treatment was confined to moving these two incisors into line and retroclining them slightly. This produced the situation shown in the second set of models, which was in fact rather more typical of a bilateral cleft, with the Class II Division 2 incisor relationship brought about by rotation of the whole primary palate. Bilateral expansion of the upper arch was then carried out, followed by fully banded therapy to produce the final result shown in the lower models which were taken some years out of retention. The intra-oral view is shown in Figure 15.8D.

We have already commented on the fact that antero-posterior growth of the maxilla frequently lags behind that of the mandible. In this type of bilateral cleft this feature is an advantage. It will be seen from the superimposed tracings in Figure 15.8C, that as the mandible has grown downwards and forwards the retroclination and deep overbite involving the upper central incisors has disappeared with comparatively minor help from the fixed appliance. In this case the condition was somewhat overdone so that in the final models the apices of the upper central incisors are too far lingually and the incisors rather over-proclined. Because of this differential growth an apparently hopeless position of the upper central incisors, will often respond to treatment better than one would hope.

BONE GRAFTING

Following conventional surgery the parts of the maxilla are joined only by soft tissue. Contraction of this is largely responsible for the collapse inwards of the segments. Not surprisingly there have been a number of techniques for bone grafting the maxilla to restore its continuity. Grafting in infancy has already been seen to interfere with subsequent maxillary growth, and its originator, Johanson, was the first to abandon it. The same author advocated grafting in the late adolescent period, using cortical bone from the ileac crest, inserted from the labial sulcus opposite the cleft, and extending to the posterior margin of the hard palate. While good results were reported, the technique was extremely demanding and not widely used.

More recently Abyholm and his team in Oslo have used a technique whereby cancellous bone is 'scooped out' from within the ileac crest, and the compact bone then replaced, reducing subsequent pain in this region. The region of the cleft is then prepared, the ends of existing bone freshened, and the cancellous 'mush' packed in as far as possible towards the base of the ala of the nose.

Not only have good results been demonstrated by this method but Semb (see Abyholm et al., 1981) has analysed the results of all cases which had then been treated, and shown a very satisfactory outcome. It would seem that the operation is best carried out at 10–11 years, before the eruption of the permanent canines, but when intercanine growth is largely complete. It is then possible, in many cases, to move adjacent teeth into the grafted area and, often, to close all spaces. Prior to the operation, that is in the late mixed dentition, the arch is expanded to eliminate all crossbite, and it would seem that permanent retention is not necessary.

Techniques for the treatment of clefts of the lip and palate cannot be fully assessed until facial growth is complete, and many apparently major advances have failed to pass this test, but this bone-grafting technique would seem to present no problems apart, perhaps, from a tendency to resorption of the roots of adjacent teeth, just below the alveolar margin. This is largely avoided if surgery is carried out before the canine erupts.

LATER SURGERY

Following the completion of orthodontic treatment, but usually before the construction of any permanent prosthesis, the patient is again seen on a combined clinic with the plastic surgeon and possibly the oral surgeon. Minor corrections of the lip may be carried out, together with closure of any remaining palatal fistulae. In the case of David (Fig. 15.8A) the upper lip at the end of treatment was obviously defective. This was repaired by the Abbé flap operation. In these cases the lower lip is often very full, so a segment of tissue may be taken from the lower lip and inserted into the philtrum region of the upper lip. It remains attached to the lower lip to ensure the blood supply, for 2–3 weeks. During this period the patient's lip is divided in two by an isthmus of lower lip, and feeding is clearly difficult. When the upper lip has healed, the attachment to the lower lip is severed. This operation tends to be a last resort, at best leaving an additional scar in the

lower lip, and usually a rather immobile upper lip.

Having replaced the philtrum with fresh tissue, the previous defective philtrum may be used to lengthen the columella of the nose, especially, as here, in bilateral clefts. This should be delayed until after puberty, when the adult size and shape of the nose can be assessed.

Finally, if the skeletal appearance is unsatisfactory, various forms of orthognathic surgery, as detailed in the next chapter, are available. In cases of a retroposed maxilla, fortunately less common nowadays, the maxilla may be advanced. This has the disadvantage that if the soft palate is also advanced, contact between soft palate and pharynx, already tenuous, may become impossible. This 'velo-pharyngeal incompetence' produces a very typical and unpleasant nasal speech, which is difficult to correct. Mr David James has employed a procedure to avoid this. The mucosa over the hard palate is lifted and the maxilla brought forward, leaving the palatine bone and attached soft palate in its original place. The mucosa is then replaced, leaving a raw area at its anterior end, which duly epithelialises.

CONCLUSION

Clefts of the lip and palate involve perhaps the most worthwhile type of orthodontic treatment which we carry out. In some ways they are the most frustrating. Patients are frequently uncooperative and lacking in dental consciousness. The parents may be over-protective, or the child may compensate for his abnormality by becoming aggressive. Happily, in the majority of cases it is possible to achieve a result which if not perfect is nevertheless satisfying. It is emphasised that a team approach is desirable, with a group of specialists who are on personally friendly terms seeing the patient together at suitable intervals. Surgery and orthodontic treatment should be arranged so as not to interfere with each other. The orthodontist should bear in mind that while his work in correcting the occlusion is important, probably the most important task is the production of an acceptable facial appearance by the surgeon, followed by the production of acceptable speech by the speech therapist.

SUGGESTED READING

Abyholm F E 1978 Cleft lip and palate in a Norswegian population. II. A numerical study of 1555 CLP-patients admitted for surgical treatment 1954–75. Scandinavian Journal of Plastic and Reconstructive Surgery 12: 29–38

Abyholm F E, Bergland O, Semb G 1981 Secondary bone-grafting of alveolar clefts. Scandinavian Journal of Plastic and Reconstructive Surgery 15: 127–40

Bishara S E, Martinez de Arrondono R S, Vales H P, Jakobsen J R 1985 Dento-facial relationships in persons with unoperated clefts: comparisons between three cleft types. American Journal of Orthodontics 87: 481–507

Gorlin R J, Pindborg J J, Cohen M M 1976 Syndromes of the head and neck (see especially Section 22). McGraw-Hill, New York

Matthews D, Grossmann W 1964 Restoration of the collapsed maxillary arch by rapid expansion and bone grafting. Cleft Palate Journal 1: 430–40

Olin W H 1966 Cleft lip and palate rehabilitation. American Journal of Orthodontics 52: 128–44

Robertson N R E 1970 Recent trends in the early treatment of cleft lip and palate. Transactions of the British Society for the Study of Orthodontics 56: 184–97

Robertson N R E 1974 Deciduous occlusion in children with repaired complete clefts of the lip and palate. British Journal of Orthodontics 1(2): 5–10

Robertson N R E, Jolleys A 1968 Effects of early bone-grafting in complete clefts of lip and palate. Plastic and Reconstructive Surgery 42: 414–21

Smith D I 1967 Cleft lip and palate in one of monozygotic twins. Transactions of the British Society for the Study of Orthodontics 111–115

Subtelny J D 1966 Orthodontic treatment of cleft lip and palate, birth to adulthood. Angle Orthodontist 36: 273–92

16

The surgical correction of malocclusion

Major oral surgery has been advocated for many years in the correction of gross Class III abnormalities with mandibular prognathism. Indeed, Angle himself carried out two such operations, of which one was successful. In recent years, this practice has been widely extended to involve the correction of many forms of skeletal abnormality and the Americans have named this orthognathic surgery. It is normally carried out when growth has effectively ceased and for this reason it is possible at an earlier age in girls than in young men. It can also be undertaken somewhat earlier for Class II skeletal patterns, where growth tends to improve the condition rather than Class III skeletal patterns, where further growth may cause a relapse. It should be emphasised that facial surgery of this magnitude involves some risk of morbidity and even mortality and should only be undertaken in co-operation with a skilled and experienced oral surgeon.

As already indicated, the keynote to success lies in co-operation between the surgeon, orthodontist and, especially in the earlier stages after operation, the nursing staff. The orthodontist clearly enters into this in ensuring a good occlusion following the operation, by localised tooth movements. In addition he can give valuable assistance in planning the operation where his knowledge of facial form and growth and the use of lateral skull radiographs can be helpful. Frequently, immobilisation of the jaws following their planned fracture can be carried out using orthodontic bands or bonds either cemented especially for the purpose or used in conjunction with orthodontic treatment before or after surgery. It is not proposed in this chapter to enter into the subject at all thoroughly: books can and have been written on this topic. It

is intended rather to give the reader some knowledge of the problems involved and the success which may be achieved.

SURGICAL PROCEDURES

Least of all would I attempt to indicate the surgical techniques involved in surgical correction of deformity. It is helpful for the orthodontist to have some idea of the types of procedures which are involved but it should be borne in mind that all of these can be modified to suit both the individual case and the whim of the surgeon. In this section only the barest outlines will be given.

Operations on the maxilla

Maxillary osteotomies may be performed either to advance or to retract the whole or part of the maxilla, or to move it upwards or downwards. The principal operations used are listed below.

Le Fort I

There are three operations on the maxilla named after Le Fort, the name being used because they involve the production of a fracture of the type classified by that author. Le Fort I (Fig. 16.1A) involves separating the alveolar region from its bony base, the incisions being made above the roots of the teeth, and once the alveolar region has been freed it may be moved anteriorly, upwards with removal of some intervening bone, or downwards with insertion of a bone graft. This is a very satisfactory operation and it is not difficult to raise

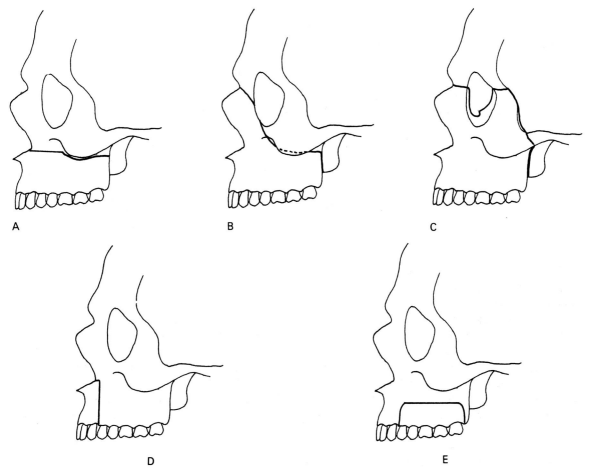

Fig. 16.1 Diagrammatic representation of operative procedures on the maxilla. A, Le Fort I maxillary osteotomy. B, Le Fort II operation. C, Le Fort III operation. D, Wassmund segmental maxillary osteotomy. E, Schuchardt operation.

or lower one end of the alveolus more than the other so that a tilting action may be achieved.

Le Fort II (Fig. 16.1B)

In this operation the incisions are made somewhat higher in the anterior region, passing through the bridge of the nose and the lower border of the orbit so that the anterior part of the face may also be corrected. It is normally used for advancement of the maxilla in cases of gross maxillary retrognathism.

Le Fort III (Fig. 16.1C)

This is an heroic operation in which the whole of

the face is separted from the cranium, the cranial cavity being entered. It carries some risk of mortality and should only be undertaken in dire straits. It is most frequently used for the correction of Crouzon's syndrome where the sutures of the maxilla fuse early so that antero-posterior maxillary growth ceases. This makes it impossible for the patient to close his eye-lids with inevitable blindness unless some operation is undertaken.

Wassmund operation (Fig. 16.1D)

In this operation only the anterior part of the alveolar regions is separated from the posterior part by vertical incisions, usually posterior to the upper canines and across the palate, together with horizontal incisions above the root apices. It is most frequently used for the reduction of an overjet where there is a prominence of the premaxillary area, and in this case the first premolar would probably be extracted and a segment of bone removed. It could also be used for advancement of this area with the insertion of a bone graft but this leaves a somewhat unsatisfactory alveolar region.

Schuchardt operation (Fig. 16.1E)

This operation is used in the correction of anterior open bite. The posterior alveolus is separated from the rest of the maxilla, bone removed and the posterior segment impacted upwards into the maxillary antrum. Popular some years ago, this operation suffered a period of unpopularity but appears once again to be becoming fashionable.

Operations on the maxilla are usually satisfactory and healing is rapid. Segmental operations in either jaw have the advantage that prolonged inter-maxillary fixation is avoided but tend to produce a less satisfactory occlusion.

Operations on the mandible

The earliest mandibular operation was the body ostectomy. In its simplest form, this consists of the removal of a segment of the horizontal ramus of the mandible (Fig. 16.2A), either taking advantage of a natural space in the dentition or extracting a suitable tooth. It is used for shortening the mandible in cases of mandibular prognathism. The obvious problem lies in the danger of severing the inferior dental nerve and associated vessels. These should be dissected out and a recess made in the adjacent bone into which they can be 'tucked'. Clearly this is easier said than done. This operation also carries the risk of delayed union or even non-union and to overcome this, modifications have been devised. The stepped ostectomy, and the angle ostectomy (Fig. 16.2B and C) are examples of this which serve to bring a larger area of bone into contact.

The body ostectomy has largely given way to more sophisticated procedures on the vertical ramus but is still useful at times where a very large reduction in mandibular length is required or

where gaps in the dentition may conveniently be eliminated by this method.

Horizontal section of the vertical ramus

The vertical ramus may be divided horizontally above the lingula and the lower segment slid backwards, or even theoretically forwards. It may be carried out either as an open operation or following the technique of Kostecka, as a blind procedure. The latter involves inserting a Gigli saw around the medial side of the vertical ramus through small incisions, and using this to section the bone. The risks of unintentionally severing other structures are obvious. Horizontal section of the vertical ramus has proved particularly unsatisfactory with a high risk of relapse towards an open bite, and of non-union, and should no longer be employed.

Sagittal splitting

This procedure was originally devised by Obwegeser but the technique illustrated in Figure 16.2D is the modification by Dal Pont. A horizontal cut is made above the lingula on the medial side of the mandible with a fine burr. A vertical cut is then made on the lateral side of the bone below the molar teeth, in each case only going through the cortical bone. These two cuts are then connected along the anterior margin of the vertical ramus. An osteotome is inserted and used to split the outer plate, attached to the condyle, from the inner plate which is attached to the body of the mandible. If successful on both sides of the mouth, the body may then be advanced, retracted or a tilting action may be used to close an open bite. In skilled hands this is a very satisfactory operation but it should be borne in mind that splitting does not always occur as cleanly as one would wish, and indeed some individuals appear to have no cancellous bone within the mandible in this region.

Vertical sub-sigmoid osteotomy (Fig. 16.2E)

This is another operation for reduction of mandibular prognathism which has many modifications. In its simplest form, the mandible is divided by

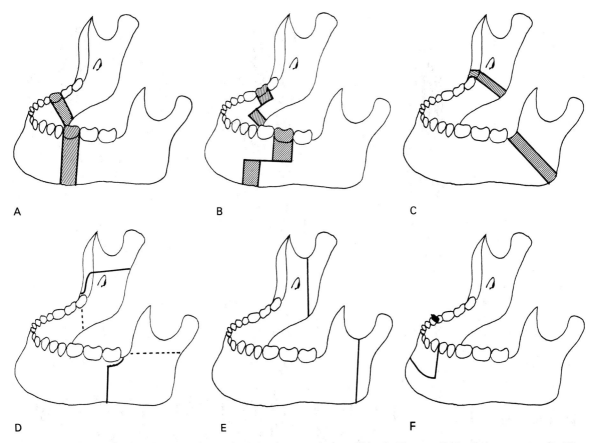

Fig. 16.2 Diagrammatic representation of operative procedures on the mandible. A, The mandibular body ostectomy. B, The stepped ostectomy. C, The angle ostectomy. D, The sagittal split (Dal Pont's modification). E, The vertical sub-sigmoid osteotomy. F, The Köle segmental operation.

a vertical cut from the sigmoid notch to the angle of the mandible, passing behind the lingula and therefore the inferior dental nerve. The posterior portion of the vertical ramus is then overlapped on the lateral side of the anterior portion. The cortical bone may be removed to improve union, although in practice this seems to be unnecessary. It is normally carried out from an extra-oral approach, unlike the previous operation, and this has the disadvantage of leaving a scar. An intra-oral approach has been devised but has not proved popular. It is clearly only useful for limited retraction of the mandible.

The Köle operation (Fig. 16.2F)

This again is a segmental operation where vertical cuts are made, usually distal to the lower canine

teeth and connected by means of a horizontal cut, passing below the roots of the lower incisors. The alveolar segment may then be raised, with a bone graft, lowered, advanced or retracted.

Chin operations

A wide variety of operations may be carried out to improve the appearance of the chin. A segment may be removed from the anterior aspect in order to reduce the prominence in cases of mandibular prognathism, or from the inferior aspect in patients with a large lower facial height. These are known as reduction genioplasties. In the latter case, the bone removed may sometimes be used as a graft in treatment of an open bite by elevating the lower labial segment of teeth by the Köle procedure. Alternatively, bone grafts may be added to the chin in order to make it more prominent. The use of artificial materials such as Silastic is not usually successful, since the underlying bone resorbs and the prominence of the chin is lost, although the more porous material 'Proplast', is apparently more satisfactory. Finally, a selection of sliding genioplasties is available, whereby the inferior margin of the chin may be slid forward to increase the prominence thereof. An example of this is illustrated in Figure 16.5. Genioplasties are usually carried out in association with other surgery but may occasionally be sufficient by themselves.

PLANNING

When the surgeon and patient meet in the operating theatre all the planning procedures should have already been carried out. Ideally, the surgeon should merely work to a precise plan agreed beforehand, giving the amount of movement required, or bone removed, in millimetres. In this he may be aided by models, templates and lateral radiographic tracings. At this stage he should not have to think.

The thinking should have been carried out on previous occasions and in this the orthodontist usually collaborates with the surgeon in planning what is required. Study models are clearly useful and indeed surgery may be carried out on the models to simulate the operation. Lateral radiographs and tracings thereof are also valuable as are life size photographs. It is desirable that the photograph should be of the same size as a tracing of the radiograph and this may best be achieved by placing the tracing on the easel of the enlarger and then enlarging the image of the photograph to coincide with the tracing as closely as possible. Occasionally, in particularly difficult cases, a model of the mandible may be produced in plastic so that the operation may first be carried out on this model.

The cephalometric radiograph may be analysed in the usual way with a series of angles and distances and indeed a routine cephalometric analysis should always be carried out. More useful, however, is the employment of a template which may be superimposed on the radiograph and indicate where the abnormality lies. Such templates are commercially available as inserts in the book by Broadbent and others (1975). These represent ideal facial forms in both lateral and postero-anterior view at a series of ages up to 18 years. Unfortunately, they have not been differentiated by sex but nevertheless are sufficiently useful for our purpose. Alternatively, the operator may produce suitable outlines, by tracing the radiographs of selected individuals, whose appearance is pleasing. It should be emphasised that the use of radiographs is not intended to be a precise procedure but a guide to the final facial form. The latter will always be a compromise between the desirable and the possible and even the desirable for the individual patient may not coincide with Dr Broadbent's ideals. An alternative type of template is to be found in 'Jacobson Proportionate Templates' published by Nola Orthodontic Specialties in America. These have the advantages of providing templates for both Caucasian and Negroid patients.

Surgery may also be carried out on the life-size photographs to indicate the likely final appearance. These prognostic photographs are usually somewhat too successful and they should not be shown to the patient since this may later give rise to disappointment. It should be borne in mind that soft tissues do not follow the hard tissues and teeth in precise ratios. The nose and soft tissue pogonion tend to follow their underlying bony structures almost completely, as do the soft tissue areas overlying points A and B. The lips themselves behave in variable fashions as the teeth are moved and in this respect the orthodontist's experience may be of value. On average they tend to follow the teeth, perhaps 60 to 70 per cent, but with very wide variations.

Planning is best illustrated by considering some actual examples:

Bronwen

This lady presented at the age of 22 years complaining of mandibular prognathism and a gross Class III malocclusion (Fig. 16.3). It will be seen that the angle SNA was reduced and the SNB increased. The lower incisors were markedly retroclined. A genioplasty to remove the anterior part of the chin had previously been carried out with results which were not acceptable to the patient. The lateral radiograph was superimposed on Broadbent's standards as shown in Figure 16.3C and this indicated that the mandible was somewhat anteriorly positioned, while the maxilla was retroposed. It is not uncommon to find in severe Class III conditions that the abnormality lies partly in both jaws. When superimposed on bony outlines of the two jaws individually (Fig. 16.3D), it was seen that the jaws themselves were of reasonably normal size. In Class III cases one frequently finds that the models will occlude reasonably well in a normal relationship and that very little preliminary orthodontic treatment is necessary. Figure 16.3E shows the result which might be expected from a Le Fort I advancement of the maxilla and this would clearly leave a rather aggressive looking individual which might be

desirable in a man but not in a woman. Figure 16.3F shows the proposed result of moving the mandible posteriorly and it was felt that this would produce an acceptable result with operation confined to one jaw.

The plaster models were therefore placed in the original occlusion and a pencil mark inscribed on upper and lower molar teeth opposite each other. The lower model was then moved backwards to simulate a normal occlusion and a second pencil mark made on the upper model. The distance between these two pencil marks indicated to the surgeon the amount of posterior movement required, which coincided well with the amount planned from lateral radiographs in Figure 16.3E. In severe Class III malocclusions, it is common to find that the lower incisors are very retroclined, and it is desirable to procline the teeth to a more normal angle before carrying out the surgery. This

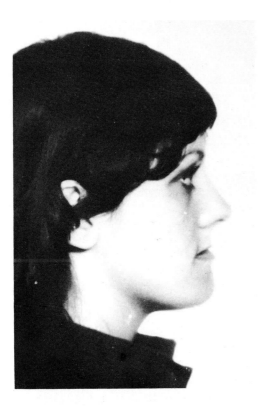
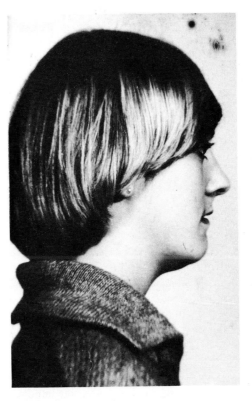

A

Fig. 16.3 Bronwen: A, Photographs before and 4 years after surgery. B, Study models before and after treatment and 4 years later. C, Lateral skull tracing superimposed on template of ideal face. D, Maxilla and mandible superimposed on ideals. E, The projected result of maxillary advancement. F, The projected result of mandibular osteotomy (C, D, E and F overleaf).

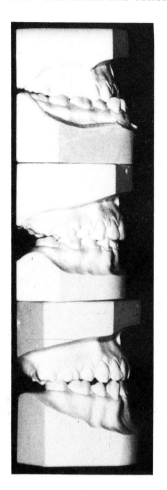
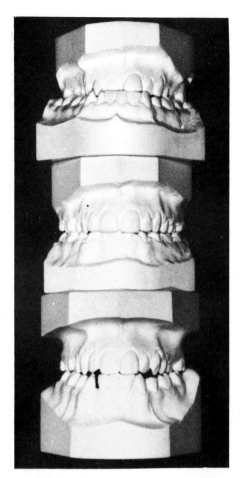
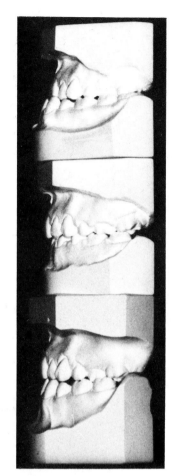

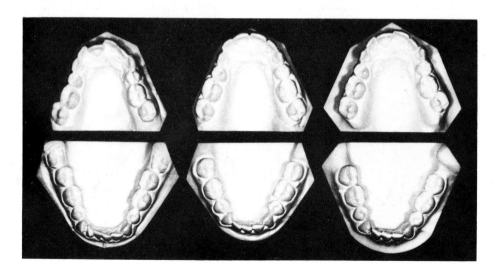

B

Fig. 16.3 (*cont'd*)

is known as 'decompensation' and of course adds to the amount of orthodontic and surgical treatment required but tends to produce a somewhat more acceptable profile and occlusion.

There is sometimes controversy as to whether the orthodontic treatment should be carried out before or after the surgical procedures. The answer would seem to be that it depends on the case. In this patient the teeth in both arches were banded (Fig. 16.4A) and alignment of the teeth

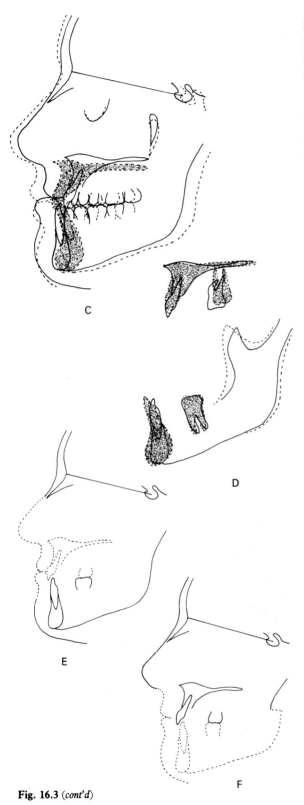

C

D

E

F

Fig. 16.3 (*cont'd*)

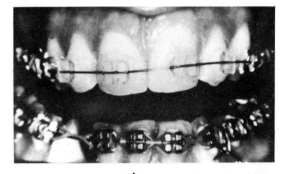

A

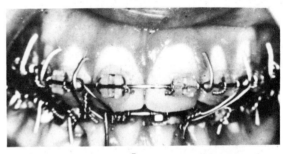

B

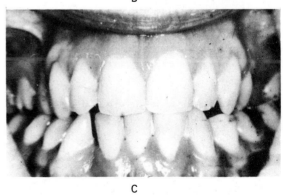

C

Fig. 16.4 A, Appliances used in the final stages of presurgical orthodontic treatment for Bronwen. B, Heavy rectangular archwires used to intermaxillary fixation. C, Intra-oral photograph 4 years after operation.

carried out with the extraction of the displaced lower right canine and some expansion of the upper arch. Almost always a small amount of orthodontic treatment is required following surgery and in Class III cases particularly, presurgical orthodontic treatment may not be necessary. In many surgical cases fairly extensive preliminary orthodontic treatment is required which may well last for 12 months or longer. It is sometimes difficult to persuade the surgeon, who is used to completing his treatment within an afternoon, that this is necessary or desirable.

Finally, the bands on the teeth were used to suport heavy rectangular archwires (Fig. 16.4B) which in turn were used for inter-maxillary fixation following the sagittal split procedure, to produce the result shown in Figure 16.3.

Christina

This patient presented a much more serious problem. As will be seen from Figure 16.5, she had a very severe Class II skeletal pattern with a steep mandibular angle and large lower facial height. Her lips were grossly incompetent and in addition her dentition was neglected and oral hygiene non-existent. She was originally referred for orthodontic treatment and was dismissed with the information that this was not practicable. However, she persevered on two further occasions and we then told her of the possibility of an operation which could only be carried out if her teeth were put in order and her oral hygiene improved. In this she proved surprisingly co-operative and it was therefore decided to plan a suitable operation. The models were mounted on an articulator (Fig. 16.6A) and the upper model was moved posteriorly; a movement which is possible with this particular machine. This produced an even greater anterior open bite and also a posterior crossbite (Fig. 16.6B). It was therefore decided to expand the maxilla bilaterally by

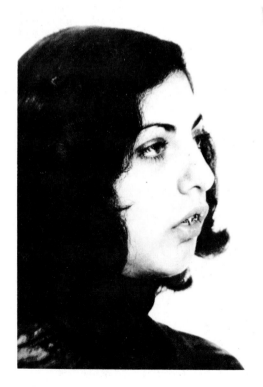
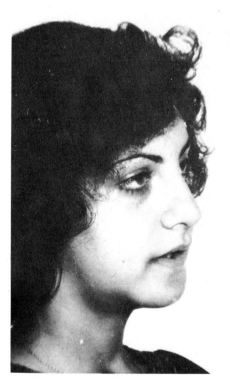

A

Fig. 16.5 Christina: A, Photographs before and after surgery. B (opposite) Study models before treatment, after orthodontic treatment but before surgery and 6 months after surgery.

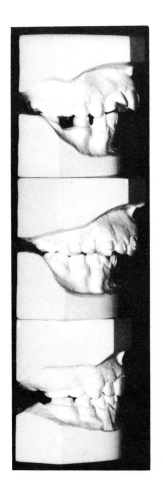
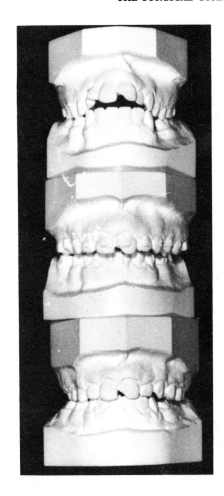
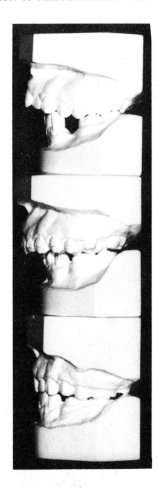
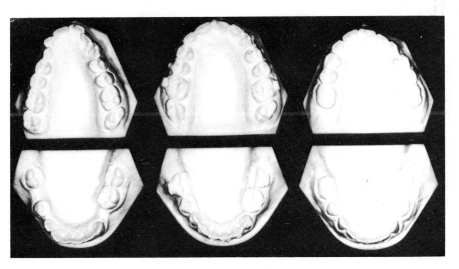

B

Fig. 16.5 (*cont'd*)

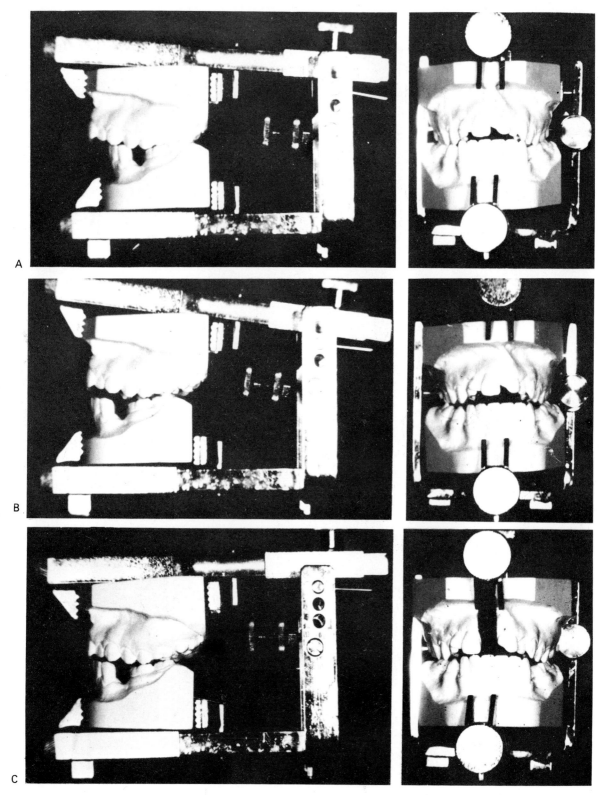

Fig. 16.6 Planning treatment of Christina with study models. A, Original condition. B, Following posterior movement of maxillary arch; note open bite. C, Following expansion and raising of upper model.

cutting the model down the centre and bringing the posterior segments into occlusion, filling in the intervening area with wax (Fig. 16 .6C). At the same time, the upper model was raised in the condyle region in order to produce a better occlusion.

Simultaneously with this, attention was given to the lateral radiographs. Figure 16.7A shows Christina's lateral skull radiograph superimposed on a template from Broadbent's book and this confirmed the impression of an unduly high maxilla and mandible with clearly a backward rotating lower jaw. The jaws themselves were of normal length, although the alveoli had over-developed in a vertical direction. A postero-anterior radiograph was also used and superimposed on Broadbent's templates (Fig. 16.7B) and this confirmed the suggestion of asymmetry in the

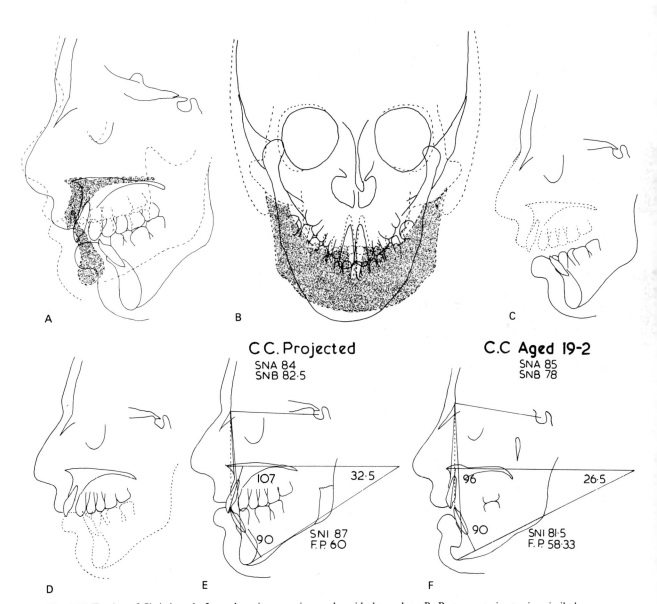

Fig. 16.7 Tracing of Christina. A, Lateral tracing superimposed on ideal template. B, Postero-anterior tracing similarly superimposed. C, The result of raising the maxilla and D, auto-rotation of the mandible. E, The final projected result with forward slide following sagittal split. F, The result achieved with advancement genioplasty.

mandible, although this was not sufficient to complicate an already difficult case.

As a first move it was proposed that the maxilla should be raised by means of a Le Fort I osteotomy. It was finally decided that this should involve 3 mm raising anteriorly and 7 mm posteriorly and our surgical colleagues can carry out this type of procedure with remarkable accuracy. The proposed result is shown in Figure 16.7; Figure 16.7C shows the raising of the maxilla and Figure 16.7D the result following auto-rotation of the mandible upwards. It will be seen that this still leaves a severe Class II skeletal pattern. The tracing of the mandible was then advanced as indicated from the models to produce the projected result shown in Figure 16.7E. It will be seen from the superimposed outline of the template that the result planned would approximate reasonably well to the ideal. At the ensuing conference, the surgeon suggested that a sliding genioplasty should be added to increase the chin prominence.

In this case substantial preliminary orthodontic treatment was carried out. Initially, the maxillary arch was expanded using rapid maxillary expansion. This procedure is not always satisfactory in adults since the inter-maxillary suture fuses at varying ages between about 17 and 30 years. Since Christina was under 17 years it could safely be undertaken and was followed by fully banded appliance therapy in both arches to retrocline the upper incisors and close the spaces where teeth had been lost as far as possible. Here again, the bands with heavy arch-wires were used for fixation (Fig. 16.8A). The maxilla was then raised using the Le Fort I operation, followed by sagittal splitting of the mandible to bring forward the anterior segment into a normal relationship. Finally a forward sliding genioplasty was carried out. The result of this operation both facially and dentally, are shown in Figures 16.5 and 16.8.

Anne

This patient also presented with a gross overjet but was in other respects quite different from Christina (Fig. 16.9). Indeed, perhaps the main point of similarity was a complete indifference to oral hygiene but in this case it proved to be a

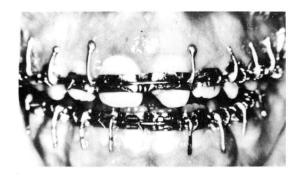

A

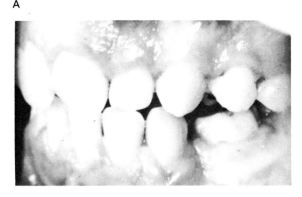

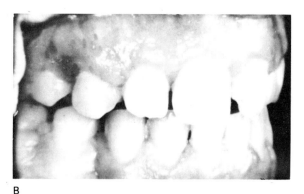

B

Fig. 16.8 A, The stabilising archwires used for fixation, immediately before band removal. B, Intra-oral view of Christina after operation.

constant problem. Both the cephalometric analysis and the superimposition on the template, showed that the mandibular retrusion in this case was moderate and the abnormality consisted partly of proclination with spacing of the upper incisors and partly of a prominence of the premaxillary area. The condition could probably have been treated orthodontically had the patient been more dentally aware but it was felt that any such treatment

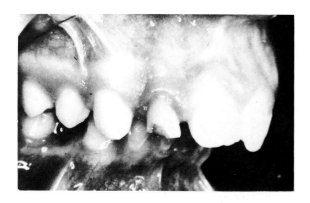

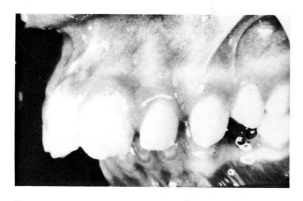

A

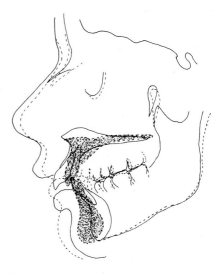

C

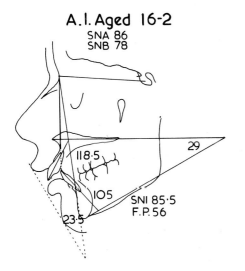

B

Fig. 16.9 Anne: A, Intra-oral photograph before treatment. B, Lateral skull tracing. C, Tracing superimposed on ideal face. D, Projected final result.

D

should be limited and that the major part of the correction should be carried out surgically. The obvious operation was the Wassmund segmental operation on the premaxillary area and it was decided to simulate this on duplicate study models (Fig. 16.10). Before doing this, a separating medium was applied to the upper study model and a plaster base prepared for it. The plaster teeth were then separated from the mould and set further lingually in wax, simulating orthodontic treatment to close the spaces (Fig. 16.11). The upper first premolars were removed from the

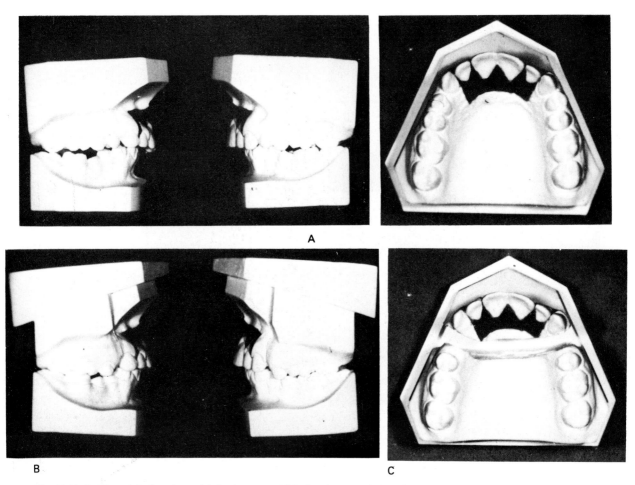

Fig. 16.10 A, The original study model for Anne on which the plaster teeth have been separated and set lingually in wax to close spaces. Note plaster base. B, The occlusion following model surgery, with new plaster base to position two parts of upper model. C, The two pieces of the upper model replaced in original base to show amount of plaster (and therefore bone) to be removed.

model and a segment of plaster also removed sufficiently wide for the labial segment to be taken back into a normal occlusion with the lower incisors. The overbite was not quite complete and from consideration of the lip line, it was decided that it would not be necessary to set down the lower incisors by the Köle procedure (which would have been quite practicable) but rather to move the upper segment upwards in addition to its retraction. The result of this model surgery is seen in Figure 16.10. The upper model is again held together by means of a plaster base and this photograph was taken in the inverted position otherwise the fragments would have fallen apart. Having decided on the result to be achieved, the

two parts of the upper model were then replaced in the original plaster base and the space between the two parts indicated to the surgeon the amount of bone which it would be necessary to remove. The projected result is shown in a lateral skull tracing in Figure 16.9 and here again it has been decided to increase the mandibular prominence slightly by means of a sliding genioplasty. As a final planning measure, the patient's life-sized photograph was trimmed to carry out the results indicated by superimposition on the projected tracing. This is shown in Figure 16.11B and will clearly produce a pleasing appearance, although as indicated previously, this may be somewhat over-optimistic.

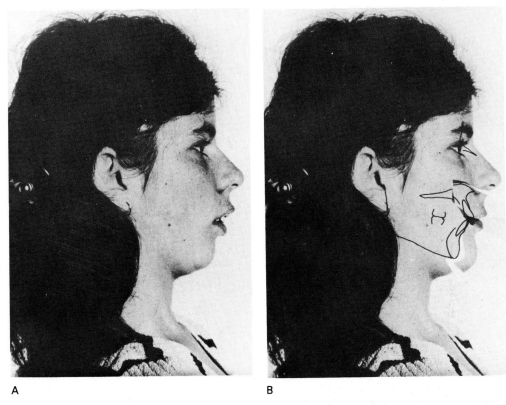

A   B

Fig. 16.11 A, Lateral photograph of Anne before treatment. B, Projected final result produced by superimposing segments of photograph on projected tracing.

Facial and intra-oral photographs of Anne are shown in Figure 16.12A and B.

These cases have indicated the quite extensive procedures necessary in planning and also to some extent the orthodontic procedures which are usually carried out. Orthodontic bands have considerable advantages in fixation since this allows the occlusal surfaces of the teeth to be brought into a good relationship. Alternatives are the arch bar and while some surgeons still prefer cast silver splints, these have disadvantages in achieving a good occlusion. Many American surgeons favour the use of an acrylic wafer between the teeth to ensure that they are brought into the desired relationship before fixation is carried out, a procedure which is becoming increasingly popular in the United Kingdom.

RELAPSE

Unfortunately, the problem of relapse exists following surgical orthodontics as following the more conventional approaches and is in many ways less understood. It is possible for the teeth to relapse through the bone in much the same way as one would expect following similar orthodontic treatment, and the same rules apply in ensuring stability. In addition, the bone itself may relapse along the line of union. This usually occurs at a fairly early stage following the operation and indeed it has been observed to occur while the teeth are still immobilised, with the teeth moving a corresponding distance in the opposite directions through the bone. Generally speaking, it is not a serious problem in cases with a deep overbite and particularly in cases of mandibular prognathism provided the more modern types of operation are employed. It is at its worst in cases involving anterior open bite and a long lower face but even at the worst, relapse is not usually complete and a worthwhile permanent improvement, if not perfection, can be achieved.

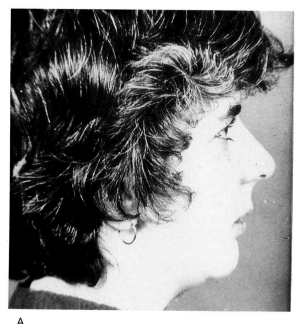
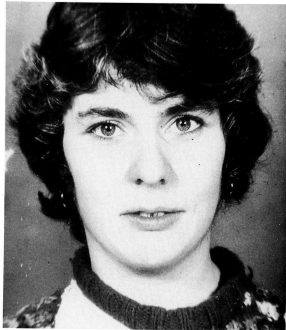

A

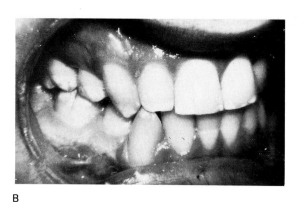
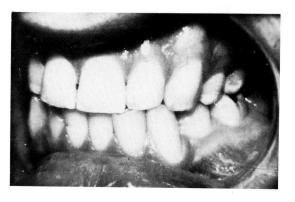

B

Fig. 16.12 Anne 4 years after treatment. A, Photographs. B, Intra-oral photographs.

SUGGESTED READING

Barton P R 1977 Assessment of stability following corrective orthodontic surgery. Proceedings of the Royal Society of Medicine 70: 432–40

Bell W H, Dann J J 1973 Correction of dentofacial deformities by surgery in the anterior part of the jaws. American Journal of Orthodontics 64: 162–86

Broadbent B H Sen, Broadbent B H Jr, & Golden W H 1975 Bolton Standards of Dentofacial Developmental Growth. Mosby, St. Louis

Converse J M, Coccaro P J 1975 Diagnosis and treatment of maxillo-mandibular dysplasias. American Journal of Orthodontics 68: 625–44

Hershey H G, Smith L H 1974 Soft tissue profile changes associated with surgical correction of the prognathic mandible. American Journal of Orthodontics 65: 483–502

Killey H C, Seward G R, Kay L W 1971 An outline of oral surgery, Part II. John Wright, Bristol, ch XV

Lines P A, Steinhauser E W 1974 Diagnosis and treatment planning in surgical orthodontic therapy. American Journal of Orthodontics 66: 378–97

Proffit W R, White R P 1970 Treatment of severe malocclusions by correlated orthodontic-surgical procedures. Angle Orthodontist 40: 1–10

Appendix

Cephalometric definitions

The following definitions of cephalometric terms are taken from the British Standard Glossary of Dental Terms (BS. 4492) by kind permission of The Director General, British Standards Institution.

Term	Definition
Soft tissue points	
Nasion (soft tissue)	The deepest point of the concavity between the nose and forehead in the mid-line
Subnasale	The point where the lower margin of the columella meets the upper lip in the mid-line
Labrale superius	The uppermost point on the vermilion margin of the upper lip in the mid-line
Stomion	The most anterior point of the line of contact of upper and lower lips in the mid-line
Labrale inferius	The lowest point on the vermilion margin of the lower lip in the mid-line
Supramentale (soft tissue)	The deepest point in the concavity between the lower lip and chin in the mid-line
Pogonion (soft tissue)	The most anterior point on the soft tissue outline of the chin in the profile view
Menton (soft tissue)	The most inferior point on the soft tissue outline of the chin
Body landmarks	(Where bilateral points give rise to a double outline, the mid-point between the two points should be taken)
Nasion (bony)	The most anterior point of the frontonasal suture, as seen in the lateral skull radiograph
Orbitale	The lowest point on the infra-orbital margin
Anterior nasal spine (ANS)	The tip of the anterior nasal spine, as seen in the lateral skull radiograph
Subspinale (point A)	The deepest midline point between the anterior nasal spine and prosthion

Term	Definition
Prosthion	The most anterior point of the alveolar crest in the premaxilla, usually between the upper central incisors
Incision (upper)	Tip of the crown of the most anterior upper central incisor
Incision (lower)	Tip of the crown of the most anterior lower central incisor
Infradentale	The most anterior point of the lower alveolar crest, situated between the central incisors
Supramentale (point B)	The deepest point in the bony outline between the infradentale and the pogonion
Pogonion	The most anterior point of the bony chin
Gnathion	The most anterior and inferior point on the bony outline of the chin, situated equidistant from pogonion and menton
Menton	The lowest point on the bony outline of the mandibular symphysis
Sella	The centre of the sella turcica, determined by inspection
Basion	The lowermost point on the anterior margin of the foramen magnum. If this is obscured, the most superior point of the anterior margin of the base of occipital condyles may be substituted
Bolton point	The highest point in the retrocondylar fossa, posterior to the foramen magnum
Condylion	The highest point on the bony outline of the mandibular condyle
Articulare	The point of intersection of the dorsal contours of the posterior border of the mandible and the temporal bone
Porion	The uppermost point of the cartilaginous external auditory meatus, usually regarded as coincidental with the uppermost point of the ear-rods of the cephalostat
Pterygo-maxillare (PTM)	The lowest point of the outline of the pterygo-maxillary fissure
Posterior nasal spine (PNS)	The tip of the posterior spine of the palatine bone in the hard palate
Gonion	The most lateral external point at the junction of the horizontal and ascending rami of the mandible. On a tracing of a lateral skull radiograph, it is found by bisecting the angle formed by tangents to the posterior and inferior borders of the mandible
Planes and lines	(It is customary to refer to most of the lines on tracings of lateral skull radiographs as 'planes'. Although not strictly correct, this practice is well established and will be used here)
SN plane	A line joining sella and nasion
De Coster's line	The outline, in a cephalometric tracing, of the upper border of the anterior base of skull in the midline, used sometimes in the superimposition of tracings

Term	Definition
Frankfort plane	A line joining porion and orbitale
Maxillary plane	A line joining anterior and posterior nasal spines. If either of these is distorted or unclear, an alternative point may be used, produced by bisecting the root of the appropriate spine
Occlusal plane	A line drawn to represent the occlusal line of the teeth. There are various definitions: 1. A line drawn which passes mid-way between the incisal edges of upper and lower central incisors, and which also passes mid-way between the tips of upper and lower cusps of the first permanent molar 2. A line joining the tips of the cusps of the upper first molars to the incisal edge of the upper central incisors 3. A line joining the tips of the cusps of the lower first permanent molars to the incisal edges of the lower central incisors 4. A line drawn along the occlusal surface of the premolars and molars. This is sometimes called the functional occlusal plane
Mandibular plane	A line representing the lower border of the horizontal ramus of the mandible. Again there are several definitions: 1. A tangent to the lower border of the mandible 2. A line joining gnathion and gonion 3. A line joining menton and gonion
Bolton plane	A line joining nasion to Bolton point
Facial plane	A line joining nasion to pogonion
Y axis (of growth)	A line joining sella to gnathion

Index

293